Austerity!

Mini Book Series

VOLUME XXXIII

By

Ronald Pattinson

1st edition

Published in July 2018 by

Kilderkin
171 hs Warmondstraat, Amsterdam, Noord- Holland

ISBN 978-94-90270-33-9

Table of Contents

Mini Book Series

This series started out really as a joke. A few slim volumes assembled from blog posts, a handful of copies printed and handed out to friends. Then my son Andrew suggested I sell them. The rest, as they say, is a mystery.

The original eleven volumes have all since been greatly expanded, leaving the designation Mini Book highly dubious. Even the thinnest numbers more than 100 pages. The thickest over 700.

Those eleven volumes have been joined by another 17 or 18. I think. I missed a couple of volume numbers by mistake and there are two different vol. X and vol. XI. I'll probably sort it all out some day. Hopefully before I die.

Inevitably there will be more volumes. Several are half-finished. Well, more like quarter- or eighth-finished some of them. They'll see the light of day sometime. I can't keep them locked in the cellar with just the odd crust to sustain them forever.

Ron Pattinson, Amsterdam 12th August 2016.

Foreword

The years immediately following WWII were fascinating, in terms of brewing. It's when British beer took on its current form. At least the traditional end of British brewing.

After a few years average OG settled at 1037°, where it remained for several decades. British drinkers had become accustomed to sub-4% ABV beer and that's mostly what they drank. Not that that meant all British beer of the period was of a similar strength. There were still occasional beers at pre-WW I gravities. Barclay's Russian Stout and Bass No. 1, for example.

While draught beer was being whittled down to just Bitter and Mild, with perhaps an Old Ale in the winter, there was a wide range of styles available in bottled form To put it bluntly: beers weren't as dull as you probably think.

This book covers the austere years immediately following WW II and the boom times of the late 1950s and the 1960s. The state of the economy had a profound effect on the brewing world, directly and indirectly. It determined how much money drinkers had in their pockets and whether there was foreign exchange available to import machinery.

The bulk of the book is made up of homebrew recipes. Though there is an introductory section detailed brewing practices, ingredients and beer styles. Its purpose is mostly to explain why and how the beers in the recipes were brewed.

Amsterdam 18th May, 2018.

I General

War and austerity

The years immediately after WW II were tough ones in Britain. The country was bust and the supply situation was even worse than in the war years.

The 1940s

Brewers faced another decade of difficult times after the war ended. Beer strengths continued to fall and tax was increasing:

> "Beer.—The basic Excise duty on beer before April, 1948, was £7 19s. 9d. per barrel plus 5s. 11d. per degree. The Budget raised the duty to £8 18s. 10d. per barrel up to a gravity of 1027 degrees, plus a surtax of 6s. 7.5d. per degree above that strength. Corresponding changes were made in the Customs duties on imported beer. The increase in duty was approximately equivalent to 1d. per pint on beer of average strength."
> "Brewing Trade Review, 1950", page 53.

That price increase put up Mild from 11d to 12d per pint. Quite a large percentage rise.

The supply of raw materials had scarcely improved, either:

> "The shortage of cereals and other brewing materials made it necessary to continue during 1947-48 the control imposed by the Ministry of Food on 1st May, 1946. Up to 31st December, 1947, the permitted rate of output of each brewer was equivalent in terms of standard barrels to 85% of production in the year ended 31st March, 1946. In order to save sugar the permitted rate of output was further reduced to 82% on 1st January, 1948. Owing to an uneven demand for beer during the summer months a redistribution of production was necessary and this was achieved by reducing from 1st January, 1949, the permitted level of production of each brewery to 78% of its standard barellage in the corresponding period of 1945-46 and arranging centrally for the balance of 4% to be allocated to brewers who could not meet their demand within 78%."
> "Brewing Trade Review, 1950", page 53.

Note that they were restricting beer output to a percentage of the 1945 figure. Which itself would have been fixed as a percentage of production in the last peacetime year. It must have been depressing for brewers to have their output still limited years after war's end.

Unsurprisingly, there was a considerable fall in the amount of beer drunk:

> "As a result of all these factors the quantity of home-produced beer retained for consumption in the United Kingdom in 1948-49 amounted to 27.05 million bulk barrels compared with 30.01 million barrels in 1947-48, the average strength being about the same as in the previous year. The quantity and strength of imported beer changed very little between the two years; imports from Continental countries continued during 1948-49 and substantial supplies continued to come from Eire."
> "Brewing Trade Review, 1950", page 53.

Some numbers to demonstrate how hard the years immediately after WW II were. Because what works better than numbers? Especially when you've used up all the day's supply of words. I don't know about you, but I don't have an infinite quantity of them. I often stop mid-sentence in the evening when they're all used up.

The numbers show the remarkable success of British brewing during WW II. Output rose. Surprisingly both in terms of bulk and standard barrels. That the latter rose, means it was a genuine rise, because the standard barrel takes gravity out of the equation. But note the sharp drop in 1947 – 3.3 million standard barrels. The result, as we've already heard, of shortages in raw materials, which prompted the government to lower production quotas.

Keeping average gravity at a little under 1035° for the final years of the war was quite an achievement. Only possible because of a massive increase in British-grown barley during the war. But in 1947 average OG fell more than two points. It must have been depressing for both brewers and drinkers.

Home-made Beer : Quantities charged with duty, Average Gravities and Net Receipts

Year (ended 81st March)	Quantities charged with duty			Net quantities duty-paid		
	Bulk Barrels	Standard Barrels	Average Gravity	Bulk Barrels	Standard Barrels	Net Receipts £
1939	24,674,992	18,364,156	1,040.93	24,187,883	17,935,568	62,370,034
1940	25,366,782	18,738,619	1,040.62	25,092,090	18,495,567	75,157,022
1941	26,203,803	18,351,113	1,038.51	25,773,766	18,121,618	133,450,205
1942	29,860,796	19,294,605	1,035.53	29,351,341	19,018,940	157,254,430
1943	29,296,672	18,293,919	1,034.34	28,971,014	18,044,678	209,584,343
1944	30,478,289	19,193,773	1,034.63	30,129,031	18,945,565	263,170,703
1945	31,332,852	19,678,449	1,034.54	31,031,814	19,475,061	278,876,870
1946	32,650,200	20,612,225	1,034.72	32,698,011	20,580,907	295,305,369
1947	29,261,398	17,343,690	1,032.59	29,226,070	17,427,961	250,350,829
1948	30,408,634	18,061,390	1,032.66	30,007,139	17,744,616	264,112,043
1949	26,990,144	16,409,937	1,033.43	27,048,281	16,319,126	294,678,035

Source:
Brewing Trade Review, 1950, page 51.

Looking at the next table, we can see that malt usage peaked in 1941, after which considerable amounts of unmalted grain and maize products were used. Only to fall back again after 1946. Sugar shows a complicated trajectory, its use falling in the early war years, increasing at the end, then dropping again post-war.

Home-made Beer : Quantities of Materials used and of Beer produced								
Year (ended with Sept.)	**Malt**	**Unmalted Corn**	**Rice, Rice Grits, Flaked Rice, Maize Grits, Flaked Maize etc.**	**Sugar including its Equivalent of Syrups, Glucose and Saccharum**	**Hops**	**Prepa - ration s of Hops**	**Hop Subst itutes**	**Beer Produced**
	Cwt.	**Cwt.**	**Cwt.**	**Cwt.**	**Cwt.**	**Cwt.**	**Cwt.**	**Bulk Barrels**
1939	9,884,803	9,910	734,771	1,986,478	285,715	113	13	25,691,217
1940	9,857,838	7,912	363,588	1,532,776	265,512	132	108	24,925,704
1941	10,988,413	11,897	246,757	1,397,642	251,354	186	166	28,170,582
1942	10,918,102	52,646	382,207	1,411,422	223,007	246	71	29,584,656
1943	10,287,322	40,592	1,238,181	1,400,573	231,589	250	96	29,811,321
1944	10,621,168	143,183	1,241,121	1,458,647	243,900	277	137	31,180,684
1945	10,435,212	245,751	1,332,032	1,784,064	244,822	714	139	31,990,344
1946	9,976,998	137,750	1,132,748	1,790,021	226,197	1,414	168	31,066,950
1947	9,454,253	92,974	614,335	1,601,186	217,759	1,423	191	30,103,180
1948	9,499,294	69,939	606,881	1,443,558	231,470	630	547	28,813,725
Source: Brewing Trade Review, 1950, page 51.								

Looking at the second table, we can see that malt usage peaked in 1941, after which considerable amounts of unmalted grain and maize products were used. Only to fall back again after 1946. Sugar shows a complicated trajectory, its use falling in the early war years, increasing at the end, then dropping again post-war.

All those changes would have had an impact on brewers' grists. One over which they had no control. Given reliable supplies, the raw materials used wouldn't have changed anything like as much. Each of those sudden changes in materials would have presented considerable challenges for brewers. How depressing must it have been for that still to be going on several years after the end of hostilities?

Raw materials for brewing weren't the only problem. All building work was strictly controlled by the government, due to shortages of building materials. Rebuilding breweries wasn't the top priority and getting permission to do so was tricky.

The 1950s

Once into the 1950s, things began to pick up. Gravities crawled up a little, average OG hitting 1037° in 1951. Where it remained for several decades.

UK beer production and average OG		
Year	bulk barrels	average OG
1948	30,408,634	1032.66
1949	26,990,144	1033.43
1950	26,513,997	1033.88
1951	24,891,746	1036.99
1952	25,156,489	1037.07
1953	24,883,227	1036.87
1954	24,582,303	1036.97
1955	23,934,215	1037.13
1956	24,551,158	1037.22
1957	24,506,524	1037.42
1958	24,647,978	1037.48
1959	23,783,833	1037.52
1960	26,115,012	1037.25
1961	27,098,240	1037.41
1962	27,495,836	1037.70
1963	27,813,506	1037.70
1964	28,964,230	1037.66
1965	29,528,050	1037.67
Sources: 1955 Brewers' Almanack, pages 50 & 80. 1971 Brewers' Almanack, pages 45 & 75.		

Worryingly for brewers, beer output and consumption continued to fall. The trend was only reversed in 1960. It's no coincidence that was also the year there was a cut in the tax on beer. Even so, beer production didn't get back to its 1948 level until 1967.

The restrictions on brewing were gradually relaxed. One of the main results of this was the replacement of flaked barley – which the government had forced brewers to use – by flaked maize, which had been the adjunct of choice before the war.

With building restrictions also relaxed, many brewers took the opportunity to enlarge or modernise their bottling plant. Bottled beer was all the rage and was one of the few growth areas. It also provided greater profit than draught beer.

In the early years of the 1950s really strong beers began to reappear for the first time since 1940. The coronation in 1953 in particular prompted the brewing of special celebratory strong beers. Some of these remained permanent fixtures.

The final years of the decade saw an upsurge of interest in Lager and many breweries, even quite small ones, starting brewing one.

The 1960s

A tax cut in 1960 saw beer production finally begin to rise from its slump. Output rose every year in the decade and the growth wasn't even stopped when tax rose again in 1963 and 1965. The future looked bright. At least for those breweries that had survived the merger frenzy.

Taxation

A feature of UK beer since WW I was a very high level of taxation. Around 50% of the retail price of a pint in the pub was tax.

The Excise duty on beer was an important source of revenue for the government. One which they sometimes milked. In the post-war period, it wasn't always a question of an ever rising tax. There were times when it was reduced. Though the long-term trend was still a rising one.

Excise duty 1945 - 1965			
Year	**Tax/Std. Brl**	**Total Tax £**	**tax per pint**
1945	286s 5.5d	278,876,870	7.42d
1946	286s 5.5d	295,305,369	7.54d
1947	286s 5.5d	250,350,829	7.13d
1948	325s 5d	264,112,043	7.24d
1949	343s 4.5d	294,678,035	9.10d
1950	343s 4.5d	263,088,673	8.27d
1951	321s	249,146,244	8.34d
1952	321s	248,165,812	8.22d
1953	321s	243,372,425	8.15d
1954	321s	242,031,712	8.20d
1955	321s	237,452,121	8.27d
1956	321s	243,682,807	8.27d
1957	321s	245,374,441	8.34d
1958	321s	246,077,234	8.32d
1959	321s	238,722,997	8.36d
1960	277s 5d	206,221,271	6.58d
1961	277s 5d	210,149,208	6.46d
1962	277s 5d	233,510,250	7.08d
1963	305s 3.5d	241,401,536	7.23d
1964	305s 3.5d	249,948,368	7.19d
1965	329s 3.5d	284,403,388	8.03d
Sources:			
1955 Brewers' Almanack, pages 50 & 80.			
1971 Brewers' Almanack, page 45 & 75.			

The drop in excise duty in 1960 was the only significant reduction in the rate of taxation on beer in the whole of the 20th century. It only lasted a few years. By 1965 it was already above the 1959 level again.

Imports

On the face of it, the UK had a big trade deficit in beer, importing around 1 million barrels more than it exported. But it's not quite as simple as that. As more than 1 million barrels of those imports came from a country not so far away: Ireland. And the vast majority of that beer was Guinness Extra Stout.

Initially, only tiny amounts were imported from elsewhere, fewer than 50,000 barrels.

UK beer imports 1936 - 1953					
Country of Origin	**1938**	**1950**	**1951**	**1952**	**1953**
Irish Republic	836,624	1,031,159	1,025,902	1,023,031	1,088,076
Other British Countries	108	22	31	133	422
Total British Countries	***836,732***	***1,031,181***	***1,025,933***	***1,023,164***	***1,088,498***
Denmark	25,459	17,686	23,058	30,959	36,410
Germany	18,813	-	-	-	2,307
Netherlands	8,708	2,685	3,492	5,905	8,910
Belgium	821	700	1,150	2,136	2,205
Czechoslovakia	3,810	915	903	702	713
Other Foreign Countries	278	224	1,703	1,922	244
Total Foreign Countries	***57,895***	***22,110***	***30,306***	***41,624***	***50,879***
Total Bulk Barrels	**894,627**	**1,053,291**	**1,056,239**	**1,064,788**	**1,139,377**
Total Standard Barrels	**856,331**				
Source: "1955 Brewers' Almanack", page 60.					

The amount of beer coming in started to rise from the middle of the 1950s, mostly due to a jump in imports from Denmark. So loads of Carlsberg and Tuborg.

UK beer imports 1954 - 1959						
Country of Origin	**1954**	**1955**	**1956**	**1957**	**1958**	**1959**
Irish Republic	1,099,717	1,166,980	1,281,064	1,234,214	1,196,066	1,232,946
Other British Countries	408	689	100	317	486	601
Total British Countries	***1,100,125***	***1,167,669***	***1,281,164***	***1,234,531***	***1,197,152***	***1,233,547***
Denmark	45,238	77,125	98,216	139,682	154,726	209,244
Germany	4,366	6,651	7,627	10,272	9,372	13,523
Netherlands	9,560	17,707	21,540	26,549	24,564	28,473
Belgium	1,024	3,181	4,349	7,138	8,180	13,084
Norway	-	-	-	1,215	1,586	3,075
Czechoslovakia	688	16	140	1,033	935	1,164
Sweden	-	-	-	662	692	734
Other Foreign Countries	384	505	1,101	266	145	352
Total Foreign Countries	***62,160***	***105,185***	***132,973***	***186,817***	***200,200***	***260,049***
Total Bulk Barrels	**1,162,285**	**1,272,854**	**1,414,137**	**1,421,348**	**1,397,352**	**1,503,196**
Source: "1962 Brewers' Almanack", page 58.						

That the numbers fell again after 1960 is probably attributable to one factor: Carlsberg starting to brew in the UK.

UK beer imports 1960 - 1965						
Country of Origin	**1960**	**1961**	**1962**	**1963**	**1964**	**1965**
Irish Republic	1,257,695	1,329,752	1,245,451	1,215,539	1,281,126	1,215,168
Other British Countries	940	1,740	2,303	3,793	3,007	3,344
Total British Countries	***1,258,635***	***1,331,492***	***1,247,758***	***1,219,332***	***1,284,133***	***1,218,512***
Denmark	184,076	178,975	148,018	149,974	159,164	143,189
Germany	7,476	8,926	7,601	9,805	13,925	12,485
Netherlands	27,444	28,077	21,212	23,321	28,245	28,363
Belgium	8,704	8,907	8,391	5,303	5,803	5,053
Norway	3,019	2,390	2,308	3,887	4,491	6,081
Czechoslovakia	1,174	1,083	1,038	922	1,391	1,276
Sweden	1063	670	578	1,112	459	460
Other Foreign Countries	402	655	589	853	1,392	1,166
Total Foreign Countries	***233,358***	***229,689***	***189,795***	***195,177***	***214,870***	***198,073***
Total Bulk Barrels	**1,491,993**	**1,561,181**	**1,437,553**	**1,414,509**	**1,499,003**	**1,416,585**
Source:						
"1971 Brewers' Almanack", page 55.						

It's safe to assume that almost 100% of the beer imported from Continental Europe was Lager of some kind.

Exports

The UK was still exporting a reasonable amount of beer, around 200,000 to 285,000 barrels a year, which is about the same as in the 1930s. It was, however, considerably lower than the half a million barrels exported before WW I

The table is so big I've had to split in in two.

UK beer exports 1946 - 1953								
destination	**1946**	**1947**	**1948**	**1949**	**1950**	**1951**	**1952**	**1953**
Channel Islands	5,342	7,021	9,958	9,693	6,505	2,721	8,959	9,815
Gibraltar	5,698	7,077	6,958	7,609	8,530	8,693	8,183	8,325
Malta	414	521	673	897	336	624	445	484
Cyprus		2,593	2,312	2,112	2,538	4,002	2,712	2,099
British West Africa	1,574	5,797	18,044	34,626	33,811	35,593	50,636	58,049
British East Africa	1,361	2,624	7,316	13,391	4,014	4,341	1,900	1,511
Aden	50	1,284	2,327	4,200	2,684	2,006	2,897	5,927
Bahrein, Koweit, etc		594	5,141	7,813	4,099	4,039	5,073	4,756
India and Pakistan	69,278	8,130	17,075	18,076	15,333	11,890	9,451	5,617
British Malaya	26,270	6,377	10,463	12,258	11,666	14,412	6,028	5,447
Ceylon	2,648	7,686	3,565	6,669	6,363	5,605	5,656	8,624
Hong Kong	10,062	5,873	5,679	12,863	9,508	12,027	7,254	4,811
Australia		54	8,481	18,761	16,879	35,790	8,303	57
Canada		313	1,598	1,281	2,090	3,352	3,680	3,892
Bermuda	22	788	977	1,603	2,843	1,901	1,466	948
British West India Islands	251	1,045	15,087	14,009	15,459	15,213	16,112	17,123

UK beer exports 1946 - 1953								
destination	**1946**	**1947**	**1948**	**1949**	**1950**	**1951**	**1952**	**1953**
British Guiana	38	175	1,991	2,752	3,871	3,247	6,056	6,594
Anglo-Egyptian Sudan		1,843	3,069	5,747	5,291	6,805	6,277	3,035
Irish Republic	221	3,280	11,327	6,201	4,225	5,223	4,966	4,674
Other British Countries	74	972	6,470	6,719	7,153	8,927	10,260	6,570
total British	***123,303***	***64,047***	***138,511***	***187,280***	***163,198***	***186,411***	***166,314***	***158,358***
Belgium	1,405	3,414	34,288	33,786	33,362	45,733	50,237	55,240
other non-Commonwealth	62,710	42,219	32,299	33,061	24,650	43,289	50,839	71,341
total foreign	***64,115***	***45,633***	***66,587***	***66,847***	***58,012***	***89,022***	***101,076***	***126,581***
total	***187,418***	***109,680***	***205,098***	***254,127***	***221,210***	***275,433***	***267,390***	***284,939***
Source: "1955 Brewers' Almanack", pages 58-59.								

UK beer exports 1954 - 1960							
destination	**1954**	**1955**	**1956**	**1957**	**1958**	**1959**	**1960**
Channel Islands	11,307	11,486	12,505	14,301	16,006		
Gibraltar	9,648	9,147	8,291	9,110	8,552	8,243	8,440
Malta	353	344	2,220	1,778	2,366	1,684	2,119
Cyprus	1,965	3,241	10,712	8,700	20,965	14,048	9,200
British West Africa	38,051	46,050	47,811	44,705	30,079	16,656	11,928
British East Africa	1,602	639	874	929	1,243	2,044	832
Aden	5,271	4,240	5,944	5,250	8,071	7,189	10,496
Bahrein, Koweit, etc	4,691	6,176	5,714	6,227	6,686	8,608	10,092
India and Pakistan	5,347	4,625	4,961	1,518	746	889	1,262
British Malaya	3,862	3,891	2,811	2,689	3,435	4,996	6,172
Ceylon	1,938	2,425	2,574	2,534	2,307	1,638	1,306
Hong Kong	3,975	2,738	2,074	2,239	2,108	1,862	1,516
Australia	58	16	3	11	88	158	141
Canada	3,674	3,992	3,785	4,041	4,657	4,420	5,452
Bermuda	1,098	1,034	1,136	890	990	920	941
British West India Islands	15,904	18,730	20,806	21,416	20,953	19,618	16,493
British Guiana	6,809	8,565	6,273	5,680	2,414	2,527	4,347
Anglo-Egyptian Sudan	1,853	1,213	199	*	*	*	*
Irish Republic	6,251	8,450	7,300	7,039	5,684	6,394	6,589
Other British Countries	6,234	5,127	4,751	7,350	8,174	5,848	5,285
total	**129,891**	**142,129**	**150,744**	**146,407**	**145,524**	**107,742**	**102,611**
Belgium	59,006	56,346	62,776	71,507	86,318	88,077	100,200
other non-Commonwealth	59,127	26,938	25,357	21,475	16,843	17,536	19,682
total foreign	**118,133**	**83,284**	**88,133**	**92,982**	**103,161**	**105,613**	**119,882**
total	**248,024**	**225,413**	**238,877**	**239,389**	**248,685**	**213,355**	**222,493**
Source: "1962 Brewers' Almanack", pages 56-57.							

Exports to Belgium continued to grow through the 1950s, rising from 33,000 barrels to 100,000 barrels. By 1960, Belgium accounted for almost 50% of UK beer exports.

While the whittling away of the Empire is reflected in the decline in exports to "British Countries", falling from 68% of the total on 1948 to 46% in 1960. Though exports to the West Indies remained quite stable at 15,000-20,000 barrels a year.

Pubs

The vast majority of beer was consumed in pubs, but the number of pubs was in decline. New licences were virtually impossible to obtain. Some licensing authorities were still actively trying to reduce the number of licensed premises by denying renewals to houses considered "superfluous".

To some extent this decline in pub numbers was offset by an increase in the number of clubs, though after 1960 these also went into decline.

Pubs in England & Wales 1945 - 1965

	On Licenses						
	Pubs						
Year	Full	Beer / wine	Total Pubs	Registered clubs	Pubs and clubs	Off Licences	On & Off Licences
1945	55,875	17,085	72,960	15,590	88,550	21,599	94,559
1946	56,009	17,017	73,026	16,496	89,522	21,693	111,215
1947	56,305	16,927	73,232	17,470	90,702	21,848	112,550
1948	58,850	16,534	75,384	18,370	93,754	22,025	115,779
1949	58,140	15,282	73,422	18,962	92,384	22,218	114,602
1950	59,054	14,429	73,483	19,221	92,704	23,532	97,015
1951	59,757	13,664	73,421	19,511	92,932	23,669	116,601
1952	60,333	13,035	73,368	19,903	93,271	23,717	116,988
1953	60,869	12,351	73,220	20,348	93,568	23,810	117,378
1954	61,265	11,708	72,973	20,772	93,745	23,863	117,608
1955	60,670	10,574	71,244	21,164	92,408	23,548	115,956
1956	61,087	9,788	70,875	21,438	92,313	23,531	115,844
1957	61,471	8,882	70,353	21,988	92,341	23,517	115,858
1958	61,762	8,151	69,913	22,567	92,480	23,530	116,010
1959	62,039	7,416	69,455	23,232	92,687	23,571	116,258
1960	63,682	5,502	69,184	23,773	92,957	23,670	92,854
1961	64,570	4,366	68,936	24,418	93,354	23,934	92,870
1962	65,615	2,422	68,037	21,459	89,496	24,644	96,644
1963	65,627	1,823	67,450	20,663	88,113	25,258	98,667
1964	65,483	1,448	66,931	21,010	87,941	25,838	99,850
1965	65,353	1,217	66,570	21,405	87,975	26,352	101,110

Sources:
The Brewers' Society Statistical handbook 1973", page 50.
2011 Statistical Handbook of the BBPA, page 74

There were still two distinct types of public house: ones with full licenses that could sell all types of alcoholic drinks and beer houses which could only sell beer, wine and cider.

Beer houses were the legacy of the 1830 Beer Act, which had allowed almost anyone to open a pub selling only beer if they met a few basic provisions. More importantly, the license was issued directly by the Excise and not by local licensing magistrates. Unsurprisingly, thousands of beer house sprung up almost immediately.

In 1869, the special provisions for beer houses were repealed and they also came under the control of local licensing magistrates. Who promptly set about trying to close as many as possible.

The increase in fully-licensed houses between 1950 and 1965 looks to be attributable to beer houses converting to full licences.

Opening times

The hours pubs were allowed to open – "permitted hours" – had been pretty much set in stone by the 1921 Licensing Act. This Act itself was very similar to the restrictions imposed by DORA (Defence of the Realm Act) during WW I. The most important being that pubs had to close for at least two hours in the afternoon.

The early start – pubs in London opened at 6 AM in 1914 – was also a thing of the past. Opening times were approximately 11:00 to 14:30 or 15:00 and 18:00 to 22:30 or 23:00. The exact times varied from location to location. On Sunday permitted hours were 12:00 to 14:00 and 19:00 to 22:30.

In Scotland the hours were even more restricted, with closing at 22:00. On Sunday pubs were closed altogether, except for hotels which could serve "bona fide travellers", which was usually defined as someone who had travelled a minimum of several miles. In wales there was total closing on Sunday.

These restrictions remained in place in England until 1988, when afternoon closing was abolished. In Scotland afternoon and Sunday opening was allowed in 1976.

Tied Houses

The vast majority of pubs were tied for beer purchases – or more – to a single brewery. Mostly through direct ownership of the freehold or lease. But even those not directly under the control of a brewery, supposedly Free Houses, were really nothing of the kind. Most were tied through a loan agreement. Genuinely free-of-tie pubs were rare.

Many small and medium-sized breweries had little or no free trade. All their business was dome through their own tied estate. And this included off sales, which were either made in tied pubs or tied off licences.

There was, however a huge variation between breweries in the proportion of tied to free trade, as this table demonstrates:

Brewers' tied estates and free-trade distribution, 1948/9					
Brewing company	**Barrelage distributed to on/off licensed premises**		**Tied estate**	**Tenanted**	**Managed**
	Tied estate %	**free trade/clubs canteens %**	**(numbers)**	**%**	**%**
All (Brewers' Society Survey)*	***69***	***31***	***54,940***	***83***	***17***
Average of 22 Companies**	***73***	***27***	***12,914***	***82***	***18***
Barclay Perkins	88	12	1,005	96	4
Boddingtons'	99.9	0.1	209	75	25
Brakspear	93	7	141	97	3
Bristol Brewery Georges	94	6	756	98	2
Matthew Brown	87	13	550	93	7
Cameron	93	7	362	93	7
Eldridge Pope	81	19	192	92	8
J. W. Green	89	11	358	100	0
Greene King	88	12	502	82	18
Hall & Woodhouse	95	5	140	100	0
Ind Coope & Allsopp	68	32	2,697	79	21
McEwan	19	81	57	7	93
Meux	90	10	341	75	25
Mitchells & Butlers	77	23	873	14	86
Newcastle	85	15	324	59	41
Russells & Wrangham	37	63	93	90	10
H. & G. Simonds	63	37	1,222	94	6
John Smith's	74	26	842	75	25
Steward & Patteson	95	5	614	99.8	0.2
Strong	91	9	468	92	8
Tetley	64	36	378	86	14
Whitbread	51	49	808	96	4

Source:
"The British Brewing Industry 1830 - 1980" by T.R. Gourvish and R.G. Wilson, 1994, page 436.
* Barrelage data include Scotland, tied house data England and Wales only.
** Companies = earlier selection of 35, excluding Bass, Guinness and Tamplin (who made no returns) and Arrol, Colchester and Style & Winch (the subject of takeovers, but adding Simonds, Strong and Eldridge Pope.
Source: Brewers' Society, Brewing Returns, 1949, BS.

One thing that stands out is the huge difference in the trade of three London brewers: Barclay Perkins, Meux and Whitbread. The first two had the typical tied estate model, with the vast majority of their beer sold in their own pubs. While Whitbread sold almost half their beer in the free trade. I think I understand why: they had long bottled a large percentage of their beer and had managed to get their bottled products into rivals' pubs. Later clever use of the Whitbread "umbrella" got their bottles into even more other breweries' tied houses.

It's no surprise that McEwan has the lowest percentage of tied trade – just 19%. The tied house system never really took off in Scotland and most pub were, at least technically, free. In reality, most were bound to one brewer by a loan tie.

Even in the late 1940s, some breweries has assembled considerable tied estates, Ind Coope, for example. These estates only grew as more and more mergers took place in the 1950s.

Most breweries let their tied pubs to tenants rather than operating them themselves through a manager. Though there were exceptions to this, such as McEwan and Mitchells & Butlers.

State Control

Since 1916 the public houses in Carlisle had been nationalised and run by the State Management Scheme. There had been other smaller schemes in other parts of the UK, but these had all ended soon after the end of WW I. The Carlisle scheme. However, lived on.

In the early 1950s the Labour government kicked around the idea of nationalising pubs in new towns. The new urban developments on greenfield sites, mostly just outside large existing urban centres, were the scene of frantic building activity in the post-war years.

Brewers hated this idea. New towns were some of their few chances to build large, modern pubs in areas with little or no local competition. A large, captive audience with the next pub miles away. Such houses were massive potential earners. Worth surrendering the licences of two or three small, run-down inner-city pubs. Which is usually what the licensing authorities expected. Genuinely new licences just weren't issued.

Estate pubs

About the only new-build pubs were ones on new housing estates. Either in new towns or in new suburbs being built around existing towns. It was the last great wave of pub-building. Many of these pubs have since closed or even been demolished. They rarely inspired the same sort of affection as Victorian and Edwardian examples.

Their importance to brewers is reflected in the price they were valued at. In an inventory of Newark brewery Holes, made in preparation for their takeover by Courage, the Lincoln Imp, an estate pub in Lincoln that still exists, was the second most valuable in their estate. Only an historic hotel in the town centre, the Robin Hood, was worth more.

Breweries

In the 1950s the first truly national brewing companies began to form. As the coalescing groups bought more rivals, it inevitably whittled down the number of active breweries. Purchasers were rarely interested in the brewery itself, only the pubs that it owned. With new licenses almost impossible to obtain, about the only way to expand the number of outlets was to buy another brewery.

No. of UK breweries	
Year	**No.**
1945	708
1946	680
1947	648
1948	625
1949	602
1950	567
1951	539
1952	524
1953	501
1954	479
1955	460
1956	426
1957	416
1958	399
1959	378
1960	358
1964	295
1965	274
Sources: Brewers' Almanack 1955, p.68 Brewers' Almanack 1962, p.67 BBPA Statistical Handbook 2003, p. 92	

The process of amalgamation was kicked off by Canadian Eddie Taylor, who had already built a national brewing group in his homeland. Using Yorkshire brewer Hammonds at its core, he embarked on a buying frenzy across the North of England and Scotland.

By the late 1960s, seven brewing groups dominated the industry: Allied Breweries, Bass Charrington, Courage, Watney Mann, Whitbread, Scottish & Newcastle and Guinness. They were usually referred to as the Big Six, Guinness being left out because it owned no pubs.

Amalgamation was often a complex affair. Bass Charrington was formed by the merger of Charrington United Breweries and Bass, Mitchells & Butlers. The former itself the result of a merger between Hammonds United Breweries and Charrington. The latter, created when Bass and M & B merged. Hammonds United Breweries was itself the result of a series of takeovers.

Between them, the Big Six controlled over half the UK's pubs. As most beer was consumed in pubs and those pubs could only sell beer from the brewery that owned them, that gave the big brewers a stranglehold on the beer trade.

Ironically, this hold started to be broken in the 1980s when supermarkets started to shift large quantities of beer. It's ironic because the big brewers dumped beer at ridiculously low prices to the supermarkets to gain market share. All the really did was devalue their pubs as assets.

The Big Seven 1963 - 1967							
	1963			**1967**			
Company	**Tied estate**	**Nominal capital**	**Market value**	**Company**	**Tied estate**	**Nominal capital**	**Market value**
		£m	**£m**			**£m**	**£m**
Allied	9,300	90.4	177.3	Bass Charr	10,230	80.7	243
Watney Mann	5,500	43.8	103.5	Allied	8,250	128.1	235
Charr Utd	5,000	43.1	92.7	Whitbread	7,376	104.8	128
CB&S	4,800	45.3	76.3	Watney Mann	6,667	84.8	145
BM&B	4,100	33	96	CB&S	4,418	57.1	94.4
Whitbread	3,500	40.6	95.2	S&N	2,076	64.8	127
S&N	1,700	44.9	92.1	Guinness	2	26.5	102
Guinness	2	19.5	94				
Total	***33,902***				***39,019***		
Total pubs	***67,450***				***66,373***		

* Guinness's tied estate = Castle Inn, Bodiam and Guinness Club House, Park Royal.

Key:

BM&B Bass, Mitchells & Butlers
Bass Charr Bass Charrington
CB&S Courage, Barclay & Simonds
Charr Utd Charrington United
S&N Scottish & Newcastle

Source:

The British Brewing Industry 1830 - 1980 by T.R. Gourvish and R.G. Wilson, 1994, page 472.

There was also consolidation on a regional level, where breweries like Greene King, Greenall Whitley and Marstons bought up rivals for their pubs and closed their breweries.

At a much smaller level, most of the remaining home brew pubs closed between 1945 and 1965. There had still been around 2,500 publican brewers at the outbreak of WW I, but large numbers gave up in the interwar period. By 1965 they were just a handful.

II Brewing

Equipment

In 1945 most UK breweries were kitted out much as they had been in the 1920s. Not that this was necessarily by design. More from necessity.

In the Depression years of the 1930s, there was little spare cash for investment. There was only one area where there was any significant investment: bottling. Bottled beer steadily increased in popularity during the interwar years at least partly due to the variable quality of draught beer. But also because of a change in home drinking habits, as families stopped buying in casks and switched to bottled beer instead.

Obviously, during the war, shortages of materials of all kinds put a complete stop to brewery improvements and even sometimes essential repairs. The situation didn't improve after war's end. Brewers needed to acquire a permit to perform any building works and these, especially in the early years, often weren't granted. With sterling not a hard currency, any equipment imported had to be paid for in dollars. Which were in short supply.

So it came about that by the early 1950s, many breweries had seen no investment for decades. Even worse, many hadn't even been properly maintained. One of the reasons many brewers were happy to sell up when the merger madness began was that their plant was knackered. Without a large investment, it was likely to become unusable. The owners, many third or fourth generation with little interest or direct involvement in the trade, were only too happy to take the money and run.

The majority of breweries were in buildings constructed in the late 19th century, usually in the classic tower format. Water tank and cooler at the top, with, in descending order, grain and hop stores, mash tun, copper, fermenting vessels and finally racking and bottling departments. There are still traditional breweries laid out this way today.

Mash tun

Mash tuns were almost invariably circular and constructed of metal. Though there remained ones made from wood in more old-fashioned breweries. The dangers of letting wood come into direct contact with wort are pretty obvious. The exterior of the tun was commonly lagged with wood for insulation purposes.

The most common way of mixing the grain with the water was through the use of a Steel's masher. This device, invented in the middle of the 19th century, was a screw which mixed the water and malt as they flowed into the mash tun. Brewers like Fullers and Harveys still use one.

It wasn't uncommon to also have internal rakes. These were initially developed to perform the same task as a Steel's masher: do the initial mixing of grain and water. They were retained for another purpose: to mix throughout the mash the hot water added during an underlet. A technique I'll be describing a little later.

Every mash tun was fitted with a sparge arm. This was made up of pipes constructed in the form of a cross. Holes were placed in these pipes so that not only was the mash sprinkled with hot water but also so the water would propel the arm in a circular motion as it exited.

Crucial for a common method of mashing was the underlet. A pipe connected low down to the mash tun that allowed water to be added to the bottom of the mash.

Copper

In this period most coppers were just that: vessels made of copper. They could be open or closed. The former being preferred in Burton where mostly Pale Ale was brewed, as they caused the least darkening of the wort. The latter were preferred in London where large quantities of Porter and Stout had been brewed.

By this time they were mostly heated by an internal steam coil. This was preferred as it spread the heat more evenly through the wort. Though there were still some breweries, such as Caledonian, that used direct heat on the base of the copper. This was more problematic as it could scorch the wort if performed incorrectly.

Hop Back

From the copper the hot wort passed into the hop back. Which served to remove the hops from the wort. But it also had a secondary function: the hops helped to filter out particles from the wort. This was increasingly important as brewers stopped using coolers which had settled most of the matter suspended in the wort.

I've come across at least one brewery – Elgood – which added some of the hops in the hop back. How modern that sounds.

Cooling

The original device for cooling wort was a cooler, a large, shallow square tray. Handy devices that, in addition to cooling the wort, also allowed much of the gunk suspended in it to settle out.

That's why after the development of refrigerators – a system of pipes through which flowed cold water or brine and over which the wort flowed – these were used in conjunction with coolers rather than replacing them. Because coolers still had an important auxiliary role in precipitating out gunk from the wort.

By the 1940s, few breweries were still using open coolers. Instead wort flowed from the hop back to the wort receiver, whose function was to feed the refrigerators. Wort receivers were much deeper than coolers and were purely designed to hold the wort on its way to the refrigerators.

The original refrigerators had been of an open design, with the wort exposed to the air as it flowed over the cooling pipes. By the 1950's enclosed coolers, where the wort wasn't exposed to the air, were the most common.

Fermenters

Most breweries still employed open fermenters. Either round or rectangular in shape. By this time they were usually constructed of metal or were at least metal lined.

Fermenters were fitted with attemperators – a series of metal pipes through which cold brine was passed. This was one of the huge innovations of the late 18th-century, allowing brewers to precisely control the fermentation temperature. It led to improved beer quality and the possibility to brew year round.

Many of the older systems of fermentation/cleansing were still in use.

Dropping System

Common in the South of England, in the dropping system two vessels were employed. The wort started fermentation in a tall, round fermenter and after a certain length of time – which could vary between 12 hours and 2 or 3 days, depending on the brewery – was dropped into a lower, shallow, square vessel.

The idea was to remove much of the yeast, which was either left in the upper round or quickly settled out in the lower square. This vessel was often called a "settling square". The transfer between the two vessels also aerated the wort and reinvigorated the fermentation.

Yorkshire Square

As the name implies, this was popular in Yorkshire, but it was also extensively employed in the Midlands. There was a main square, usually made from slate but sometimes of metal, above which there was a second chamber. The fermenting wort was pumped to the upper chamber and then allowed to drain back down, leaving most of the yeast behind.

As with the dropping system, main purposes were to remove surplus yeast and to aerate the wort. Yeast used to operating in a Yorkshire square often struggles in a standard fermenter due to not being sufficiently roused.

There are still several breweries in the UK that employ this sort of fermenter.

Burton Union

This system was once common across the UK for brewing Pale Ales and wasn't just limited to Burton. It is not, as people today seem to think, a fermentation vessel, but a cleansing vessel. Fermentation began in a conventional open round or square and the wort was only transferred to a union after a couple of days.

A union set is a series of linked casks. In the bung-hole of each cask there's a swan-necked pipe through which yeast-laden wort rises and spills into a trough. The trough channels the wort back into the casks leaving the yeast behind. As with the other systems described above, it's mostly about cleansing, that is removing yeast.

Brewing Techniques

British brewer still mostly stuck to tried and tested techniques, mostly pioneered in the previous century.

Mashing schemes, though having progressed from the three and four mash schemes of the early 19th century, remained quite complex. Fermenting vessels had changed little since 1900 and remained resolutely unclosed, relying on the yeast head for protection from invading infection. A Victorian brewer would have felt right at home in all but h most modern brewery.

Mashing

Single mash infusions followed by sparging wasn't, as you might having expected a universally standard regime. As always, things were more complicated than that.

In Scotland, home of sparging, that was mostly the case. Though there were Scottish breweries that indulged in more complex mashing schemes. In England, more fiddling around was the rule rather than the exception.

What I call underlet mashing was a widespread practice. The mash started with an infusion with at around 148° F. After 20 to 30 minutes hotter water was added via the underlet, the rakes given a few spins to mix it thought the mash, and the temperature raised to 152-153° F. Then left to stand for 90 to 120 minutes. Variations on this method were common across England. It's effectively a sort of step mash.

A few breweries made their Lagers using a proper decoction mash, Barclay Perkins, for example. But they had a shiny, purpose-built, continental-style Lager brew house. Most breweries didn't and made their Lagers using a standard infusion mash.

Boiling

The wars and the need to save fuel had generally reduced boiling times. Though the times varied immensely between breweries and also depended on the style of beer being brewed. Very strong beers often required long boils to concentrate the wort.

Before WW I, boils of two hours and more had been common and anything under 90 minutes was unheard of. By the late 1940's, 90 minutes was the norm, but times as short as 60 minutes weren't unknown.

Fermentation

Despite being performed in open vessels, fermentation was a controlled affair. Mostly through the use of attemperators. Yeast was pitched when the wort was between 57° and 63° F, depending on the gravity of the wort. The higher the gravity, the lower the pitching temperature, as more heat would be generated during fermentation.

Most breweries aimed for a maximum fermentation temperature of 70° – 72° F. Once this had be reached after a day or two of fermentation, they'd switch on the attemperators to stabilise and then slowly lower the temperature, dropping to 58° - 60° F at the end.

Some breweries fermented Lagers at the correct cool temperature in the 40's Fahrenheit, but most pitched them at 60° F, just like their top-fermenting beers, even when they were using a genuine Lager yeast.

Parti-gyling

A technique much-beloved of UK breweries, for a whole variety of reasons. The most obvious being efficiency. It was a way of using every last drop of wort.

Parti-gyling was also a very convenient and economical way of producing low-volume beers. Fullers, for example, with a brew length of 200-300 barrels, produced OBE, their Burton Ale, in batches as small as 10 barrels. This was only possible because it was parti-gyled with a much larger quantity of Mild Ale.

Here's an example of one of those Fullers parti-gyles of OBE with Mild:

1958 Fullers OBE	
barrels	**OG**
21.75	1059.5
4.25	1013.1
1.25	1002.8
27.25	**1049.6**
Source:	
Fullers brewing record held at the brewery	

1958 Fullers Hock	
barrels	**OG**
79.25	1059.5
117.5	1013.1
2.25	1002.8
199	**1031.4**
Source:	
Fullers brewing record held at the brewery	

The three worts were hopped and boiled separately then blended post-boil to hit the required volumes and gravity for the two beers.

In Scotland, virtually everything was parti-gyled. Most breweries had a single recipe from which they produced three separate Pale Ales (60/-, 70/- and 80/-) and a Strong Ale.

Priming

With much draught beer still sold in cask form, getting it into good condition before serving was vital. Which is why many breweries primed every cask with a high-gravity (1150°) sugar solution at racking time.

The idea was to let primary fermentation run its course and then to provide some new, readily fermentable material to quickly condition the beer before sale. As most beer was consumed within a week of racking, a quick secondary fermentation was vital.

Primings could vary, depending on the type of beer. While a Pale Ale would be primed with a relatively clear solution, primings for Mild Ale often contained some sort of caramel to darken the beer.

Fining

Though very common, fining was not universal. Some Scottish breweries, for example, didn't add finings at all.

Before WW I, fining was often the responsibility of the publican, who would add them when the beer was delivered. But by the 1950s, brewers, who were generally distrusting of publicans when it came to handling beer, finings were mostly added when the beer was racked.

Ingredients

The UK was long dependent on imported ingredients to make up for the shortfall in its own shortfall and booming beer production. That had all changed by 1945. Mostly out of necessity, Britain had become self-sufficient in the raw materials for brewing for around 100 years.

Brewing materials (cwt)

year	malt	Un--malted corn	rice, maize, etc	sugar	total malt & adjuncts	hops	Preparations of hops	hop substitutes
1945	10,435,212	245,751	1,332,032	1,784,064	13,797,059	244,822	714	139
1946	9,976,998	137,750	1,132,748	1,790,021	13,037,517	226,197	1,414	168
1947	9,454,253	92,974	614,335	1,601,186	11,762,748	217,759	1,423	191
1948	9,499,794	69,939	606,881	1,443,558	11,620,172	231,470	630	547
1949	9,087,351	60,709	505,071	1,303,212	10,956,343	233,158	164	74
1950	9,094,097	56,174	454,500	1,285,877	10,890,648	232,979	114	90
1951	9,282,152	57,681	452,581	1,355,152	11,147,566	229,106	178	82
1952	9,312,437	51,992	467,189	1,385,836	11,217,454	228,512	114	177
1953	9,085,688	58,012	426,396	1,405,154	10,975,250	225,569	335	222
1954	8,629,252	52,219	462,005	1,484,605	10,628,081	216,841	286	188
1955	8,635,522	46,556	478,150	1,529,256	10,689,484	217,716	92	27
1956	8,630,145	40,038	486,838	1,544,258	10,701,279	218,820	110	42
1957	8,872,468	13,834	532,214	1,564,673	10,983,189	215,114	91	28
1958	8,642,500	10,717	543,467	1,527,997	10,724,681	208,870	102	24
1959	8,885,364	8,007	590,006	1,569,002	11,052,379	216,037	107	29
1960	9,406,860	8,994	573,252	1,650,843	11,639,949	226,371	111	24
1961	9,897,187	8,445	584,816	1,746,379	12,236,827	234,611	112	10
1962	9,965,073	10,690	608,755	1,757,756	12,342,274	226,437	180	17
1963	10,020,449	13,906	644,349	1,751,019	12,429,723	226,565	246	25
1964	10,591,938	25,861	711,729	1,834,906	13,164,434	237,356	474	37
1965	10,619,331	61,392	734,898	1,813,541	13,229,162	236,424	599	57

Sources:
Brewers' Almanack 1955, page 62
1971 Brewers' Almanack, page 54

You can see that while the use of unmalted adjuncts declined steeply after the war, the amount of sugar used was more stable. There's a simple enough explanation. Brewers were forced by the government to use flaked barley during the latter war years. The idea being that flaking consumed less energy than malting. While brewers had a limit on the amount of sugar they could use in wartime, when they would have preferred to use more.

It's probably easier to see the trends if those numbers are converted into percentages:

Brewing materials (%)			
year	**malt**	**adjuncts**	**sugar**
1945	75.63%	11.44%	12.93%
1946	76.53%	9.74%	13.73%
1947	80.37%	6.01%	13.61%
1948	81.75%	5.82%	12.42%
1949	82.94%	5.16%	11.89%
1950	83.50%	4.69%	11.81%
1951	83.27%	4.58%	12.16%
1952	83.02%	4.63%	12.35%
1953	82.78%	4.41%	12.80%
1954	81.19%	4.84%	13.97%
1955	80.79%	4.91%	14.31%
1956	80.65%	4.92%	14.43%
1957	80.78%	4.97%	14.25%
1958	80.59%	5.17%	14.25%
1959	80.39%	5.41%	14.20%
1960	80.82%	5.00%	14.18%
1961	80.88%	4.85%	14.27%
1962	80.74%	5.02%	14.24%
1963	80.62%	5.30%	14.09%
1964	80.46%	5.60%	13.94%
1965	80.27%	6.02%	13.71%
Sources: Brewers' Almanack 1955, page 62 1971 Brewers' Almanack, page 54			

You can see the trends much more clearly in that form. Malt usage increased from 75% to a peak of 83.5% in 1950, then slowly fell back down to 80%. Adjunct usage dropped quickly after the end of the war then plateaued at around 5%.

The fall in the proportion of sugar used in 1949 and 1950 probably wasn't voluntary, but as a result of government restrictions. Pre-war, it clocked in around 15% and you can see that when brewers were free to use as much as they liked in the later 1950's, it returned to around that level.

Water

Most breweries had their own water supplies, usually from a well. The makeup of these well waters varied enormously. But, well aware of the effects of water chemistry on the brewing process, brewers had become quite sophisticated in their water treatment regimes.

Adding gypsum to Burtonise water for brewing Pale Ale is an obvious one. But it didn't end there. Barclay Perkins, for example, had several different water treatment regimes. One for Mild Ales, one for Pale Ales, one for Burton Ales and one for Stout.

I'm sure they weren't alone in this. Though, sadly, often there are no details of water treatment in brewing records.

Recommended water for different types of beer						
		Grains per gallon				
	O.G.	**Calcium sulphate.**	**Magnesium sulphate.**	**Calcium chloride.**	**Sodium chloride.**	**Calcium carbonate**
Pale Ales	1035-45	14-24	4-8	2	2-4	Under 4
Pale Ales	1045-55	24-38	4-8	2-4	2-4	Under 4
Mild Ales	1035-50	5-10	4	4-8	4-8	Under 4
Stouts	1040-55	—	4	8-12	8-14	5-10
	Grain Equivalents of the Ions Present*					
		Ca"	**Mg"**	**Na'**	**Cl'**	**SO4"**
Pale Ales	1035-45	0.25-0.39	0.07-0.13	0.04-0.07	0.08-0.11	0.28-0.48
Pale Ales	1045-55	0.30-0.63	0.07-0.13	0.04-0.07	0.08-0.14	0.42-0.69
Mild Ales	1035-50	0.14-0.29	0.07	0.07-0.14	0.14-0.28	0.14-0.22
Stouts	1040-55	0.14-0.22	0.07	0.14-0.24	0.28-0.46	0.07

* Excluding Mg and Ca present as carbonates.
Source:
"Brewing Theory and Practice" by E. J. Jeffery, 1956, page 104.

Malt

While often using foreign-grown barley, the malt UK brewers employed was always produced in Britain. Though the increase in British barley production during WW II meant there was far less dependence on imported grain than there had been previously.

There were more types of base malt than you might expect. Pale malt is pretty obvious, and mild malt probably not totally unexpected. But there was also SA malt and the enigmatic high-dried malt. All had their specific uses.

Typical Malt Analyses of English Malt						
	Well-modified		Under-mod. P.A. curing	High N: Starch not fully modified.		Over-modified.
	P.A.	M.A.				
Diastatic activity	35-45	25-35	20	50	25	40
Colour 1" cell	3-5	6-8	3.5	4	12	8
Extract per 336 lb.	99-102	97-99	95	94	93	96
Cold water extract %	18—20	18-21	16	18	18	22
Moisture, % .	1.5-2.5	1.5-2.0	3	2.5	1.5	1.5
T.N. (% on dry) .	1.3-1.5	Up to 1.7	1.5	1.9	1.9	1.5
P.S.N. (% on dry)	0.52-0.56	0.52-0.58	0.45	0.53	0.5	0.63
Index of modification	40-36	34-40	30	29	27	42
Suitable for:	Best P.A.	Good M.A.	Blended for running M.A.	Draught P.A.	Dark beers	Mild ales
Prob. mashing temp.	152º	146-149	147-148	153-4	146-8	150
		(underlet)	(underlet)	(underlet)		
Flakes, % grist	10-15	10	None	15-20	5-10	15
Source: "Brewing Theory and Practice" by E. J. Jeffery, 1956, page 151.						

Barley

The acreage dedicated to barley more than doubled during the war years, as did production. Surprisingly, this trend continued after the end of the war, even accelerating in the late 1950s and early 1960s. Almost ten times as much barley was produced in 1965 as in 1939. Barley imports also fell dramatically after 1961.

Though it should be borne in mind that the bulk of this barley wasn't being used in brewing. Much was grown as animal feed and some was used to make whisky.

UK barley production 1938 - 1965				
Year ended Dec. 31.	**Acreage.**	**Production (cwt.)**	**Average Price per cwt.**	**Barley Imports (cwt.)**
1938	988,000	18,080,000	10 2	19,876,000
1939	1,013,000	17,840,000	8 10	13,740,000
1940	1,339,000	22,080,000	18 2	9,146,000
1941	1,475,000	22,880,000	24 0	1,277,000
1942	1,528,000	28,920,000	45 8	0
1943	1,786,000	32,900,000	31 5	0
1944	1,973,000	35,040,000	26 5	0
1945	2,215,000	42,160,000	24 5	2,037,000
1946	2,211,000	39,260,000	24 3	2,195,000
1947	2,060,000	32,380,000	24 0	2,257,000
1948	2,082,000	40,540,000	26 10	15,618,000
1949	2,060,000	42,580,000	25 10	9,223,000
1950	1,778,000	34,220,000	27 11	15,289,000
1951	1,908,000	38,780,000	38 10	24,270,000
1952	2,281,000	46,680,000	32 7	22,641,000
1953	2,226,000	50,420,000	30 1	28,702,000
1954	2,063,000	44,880,000	25 9	18,602,000
1955	2,295,000	58,720,000	26 0	18,554,000
1956	2,323,000	56,000,000	25 8	16,215,000
1957	2,622,000	59,140,000	23 2	20,168,000
1958	2,755,000	63,400,000	22 11	26,504,000
1959	3,057,000	80,320,000	22 7	19,939,000
1960	3,372,000	84,820,000	21 3	14,083,000
1961	3,828,000	99,480,000	19 10	19,474,000
1962	3,980,000	115,440,000	23 0	7,003,000
1963	4,713,000	131,980,000	20 8	6,978,000
1964	5,032,000	148,080,000	21 2	6,773,000
1965	5,395,000	161,243,000	22 10	5,616,000
Source: 1971 Brewers' Almanack, page 61.				

In the list of countries supplying the UK with barley there are a couple of surprises:

Barley imports by country 1941 - 1969 (1,000 cwt.)									
Year ended 31st August	**Australia**	**Canada**	**Argentina**	**U.S.S.R.**	**Iraq**	**Morocco**	**USA**	**Other Countries**	**Total**
1941*		67			664			540	1,271
1946*			2,195						2,195
1948	973		6,065					5,508	12,546
1950	2,068			9,366	2,286			4,845	18,565
1952	2,952			10,429	3,752	801		4,781	22,715
1954	2,375		2,226		1,887	260		12,993	19,741
1955	993	20,258		714	905	58		498	23,426
1956	1,394	10,490		450	352			830	13,516
1957	956	13,144		94	147			6,210	20,551
1958	1,091	15,789			1,899			8,564	27,343
1959	1,791	17,128					2,099	84	21,102
1960	1,755	13,222			285		564	26	15,852
1961	4,386	4,023			156		82	10,551	19,198
1962	3,912	3,272					73	2,053	9,310
1963	927	3,079					314	1,088	5,408
1964	2,103	4,127					30	1,135	7,395
1965	659	4,481					10	381	5,531
1966	371	1,976						171	2,518
1967	561	3,715						85	4,361
1968	14	1,274						127	1,415
1969	3,555	5,637						3,655	12,847
Source: 1971 Brewers' Almanack, page 62.									

Missing are some of the main sources of barley from before WW II: Chile and India. There's little from the USA, either, which was one of the main suppliers from the late 19th century on.

Australia and Canada are to be expected, but the USSR? I'm amazed that it would have been exporting food in the early 1950s.

The price of malting barley varied considerably over the years:

Barley price 1939 - 1960		
Year ended Dec. 31.	**Average price per quarter (400 lbs.)**	
	s	**d**
1939	31	7
1940	64	11
1941	85	9
1942	163	1
1943	112	2
1944	94	4
1945	87	2
1946	86	7
1947	85	9
1948	95	10
1949	92	3
1950	99	8
1951	138	8
1952	116	4
1953	107	5
1954	91	12
1955	92	10
1956	91	8
1957	82	9
1958	81	10
1959	80	8
1960	75	11
1961	70	10
1962	82	2
1963	73	10
1964	75	7
1965	81	7
Source: 1971 Brewers' Almanack, page 61.		

After a peak in 1951, barley prices had started to fall again. But remained far above their 1939 level. The high price in 1942 was doubtless in response to the high demand for barley from various sources during the war. In addition to its use as fodder and in brewing and distilling, barley was also employed in the national loaf, the only type of bread available.

Prices were pretty stable after 1956, only varying between 70s and 82s per quarter. That would have pleased brewers as it made it easier to plan costs.

Barley Varieties

Barley is divided into two main types: two-row and six-row. Tow-row barley was grown in the UK, Australia, Turkey and Chile. While six-row was grown in California, Australia, Morocco, Smyrna and Chile.[1]

Before WW II, British brewers were convinced that you couldn't brew good beer from exclusively UK two-row malt and that you need a percentage of six-row. Made from barley grown either in Chile or California. According to Jeffery this was because:

> "Due to the sunnier and more equable climates of these countries as compared with the British climate these barleys were more uniform in quality and this was of distinct advantage to the maltster. Further, the coarser husk of the six-rowed varieties tended to give a better filtration in the mash tun and to prevent those filtration troubles caused by the too-close packing of the undissolved parts of the malt (known to the brewer as grains'), which form the medium through which the solution containing the extractable materials is filtered off"
> "Brewing Theory and Practice" by E. J. Jeffery, 1956, page 129.

In the mid-1950s, British two-rowed barleys could be divided into two main groups:; the Goldthorpe and Chevallier types. By crossing Goldthorpe and Chevallier various new barley varieties were developed in the early 20th century. The most successful of these were Plumage-Archer, Spratt-Archer and Standwell. By the mid-1950's, Standwell had mostly disappeared but large quantities of Plumage-Archer and Spratt-Archer were still being grown. Though in 1955 just over half the malting barley grown in the UK was Proctor, an even newer variety. [2]

New varieties were being developed, mostly by cross-breeding English varieties with Scandinavian ones. The latter gave better yields and were more disease-resistant, but didn't have such good malting characteristics as English barley. By crossing, breeders were able to combine the good features of both.

Here are some of the new barley types developed in the early 1950s:

> Proctor: Plumage-Archer and Kenia.
> Pioneer: Spratt-Archer and a Scandinavian variety.
> Carlsberg: Archer variety.[3]

Pale Malt

As for the previous 150 years, the most beers used pale malt as their base. This came in various qualities, the best usually being reserved for the better type of Pale Ale. There was also a variation called PA malt, i.e. Pale Ale malt. It's obvious from the name what its intended usage was.

Mild Malt

As the name implies, mild malt was principally used as the base malt in Mild Ales. Though it does show up in other styles like Stout and even some cheaper Pale Ales. It was slightly darker than pale malt and generally made from lower-quality barley.

---

[1] "Brewing Theory and Practice" by E. J. Jeffery, 1956, page 129.
[2] "Brewing Theory and Practice" by E. J. Jeffery, 1956, page 129.
[3] "Brewing Theory and Practice" by E. J. Jeffery, 1956, page 130.

SA Malt
A base malt designed for use in Stock Ales, SA malt produced a less readily fermentable wort. Which was presumably handy if you wanted a long secondary fermentation. But no-one was ageing Ales after WW II. Yet SA malt continued to be employed. It was in most of Barclay Perkins beers in the late 1940s. Not in their Burton, but in Mild and Stouts. Bit weird, that.

It's a difficult one when devising recipes. As it isn't available commercially – at least not as far as I know – the best substitute is probably mild malt.

Crystal malt
This is a really tricky one to translate. There's no indication in brewing records of how dark crystal malt was. I assume that it varied across different maltsters, but they don't seem to have marketed it as having a specific colour number. In the recipes I've generally guessed at 60 L.

It's after WW II that crystal malt started to be used regularly in Pale Ales. Before it had been mainly limited to Mild Ale, Brown Ale, Porter and Stout.

Amber Malt
Drum-roasted and without any diastatic power, amber malt occasionally turns up in grists. Mostly in Stout, but sometimes in Mild Ale.

Brown Malt
By this period brown malt was all made the modern way, by roasting in a drum, much the same as black malt.

Chocolate Malt
Not all brewers coloured their Black Beers with black malt or roasted barley. Between the wars Whitbread dropped black malt from their Porter and Stout grists and replaced in with chocolate malt. Which is what they continued to use at Chiswell Street right up until it closed in 1974.

Black Malt
While mostly used in Stout, other beers occasionally contained small amounts of black malt. Mild Ale, for example, though it wasn't that common.

High-dried Malt
This is another tricky one. It's malt that has been kilned at a higher temperature than pale malt, but which retains its diastatic power.

Enzymic Malt
Also known as Dixon's malt after the head brewer at JW Green who invented it, turns up in many grists. I suspect as a reaction to the lack of malt made from US-grown barley, which had greater diastatic power, in post-war grists.

Oat Malt
There was the occasional brewer that used oat malt rather than the more common oatmeal.

Though I imagine many brewers had been put off oat malt after being forced to use it at one point during WW II. It wasn't a generally popular move.

Hops

In the fifty years preceding WW I, the UK was dependent on foreign hops to make up for the shortfall in the UK crop. Britain simply couldn't grow enough hops to meet the demands of the brewing industry. Two world wars changed all that.

Despite 75% of hop bines being grubbed up in 1917 to make way for food production, after WW I the UK became mostly self-sufficient in hops. Because fewer hops were needed. Less beer was being brewed and at a much reduced gravity.

Some hops were imported between the wars. Mostly either classy continental like Saaz and Hallertau, or cost-efficient hops from the West Coast of the USA.

Hops: home production and imports 1938 - 1965

Year ended 31st Dec.	Acreage	Estimated Produce	Yield per acre	Imports: Less Re-Exports	Exports: British Hops	Consumption Years ended 30th Sept. following	surplus British hops
		Cwts.	Cwts.	Cwts.	Cwts.	Cwts.	Cwts.
1938	18,460	257,000	13.9	45,287	12,580	286,716	-29,716
1939	18,812	288,000	15.3	7,840	16,050	265,512	22,488
1940	18,592	270,500	14.5	14,675	26,830	251,354	19,146
1941	18,158	262,800	14.5	31	17,209	223,007	39,793
1942	18,420	261,900	14.2	2,963	30,673	231,689	30,211
1943	19,131	285,200	14.9	198	24,941	243,900	41,300
1944	19,603	253,900	13	--	26,525	244,822	9,078
1945	19,957	282,900	14.1	574	32,337	226,197	56,703
1946	21,163	257,451	13.4	29,243	35,056	217,759	39,692
1947	22,142	289,908	13.2	7,716	31,661	231,470	58,438
1948	22,787	273,584	12	4,561	29,135	233,168	40,416
1949	22,196	250,406	11.3	900	42,301	232,979	17,427
1950	22,198	368,313	16.6	269	84,027	229,106	139,207
1951	22,460	321,824	14.3	626	107,738	228,512	93,312
1952	22,279	282,349	12.7	502	76,620	225,569	56,780
1953	21,932	272,593	12.3	1,015	64,762	216,841	55,752
1954	20,760	246,748	11.9	3,075	51,323	217,716	29,032
1955	20,453	256,821	12.1	5,836	49,049	218,820	38,001
1956	19,982	184,170	9.2	6,416	40,746	215,114	-30,944
1957	20,415	267,677	13.1	8,848	38,635	208,870	58,807
1958	21,130	302,640	14.9	5,441	42,352	226,371	76,269
1959	20,350	222,768	10.9	6,007	34,291	234,611	-11,843
1960	20,098	248,195	12.4	8,172	12,220	234,611	13,584
1961	19,681	204,306	10.3	19,235	24,914	226,437	-22,131
1962	20,319	266,812	13.1	16,489	16,070	234,611	32,201
1963	20,957	276,384	13.2	10,063	21,790	226,437	49,947
1964	20,880	252,398	12.1	12,624	24,181	226,565	25,833
1965	20,687	258,727	12.5	12,961	19,474	237,356	21,371

Sources:
1955 Brewers' Almanack, page 63, 1971 Brewers'Almanack, page 54

WW II cut off imports again. More reductions in output and gravity meant the UK had plenty of hops for domestic use after the war. Imports declined to almost zero, as you can see in the table above.

There was an initial flood of imports immediately after the end of the war, but they almost totally dried up after 1948. Imports rose during the 1950s, but remained only a small fraction of what they had been in 1939.

Other figures give an idea of the average hopping rates:

UK hop usage 1945 - 1965					
year	**hops**	**Qtrs. malt, adjuncts & sugar**	**bulk barrels**	**lbs hops per barrel**	**lbs hops per quarter**
1945	244,822	4,896,364	31,990,334	0.86	5.60
1946	226,197	4,644,176	31,066,950	0.82	5.46
1947	217,759	4,187,780	30,103,180	0.81	5.82
1948	231,470	4,113,984	28,813,725	0.90	6.30
1949	233,158	3,869,316	26,744,457	0.98	6.75
1950	232,979	3,844,529	25,339,062	1.03	6.79
1951	229,106	3,941,714	24,870,564	1.03	6.51
1952	228,512	3,970,124	25,285,589	1.01	6.45
1953	225,569	3,892,609	24,789,130	1.02	6.49
1954	216,841	3,790,128	24,153,387	1.01	6.41
1955	217,716	3,818,037	24,324,623	1.00	6.39
1956	218,820	3,824,469	24,187,096	1.01	6.41
1957	215,114	3,921,842	24,839,755	0.97	6.14
1958	208,870	3,829,560	24,129,462	0.97	6.11
1959	216,037	3,945,627	25,023,044	0.97	6.13
1960	226,371	4,155,124	26,313,796	0.96	6.10
1961	234,611	4,370,006	27,600,860	0.95	6.01
1962	226,437	4,407,051	27,736,049	0.91	5.75
1963	226,565	4,435,078	27,942,561	0.91	5.72
1964	237,356	4,693,962	29,485,128	0.90	5.66
1965	236,424	4,711,978	29,579,855	0.90	5.62
Sources:					
Brewers' Almanack 1955, page 62					
1971 Brewers' Almanack, page 54					

Looking at the quantity per barrel, it looks as if hopping rates increased. But that doesn't take into account that beer was lower gravity in the late 1940s than it was in the 1950s. The figure per quarter of fermentables takes the beer's gravity out of the equation. That shows hopping rates rising until 1956, then falling back to almost exactly their 1945 level by 1965.

Cold Storage

It can be disconcerting to see the age of hops listed in brewing records. Two, three or even older hops aren't uncommon. It would be easy to assume that such old hops would have little left in the way of alpha acid. But brewers weren't stupid. They didn't just leave hops that they weren't going to use immediately lying around at room temperature. The kept them in a cold store.

Cold Storage had a huge effect on the deterioration of hops. Especially after the first six months. Here are some numbers on the topic:

Analyses of Fuggle's hops during storage						
	cold store			warehouse		
storage period	alpha resin	beta resin	preservative value	alpha resin	beta resin	preservative value
	6.28	8.6	91.5	6.67	9.26	97.6
5 months	6.22	8.2	89.5	5.83	9.17	88.8
9 months	5.72	8.25	84.7	4.72	9.34	78.5
14 months	5.84	8.54	86.9	3.48	8.64	63.6
19 months	5.15	8.92	81.2	3.21	9.9	55.1
Source: "Brewing Science & Practice" H. Lloyd Hind, 1943, page 349						

Even after 19 months, the alpha acid content of hops held in a cold store had only declined by around 18%. Whereas the fall in those stored warm was 52%.

UK Hops

The classic 19th-century varieties – Fuggles and Goldings – remained by far the most popular hops, both for brewers and growers. Inevitably leading to minimal imports.

Though it's not quite as simple as that. Most Goldings hops weren't exactly Goldings, but related varieties of whitebine.

> "Goldings and Fuggles appear to have been the dominating types for many years, but there are now so many varieties on the market that the two original types have been swallowed up in a maze of cross breeds. With the increasing variety of names, it is more and more difficult to classify hops. We should be more accurate if, instead of calling the hops Goldings and Fuggles, we placed them under the headings of Golding type and Fuggle type. When the reason for the introduction of the various types is investigated it will be readily understood, why this complication has arisen."
> "Brewing Theory and Practice" by E. J. Jeffery, 1956, page 172.

Growers, who were unable to get a higher price for genuine Goldings, which were tricky to grow and had a poor yield, instead planted led tricky, related varieties. They looked like Goldings, but didn't have as delicate a flavour as the genuine article.

New hops were being developed. With the aim of increasing disease resistance, yield and alpha acid content.

Different regions, due to difference in climate and soil, tended to concentrate on certain hop varieties. This is useful to know when writing recipes as brewing records often only list the region where a hop was grown, not the variety.

Here's a review of the English hop growing districts and their varieties. First before the war:

Hop varieties by region in the 1930's	
Region	**main varieties**
East Kent (Canterbury, Faversham)	Goldings, Bramling, Cobb and Tutsham
Mid Kent (Medway valley, Maidstone to Tonbridge)	Fuggle's, Bramling, Tutsham, Cobb, Goldings, Tolhurst
Weald of Kent (Tonbridge to Sussex)	Fuggle's
Sussex	Fuggle's
Hampshire, Surrey	Fuggle's, Farnham Whitebine.
Hereford and Worcester	Mathon, Bramling, Fuggle's
Berkshire and Shropshire	Fuggle's, Goldings
Source: "Brewing Science & Practice" H. Lloyd Hind, 1943, page 391	

Then after it:

Hop varieties by region in the 1950's	
Region	**main varieties**
East Kent (Canterbury, Faversham)	Goldings
Mid Kent (Medway valley, Maidstone to Tonbridge)	Fuggle's, Goldings
Weald of Kent (Tonbridge to Sussex)	Fuggle's, Colegate
Sussex	Fuggle's, Colegate
Hampshire, Surrey	Fuggle's, Farnhams
Hereford and Worcester	Mathon, Cobb, Mayfield Grape, Fuggles
Source: "Brewing Theory and Practice" by E. J. Jeffery, 1956, pages 172 - 175.	

These were the principal hop varieties being grown in England during the 1950s:

English Goldings were quite small hops with a delicate aroma and few seeds. The latter two characteristics made them eminently suitable for dry hopping.

Golding Types included Bramlings, Worcester Mathons, Cobbs, and Tutshams. These were all similar to Goldings, but still distinct from them.

Bramlings ripened earlier than Goldings, but lacked their delicate aroma. Mathons were claimed to be almost as good as Goldings and were the pick of Worcester hops. Cobbs were slightly larger than Goldings, but with a coarser flavour. Tutshams were larger still and packed with flavour.

Fuggles were very variable depending on where they had been grown and at what stage they had been harvested. Ones from the Weald of Kent were coarse in flavour, but those grown on lighter soils in East Kent and Worcester had a much more delicate flavour making them suitable for some Pale Ales. Mostly, however, Fuggles were used in Mild Ale and Stout.

Farnham and Country Farnhams came from Surry and northern Hampshire. They were mostly Goldings types and their extremely delicate flavour meant that they were mostly reserved for the better class of Pale Ale.

Sussex Fuggles had much improved, better growing practices making their flavour more refined. They were generally used in Mild Ale and Stout.[4]

The types of hops grown in the UK changed surprisingly little between 1912 and 1957. The vast majority were either Fuggles or some sort of Goldings type. As the 1950s progressed, the percentage of Fuggles began to fall, replaced by newer varieties such as Pride of Kent and Northern Brewer. The proportion of Goldings, however, remained remarkably constant.

Varieties of hops grown in the UK 1912 - 1957				
1912 Varieties	**1952 Varieties**	**% of crop**	**1957 Varieties**	**% of crop**
Old Golding	Old Golding	}	Old Golding	}
Canterbury Goldings	Canterbury Goldings	}	Canterbury Goldings	}
Bramlings	Bramlings	}	Bramlings	}
Mathons	Mathons	}	Mathons	}
Hobb's Early Goldings	Early Bird Bramlings	}	Early Bird Bramlings	}
Searle's Early Goldings	Eastwell Goldings	24%	Eastwell Goldings	25%
White's Early Goldings	Rodmersham or Mercer Golding	}	Rodmersham or	}
Buss's Late Goldings	Petham Golding	}	Mercer Golding	}
Late or Wild Goldings	Cobbs	}	Petham Golding	}
Bate's Brewers	Tutshams	}	Cobbs	}
Cooper Whites	Whitebines	}	Tutshams	}
Whitebines			Whitebines	}
Green Bines				
Red Bines				
Fuggles	Fuggles	72%	Fuggles	67%
Jones	Brewer's Gold	}	Brewer's Gold	}
Grapes	Bullion	}	Bullion	}
Meophams	Northern Brewer	}	Northern Brewer	}
Henhams	John Ford	4%	John	}
Mayfield Grapes	Pride of Kent	}	Pride of Kent	8%
Colegates	Early Promise	}	Early Promise	}
Prolifics			Keyworth's Midseason	}
			Whitbread Golding	}
			Variety	}
			Bramling Cross	}
Source:				
Journal of the Institute of Brewing, Vol. 65, 1959, page 468.				

New UK Hop Varieties

Despite mostly Fuggles and Goldings types being grown, there was still active development of new hop varieties. The aim of breeding was threefold: better yield, more disease

[4] "Brewing Theory and Practice" by E. J. Jeffery, 1956, pages 173 - 175.

resistance and increased alpha acid content.

I'm slightly surprised that Brewer's Gold and Northern Brewer were still considered "new" varieties as these had originally been developed in 1919 and 1934 , respectively.

Hops entered for the new varieties Challenge Cups Competition in 1952						
			Alpha Resin	Beta Resin	Moisture	Average Alpha Resin
Grower	Variety entered		%	%	H2O	%
Chambers, Wm. & Sons	Brewers Gold	C9a	8.88	9.87	10.11	
Chambers, Wm. & Sons	Brewers Gold	C9a	7.08	5.18	9.89	7.98
Wimshurst, T. E.	College Cluster	N15BIS	5.72	7.72	9.27	
Chambers, Wm. & Sons	Early Promise	X35	6.84	7.71	8.69	
Chambers, Wm. & Sons	Early Promise	X35	6.74	6.49	8.96	
Chambers, Wm. & Sons	Early Promise	X35	5.51	9.38	7.97	
Chambers, Wm. & Sons	Early Promise	X35	6.07	8.99	9.18	
Skinner, Wm. & Son	Early Promise	X35	6.31	8.23	8.84	
Little Fowle Hall	Early Promise	X35	7.71	8.27	9.52	
Wickham, R. D.	Early Promise	X35	4.38	13.03	9.92	6.22
Wimshurst, T. E.	John Ford	WFA90	8.77	10.31	10.26	
Amos, A. & K. J.	Northern Brewer	WFB135	8.69	9.74	9.6	
Hukins, W. D.	Northern Brewer	WFB135	7.95	9.18	9.7	
Nott, J.	Northern Brewer	WFB135	9.02	10.88	10.38	
Worley, J. A.	Northern Brewer	WFB135	8.36	9.98	9.03	
Veall, H.	Northern Brewer	WFB135	8.45	8.89	9.31	8.49
Amos, A. & K. J.	Pride of Kent	170a	7.25	12.05	9.94	
Chambers, Wm. & Sons	Pride of Kent	170a	7.71	11.82	9.59	
Chambers, Wm. & Sons	Pride of Kent	170a	7.41	12.96	10.39	
Wimshurst, T. E.	Pride of Kent	170a	7.07	11.79	9.9	
Veall, H.	Pride of Kent	170a	8.04	14.36	10.14	7.50
Bomford. J. F. Ltd.	Sunshine Hop	V94	6.19	8.41	8.59	
Chambers, Wm. & Sons	Sunshine Hop	V94	7.51	9.75	7.84	6.85
Source: "Brewers' Guardian 1953", February page 74.						

All of these hops, with the exception of Early Promise, had a higher alpha acid content than usually found in Fuggles or Goldings.

Continental Hops

British brewers classed the different types of continental hops differently. The best were considered a match for the best English hops and were considered good enough for use in top-class Pale Ales, which is praise indeed. They were also considered very suitable for dry hopping, as they didn't fall apart as English hops were wont to.

Here the hierarchy of these hops is explained:

> "In order of brewing value we place first and foremost Certificated Saaz. They are usually of extreme delicacy of flavour, well managed, nicely cured and full of resins. As such, they are highly favoured for the best beers. Next comes the choicest Spalts, which nearly reach the excellence of the Saaz mentioned above. They are not quite so

delicate in flavour, however. Then may be bracketed together in about equal value the Saaz Country and Spalt Country, a little greener in colour than the choicer samples, and not quite so regular in size and development. Hallertaus may be placed next, but they require careful examination and selection because, at times, they are decidedly on the green side and not fully grown out. Following these, we place Wurtembergs, hops of some variation in colour and quality. We have seen some quite rich in resins, while others have a distinct deficiency. Lastly, we mention Poperinghes, about which we hardly dare hazard a guess why they are grown at all. They are practically devoid of resin. Their value is for freshening up old hops at the beginning of the season, because they are the first harvested. They have neither character nor flavour. We sometimes hear of Alosts, which can only be classified with Poperinghes."
"Brewing Theory and Practice" by E. J. Jeffery, 1956, page 176.

Large quantities of Belgian Poperinghe hops were used before and during WW I. They found favour for one simple reason: they were cheap. After WW II, they weren't as popular, probably because there was an ample supply of quality hops at reasonable prices.

North American Hops

The glory days for foreign hop growers were over, especially those in the USA. Who had exported massive quantities to the UK in the 50 years before WW I. In years where the English harvest was particularly poor, perhaps as much as 50% of all hops used. US hops were liked because of their high bittering and preservative qualities.

Brewers weren't so keen on their flavour. Which is why American hops were mostly used early in the boil and rarely as dry hops.

As with continental hops, there was a hierarchy in quality. Surprisingly, New York hops were considered the best. I thought that the hop industry on the East Coast had disappeared by the 1950's. Evidently not. Next in quality were Sonomas, Oregons, and Sacramentos. That is hops from Oregon and California.

One problem with American hops was the high percentage of other vegetable matter mixed in with the hop flowers. This was because they were mostly picked by machines, unlike UK hops which were still mostly picked by hand.

British Columbia, on the west coast of Canada also provided some hops, though the industry there was on a very small scale. In the early 1950s, Canada produced around 17,000 cwt. annually. Not much compared to the 500,000 cwt of the USA.[5]

Unmalted grains

In 1945 the most popular adjunct by far was flaked barley. There was a good reason for that: the government forced brewers to use it. Though they would have had to search for an alternative to their preferred adjunct, flaked maize. All maize was imported and was in short supply on account of the war.

As the supply situation eased in the 1950s, most breweries reverted to flaked maize.

[5] 1955 Brewers' Almanack, page 65.

Unmalted grains commonly made up 7-15% of the grist. Though not all breweries used adjuncts. Unlike sugar, the use of which was pretty much universal.

Unmalted wheat was also reasonably common in small amounts. Its purpose was to aid head retention.

Oats, mostly in flaked form, were used in Oatmeal Stout. Though the quantity employed was often just a token amount, only around 1% of the grist. I assume this was for legal reasons.

Sugar

Sugar had been an essential element in British beers since the late 19th century. Some styles were simply impossible to brew without its use. How could you make a Milk Stout without lactose?

Sugar mostly came in one of two forms: numbered invert sugars and proprietary sugars.

Numbered Invert Sugars

These formed the backbone of sugar usage in the first half dozen decades of the 20th century. They came in four different types, mostly distinguished by their different colour.

Numbered invert sugars	
Sugar	**SRM**
No.1 Invert	12.5-17.5
No.2 Invert	30-35
No.3 Invert	60-70
No.4 Invert	275-325

No. 1 was usually reserved for the better class of Pale Ales, No.2 was for the commoner sort of Bitter and some Mild Ales. No. 3 for the working-class end of the beer range, Mild Ale and Brown Ale. The blackest, No. 4, usually only featured in Stout.

Proprietary Sugars

Secondly, there were proprietary sugars, which were usually a mix of invert and caramel. These were often designed for use in a specific type of beer, such as Mild Ale or Oatmeal Stout. For anyone trying to recreate old beers, they're a total nightmare. No longer available commercially, their composition isn't known, either. In the recipes I've substituted combinations of invert sugars and caramel. How close I get, is anyone's guess.

Malt Extract

It was common to use a small amount of malt extract. The quantities are so small, I can only assume that it was for extra enzymes. It's often listed in brewing records as DME: Diastatic Malt Extract.

It also had other uses, as this quote explains:

> "**Malt Extract.**
> This is prepared from a malt wort evaporated in a vacuum to give a syrup of about

80% solids. (Malt extracts are also obtainable as powders, but these are not usually used in brewing.) Non-diastatic malt extracts, or those with low diastase, are suitable for adding in the copper, and enable a larger brew to be made on occasions when perhaps the existing mash tun capacity is inadequate. However, apart from this, their regular use is of value and many brewers always include a proportion in their beers. They are of use in assisting head retention and there are special grades made in such a way as to have a high proportion of those protein products which assist in head retention. Diastatic malt extracts are also used in the mash tun if the malts are deficient in diastase, or if a high proportion of flakes is to be used. As flakes do not contribute head-retaining materials, their use tends to reduce the foam-retaining qualities of the beer; the use in the copper of the high nitrogen malt extracts, already referred to, will therefore counteract this tendency.
"Brewing Theory and Practice" by E. J. Jeffery, 1956, page 167.

When you get to the recipe section you'll see just how common malt extract was.

Yeast

Few UK brewers used pure yeast strains, discouraged by problems with secondary fermentation in the late 19th century. Most had multiple strains in their pitching yeast and not always all Saccharomyces. Brettanomyces was still lurking around in many. Though, as few beers were kept for any length of time, usually being racked into casks and shipped off to pubs or bottled immediately after the end of primary fermentation.

Fullers, for example had a three-strain pitch. When they moved over to conical fermenters in the 1970s, they analysed the influence of the three different yeasts. Discovering that one was responsible for the marmalade character of their beers, they went with that.

An analysis of bottle-conditioned beers in the early 1950s found a wide range of different strains of Brettanomyces, sometimes within the same beer. With an ability to ferment a variety of sugars – many couldn't ferment maltose, some could ferment lactose – they must have created beers with very differing characters.

III Beer Styles

Introduction

The beer styles of this period, both in their form and strength, are very much like those of today. Though some have lost much of their popularity and become quite rare. Brown Ale and Light Ale, once mainstays in every brewer's range, are now very thin on the ground. Mild has not fared well, either. Though, weirdly, Milk Stout is making a comeback.

Draught Beer

A typical brewery produced two to five draught beers and half a dozen bottled ones. Bitter and Mild made up the vast majority of draught beer, supplemented by a little Stout (mostly restricted to London and Norther Ireland) and the occasionally stronger beer in the winter.

At the start of the period, draught beer was almost exclusively in cask form. About the only exception was the small amount of Lager sold on draught, which was served by top-pressure. In the 1950s, in a reaction to dodgy cask beer and the popularity of bottled beer, more and more breweries began producing keg beer. The initial keg products were mostly premium Bitters, but soon there were keg versions of other draught beers such a Mild.

There was a third type of draught: bright beer. This was filtered and artificially carbonated, but not pasteurised. Served through electric pumps rather than on top pressure, it had some of the advantages of both cask and keg. Mostly it was limited to the North and the Midlands.

Bottled Beer

There was more variation in bottled beer, both in terms of styles and strengths. Stronger beers just didn't sell in large enough quantities to be sold on draught. Other beers, such as Brown Ale and Light Ale, were considered bottled products. And some, like Sweet Stout, were only really practical in bottled form.

Bottled beer was all the rage in the 1950's. It was the only type of beer whose sales were increasing. Making it vital for brewers to have good bottling facilities and the right range of bottled products. In 1900, only about 5% of beer was bottled. By 1939 it had risen to 25%, though its growth was temporarily halted by the advent of war. In 1954, it hit 35%.[6]

Undoubtedly the percentage of bottled beer would have been higher, had it not been for WW II. There was a shortage of glass for bottles and even wood for crates, which limited the amount a brewer could produce. (During the war Barclay Perkins regularly sent letters to their tenants warning them they would only get bottled beer delivered if they returned the empty bottles and crates.) Plus bottling used more energy than producing draught beer, which was another important consideration.

Around a third of beer was in bottled form. That's even more significant when you realise 70-80% of beer was consumed in pubs at the time. There must have been a lot of customers drinking either bottled beer or draught and bottled beer mixed. The situation now is much more complicated. A much higher proportion of drinking goes on at home, so that naturally boosts the amount of bottled or canned beer sold. On the other hand, bottled beer is much less often consumed in pubs.

[6] "Brewing Theory and Practice" by E. J. Jeffery, 1956, page 330.

Bottled sales continued rising until around 1960. The advent of keg beer made bottled beer less attractive. Keg was a similar product, but cheaper in price. The percentage of bottled (and by then canned, too) sales only began to rise again with a change in drinking habits after 1980 when beer was increasingly drunk at home.

Bottle-conditioning, already a minority sport since WW I, was on its way out in the 1950s. It was mostly restricted to Old Ales, strong Stouts, Burton Pale Ales and Guinness Extra Stout. By 1970, there would only be half a dozen left.

Most bottled beer – and certainly all the lower-gravity stuff like Light Ale and Brown Ale – was brewery-conditioned in one way or another. As was Sweet Stout for safety reasons. Some contained so many fermentable sugars any live yeast would have turned them into bombs.

The older method of producing bright bottled beer was called chilling and filtering. Beer was chilled in a tank to drop out any potential protein haze, then filtered and bottled with artificial carbonation.

Mild Ale

Still by far the nation's favourite at the start of this period, as the 1950's progressed Mild's popularity started to slip. By the decade's end, a serious decline was setting in. One that would accelerate in the 1960s.

By 1945 Dark Mild had become the norm, though there were still pale versions and some were only semi-dark. Intriguingly, London Milds were, on average, darker in colour and less well attenuated than those from other parts of the country.

Best Mild

In the North of England – in particular the Northwest and parts of Yorkshire – it was common for a brewery to have both a Mild and a Best Mild. They weren't usually hugely different in gravity, perhaps 1030° and 1033°. Quite often, they'd be different in colour. Usually Ordinary would be dark and Best pale. Though Lees did it the other way around.

Mild and Best Mild 1950 to 1959

Year	Brewer	Beer	Price per pint	OG	FG	ABV	App. Atten-uation	colour
1951	Taylor Walker	Ale	12d	1031.7	1006.9	3.22	78.23%	100
1951	Taylor Walker	Mainline	15d	1035.2	1007.6	3.58	78.41%	100
1951	Watney	Ale	14d	1032.8	1007.4	3.30	77.44%	105
1951	Watney	Best	20d	1043.1	1008	4.57	81.44%	110
1959	Ramsdens	Mild	12d	1029.2	1004.7	3.06	83.90%	45
1959	Ramsdens	Best Mild	13d	1035.5	1006.5	3.63	81.69%	35
1959	Websters	Mild	12d	1032	1005.7	3.29	82.19%	50
1959	Websters	Best Mild	13d	1034.9	1004.4	3.81	87.39%	20

Source: Whitbread Gravity book held at the London Metropolitan Archives, document number LMA/4453/D/02/002.

Talking of Lees, they're the brewery that gives a lie to my next statement. Dark Mild wasn't coloured with malt but with sugar. What I naively thought was the flavour of darker malts really came from sugar. More specifically, No. 3 invert sugar. I realised that the first time I tasted No. 3. With all its rich, dark fruit flavours. Yep, that's the Dark Mild flavour.

While most breweries were content to produce Mild from base malt, a bit of crystal malt, flaked maize and No. 3 invert, Lees threw everything in their Best Mild: six malts and five types of sugar. The crazy bastards.

There was the occasionally truly stronger Mild, Watney Best Mild, for example. But that was one of a very few to break the 1040° line. Whitbread attempted to introduce a stronger Mild in the mid-1950s, XXX, but it wasn't a success, despite newspaper advertising support.

London Mild

Mild was still very popular in London. Though its popularity began to collapse in the 1950's as Bitter became the capital's new favourite style. The first time I drank in London in the mid-1970's, cask Mild had all but disappeared. And many pubs didn't sell Mild at all, not even keg.

The immediate post-war years are also when average gravity hit a new nadir, though not quite as low as during WW I. Mild, as a cheap mass drink, suffered the most in terms of reduced gravity. You can see the average gravity of all the Milds in the table is just over 1030. The strongest is Truman Best Mild at 1042.5°. But it did cost about 50% more at 19d a pint. The next highest gravity is just 1033.7°. For Mainline, a beer sold as a strong Mild.

There's a reason why none of the beers has an OG under 1027°. The minimum tax on a barrel of beer assumed an OG of 1027°. A beer with a lower OG still paid that rate of tax, so it made no economic sense to have a beer weaker.

All but one example is a dark Mild. And most are pretty dark. Certainly darker than many Milds were pre-war. When many were what I'd call semi-dark, with colour values of 40-50° Lovibond. I'd reckon 80° Lovibond to be about the minimum for a properly dark Mild.

Attenuation isn't great, averaging just over 70%. I reckon they were leaving the FG reasonably high so the beer didn't taste too watery. But it does mean that the average ABV is below 3% ABV. Meaning you'd need to be very determined to get more than mildly intoxicated.

1940s

There are examples from 11 different London breweries in the table. And not all the breweries of the day are represented. Until recently, it would have seem weird that so many different beers of one style were brewed in the capital. Then London's brewing industry was reborn in a very happy development. Though for all the number of brewers today, I bet there aren't 11 regularly brewing Mild in the capital.

London Mild Ale 1946 -1949								
Year	**Brewer**	**Beer**	**Price per pint d**	**OG**	**FG**	**ABV**	**App. Atten-uation**	**colour**
1946	Barclay Perkins	Ale	13.5	1031.1	1008.8	2.89	71.70%	19.5
1946	Charrington	X	11	1028.7	1008.4	2.63	70.73%	120
1946	Courage	X	11	1030.4	1006.8	3.06	77.63%	90
1946	Mann Crossman	X	12	1032.5	1011.5	2.71	64.62%	100
1946	Meux	X	11	1028.1	1008.8	2.5	68.68%	105
1946	Taylor Walker	X	11	1028.4	1009.9	2.39	65.14%	100
1946	Taylor Walker	Mainline	12	1032	1010.9	2.73	65.94%	85
1946	Truman	X	11	1030.1	1010.8	2.49	64.12%	130
1946	Watney	X	11	1030.8	1006.5	3.15	78.90%	
1946	Wenlock	X	11	1029.8	1010.4	2.51	65.10%	80
1946	Whitbread	XX	11	1030.8	1012.1	2.41	60.71%	85
1948	Barclay Perkins	XX	14	1031.4	1011.3	2.6	64.01%	108
1948	Charrington	XX	14	1028.9	1007	2.84	75.78%	105
1948	Courage	XX	14	1031.3	1005.1	3.41	83.71%	55
1948	Mann Crossman	XX	14	1032.3	1009.3	2.98	71.21%	110
1948	Meux	XX	13	1028.1	1006	2.87	78.65%	215
1948	Taylor Walker	Mainline	15	1033.7	1012.1	2.79	64.09%	95
1948	Taylor Walker	XX	13	1026.8	1006.9	2.58	74.25%	80
1948	Truman	XX	13	1028.9	1007.7	2.75	73.36%	95
1948	Truman	B MA	19	1042.5	1010.4	4.17	75.53%	105
1948	Watney	Best Ale	13	1031.5	1010.3	2.74	67.30%	95
1948	Whitbread	XX	13	1029.1	1006.5	2.93	77.66%	85
1949	Charrington	MA	12	1029.4	1010.3	2.47	64.97%	130
1949	Courage	MA	12	1028.3	1007.5	2.69	73.50%	100
1949	Mann Crossman	Mild Ale	13	1032	1004	3.64	87.50%	100
1949	Meux	XX	12	1028.4	1005.3	3	81.34%	190
1949	Taylor Walker	MA	12	1029.7	1009.5	2.61	68.01%	75
1949	Truman	MA	12	1029.7	1005.8	3.1	80.47%	85
1949	Wenlock	MA	12	1031.1	1011.7	2.5	62.38%	85
1949	Whitbread	Best Ale	13	1032.5	1009	3.04	72.31%	100
	Average		***12.6***	***1030.6***	***1008.7***	***2.84***	***71.64%***	***100.9***

Sources:
Whitbread Gravity book held at the London Metropolitan Archives, document number LMA/4453/D/02/002.
Truman Gravity Book held at the London Metropolitan Archives, document number B/THB/C/252
Whitbread brewing records

1950s

Let's move forward a little in time, to the early 1950s, and take a look at the standard-strength Milds being brewed by London's large brewers.

Large London brewery Ordinary Mild Ale 1950 - 1954								
Year	Brewer	Beer	Price per pint d	OG	FG	ABV	App. Atten-uation	colour
1950	Barclay Perkins	Ale	13	1031.8	1006.8	3.24	78.62%	95
1950	Charrington	MA	12	1029.6	1007.1	2.92	76.01%	120
1950	Courage	MA	13	1032.4	1006.7	3.34	79.32%	120
1950	Ind Coope	MA	12	1027.9	1008.9	2.46	68.10%	67
1950	Mann Crossman	Mild Ale	13	1031.8	1005.8	3.38	81.76%	95
1950	Meux	XX	12	1026.9	1005.6	2.76	79.18%	152
1950	Taylor Walker	MA	12.5	1028.9	1006.1	2.96	78.89%	80
1950	Truman	MA	13	1031.9	1008	3.10	74.92%	95
1950	Watney	Best Ale	13	1031.2	1006.3	3.23	79.81%	105
1950	Whitbread	Best Ale	13	1031.7	1010.5	2.80	66.88%	110
1951	Barclay Perkins	Ale	14	1033.8	1007	3.48	79.29%	120
1951	Charrington	Ale	13	1033.5	1007.3	3.40	78.21%	110
1951	Courage	Ale	13	1034.5	1010.3	3.13	70.14%	110
1951	Ind Coope	Ale	12	1029.4	1008	2.77	72.79%	50
1951	Mann Crossman	Ale	13	1034.5	1006.5	3.64	81.16%	90
1951	Taylor Walker	Ale	12	1031.7	1006.9	3.22	78.23%	100
1951	Truman	Ale	13	1033.9	1006.3	3.59	81.42%	100
1951	Watney	Ale	13	1032.7	1006	3.47	81.65%	110
1951	Watney	Ale	14	1032.8	1007.4	3.30	77.44%	105
1953	Mann Crossman	Best Ale	14	1032.9	1009.2	3.07	72.04%	110
1953	Truman	Ale	14	1034	1008.1	3.36	76.18%	90
1953	Watney	Ale	14	1033	1010.1	2.96	69.39%	95
1953	Whitbread	Best Ale	14	1032.7	1010.5	2.87	67.89%	100
1954	Barclay Perkins	XX	14	1029.4	1005.2	3.14	82.31%	110
1954	Charrington	Ale	13	1030.7	1009.6	2.73	68.73%	120
1954	Courage	Ale	14	1032.6	1006.2	3.43	80.98%	125
1954	Mann Crossman	X	14	1032.9	1007.5	3.30	77.20%	115
1954	Meux	Mild Ale	14	1031.2	1007.3	3.10	76.60%	120
1954	Taylor Walker	T.W.X.	13	1031.7	1010.3	2.77	67.51%	100
1954	Truman	LM	14	1034	1007.8	3.40	77.06%	95
1954	Watney	XX	14	1032.3	1011.4	2.70	64.71%	110
1954	Whitbread	Best Ale	14	1032.9	1009.9	2.98	69.91%	105
	Average		***13.2***	***1031.9***	***1007.8***	***3.12***	***75.45%***	***104.0***

Sources:
Whitbread Gravity book held at the London Metropolitan Archives, document number LMA/4453/D/02/002.
Whitbread brewing records

There were still quite a few large breweries in London in the 1950's. And all produced Mild. Or to be even more specific, Dark Mild Ale. Because there isn't a pale one in the list. The lowest colour value is 50, which is a dark amber. Pretty well all the others are dark brown. The average is 104. Or quite dark.

The average OG has increased a little - 1.3 points – despite me having stripped out Best Mild to a separate table. So I'd reckon the real increase is more like 2 points. Combine that with a slightly lower average FG and it allows the ABV to tentatively poke its head above 3%. Hurray, you could now actually get drunk on Mild.

A few examples are still under 1030°. But in the case of Ind Coope this can be explained by the fact that they also brewed a stronger Mild. Which appears in a later table.

The price has increased a little, form 12.5d in the late 1940's to 13.3d. That's about 6p in modern money. It wouldn't even get you a sip of Mild today. If you could find Mild, that is. There's bugger all of it about nowadays.

Next it's the turn of smaller London breweries:

Small London brewery Ordinary Mild Ale 1950 - 1953

Year	Brewer	Beer	Price per pint d	OG	FG	ABV	App. Atten-uation	colour
1950	Wenlock	Ale	12	1030.6	1008.4	2.88	72.55%	100
1951	Wenlock	X	12	1032.83				88
1953	Wenlock	Amber Ale	14	1031.6	1006.5	3.26	79.43%	100
1950	Beasley	Ale	12	1031.43				56
1953	Beasley	X	13	1031.47				116
1953	Cannon	X	13	1031.84				96
1951	Friary	Mild Ale	14	1029.9	1004.5	3.30	84.95%	85
1950	Friary Holroyd	X	12	1033.47				82
1951	Fullers	Mild Ale	14	1031.2	1008.9	2.89	71.47%	90
1950	Hammerton	Ale	12	1030.41				94
1950	Harman's	X	12	1032.07				84
1950	Young & Co	X	12	1033.07				68
1953	Young & Co	X	13	1030.73				60
	Average		***12.7***	***1031.6***	***1007.1***	***3.08***	***77.10%***	***86.1***

Sources:
Whitbread Gravity book held at the London Metropolitan Archives, document number LMA/4453/D/02/002.
Truman Gravity Book held at the London Metropolitan Archives, document number B/THB/C/252

To be honest, there's not much difference with the large brewery Milds. That isn't really a surprise, as they were serving the same market. An average OG just over 1030°, about 3% ABV, around 75% attenuation. The only significant difference is the colour, which is a full 20 points lower. Oh, the price. That's lower, too. About 0.75d.

Now for the stronger Milds from London's large breweries:

Large London brewery Best Mild Ale 1950 - 1954								
Year	**Brewer**	**Beer**	**Price per pint d**	**OG**	**FG**	**ABV**	**App. Atten-uation**	**colour**
1950	Charrington	Best Mild Ale	14	1037.4	1010.4	3.50	72.19%	105
1950	Ind Coope	Mild Ale	15	1039.2	1009.6	3.84	75.51%	75
1951	Ind Coope	XXX	14	1034.76				
1951	Taylor Walker	Mainline	15	1035.2	1007.6	3.58	78.41%	100
1951	Watney	Best	20	1043.1	1008	4.57	81.44%	110
1952	Ind Coope	X	13	1036.69				102
1954	Ind Coope	Strong Mild Ale	19	1043.5	1010.7	4.26	75.40%	110
1954	Taylor Walker	Mainline	15	1036.5	1014.5	2.84	60.27%	95
1954	Taylor Walker	Main Line Special	27	1044.5	1017.5	3.48	60.67%	125
	Average		***16.89***	***1039.0***	***1011.2***	***3.72***	***71.99%***	***102.8***

Sources:
Whitbread Gravity book held at the London Metropolitan Archives, document number LMA/4453/D/02/002.
Truman Gravity Book held at the London Metropolitan Archives, document number B/THB/C/252

All these stronger are Milds are from large breweries. I don't know if that's just the vagaries of my sample, which is pretty small in size. Or if it was generally the bigger boys that bothered with more than one cask Mild. Because that's one thing all these beers have in common: they had a weedier younger brother with an OG of around 1030°. No brewery produced just a strong Mild.

Taylor Walker were unusual in having particularly strong branding for their Best Mild, Mainline. A beer which they pushed quite a bit. And, unusually for a Mild, was found in both draught and bottled form. Main Line Special in the table is the bottled version, which you can see was considerably stronger than its draught counterpart.

The gravity averages 7 points higher than for Ordinary Mild, while the ABV is more than 0.5% higher. Watney's Best comes in at over 4.5% ABV, which would have been a very reasonable strength for a Best Bitter in the early 1950's.

Once again, they're pretty dark beers. Not quite as dark on average as the Ordinary Milds from large breweries, but darker than the ones from small brewers. The lesson? Londoners liked their Mild dark.

Let's take a look at London Mild in the remainder of the 1950s. The price for Ordinary Mild has crept up from around 13d to 14.5d. While the average price for Best Mild has gone up by about 2.5d. It still looks dirt cheap compared to modern prices. On a happier note, average OG and ABV for Ordinary Mild have increased slightly. Only two examples are under 3% ABV. Which is good news for pissheads.

All the veers, both Ordinary and Best Mild, are pretty dark, with the lowest colour value 70. None are even vaguely close to being pale.

Whitbread's Best Mild, XXX, didn't last long, only being brewed in 1954 and 1955. That's despite being pushed by Whitbread in print adverts. Obviously, it was parti-gyled with their deceptively named Ordinary Mild, Best Ale.

Not much more else to say. Other than that these look very much like the Mild Ales of my youth: around 3% ABV and dark brown. It wasn't until the last ten years that I came to realise that this type of Mild was only about as old as me.

It's a sobering thought. And an indication of a common way of thinking. We assume that things which were common when we were young had been around forever.

London Mild Ale 1955 - 1959

Year	Brewer	Beer	Price per pint d	OG	FG	ABV	App. Atten-uation	colour
1955	Truman	X		1033.6				82
1955	Whitbread	Best Ale		1030.4	1009.5	2.76	68.75%	95
1957	Barclay Perkins	XX	15	1031.4	1005.8	3.33	81.53%	100
1957	Charrington	Mild Ale	14	1032.6	1007.4	3.27	77.30%	110
1957	Courage	Mild Ale	15	1032.5	1006.4	3.39	80.31%	115
1957	Ind Coope	Mild Ale	15	1032	1006.6	3.30	79.37%	70
1957	Mann	Mild Ale	15	1033	1004.7	3.68	85.76%	105
1957	Truman	Mild Ale	15	1032.4	1008.2	3.14	74.69%	95
1957	Watney	Mild Ale	15	1032	1007.6	3.16	76.25%	100
1957	Wenlock	Mild Ale	15	1031.8	1006.4	3.30	79.87%	95
1957	Whitbread	Mild Ale	14	1032.4	1011.4	2.71	64.81%	95
1958	Whitbread	Best Ale	15	1033.1				
1958	Young & Co	Mild Ale	14	1031.6	1005.8	3.35	81.65%	75
1959	Fullers	Mild Ale	12	1032.2	1006.6	3.32	79.50%	90
	Average		***14.5***	***1032.2***	***1007.2***	***3.23***	***77.48%***	***93.9***
1955	Taylor Walker	Main Line	27	1044	1014.5	3.82	67.05%	115
1955	Whitbread	XXX		1034.8	1010.0	3.28	71.26%	115
1957	Ind Coope	Mild Ale	15	1034.9	1008.4	3.44	75.93%	95
1957	Taylor Walker	Mainline	16	1037.4	1010.4	3.50	72.19%	100
	Average		***19.3***	***1037.8***	***1010.8***	***3.51***	***71.61%***	***106.3***

Source:
Whitbread Gravity book held at the London Metropolitan Archives, document number LMA/4453/D/02/002.

1960s

And finally, London Milds in the early 1960s. The most surprising thing is that the average price has dropped from 14.5d to 13.8d per pint. Though not so surprising when you remember that the tax on beer was reduced in 1960.

On the other hand, the average OG has fallen a little. And the rate of attenuation is lower, too. Which has pushed the average ABV down below 3%. The high finishing gravities must have left these as quite sweet beers, due to all the residual sugar.

London Mild 1960 - 1965								
Year	**Brewer**	**Beer**	**Price per pint d**	**OG**	**FG**	**ABV**	**App. Atten-uation**	**colour**
1960	Charrington	Mild	12	1033.5	1012.6	2.70	62.39%	
1960	Courage	Mild	12	1031.7	1010.8	2.70	65.93%	
1960	Friary Meux	Mild	12	1031.1	1006.5	3.20	79.26%	
1960	Truman	Mild	12	1033.2	1009.3	3.10	72.14%	
1960	Watney	Mild	12	1031.1	1011.7	2.50	62.38%	
1960	Whitbread	Mild	12	1031.4	1011.3	2.60	64.01%	
1961	Whitbread	Best Ale		1030.4	1009.7	2.74	68.09%	110
1962	Charrington	Mild Ale	14	1032.8	1010.2	2.92	68.90%	100
1962	Courage	Mild Ale	14	1033	1008.8	3.14	73.33%	105
1962	Friary Meux	Drum Mild	14	1029.1	1006.3	2.85	78.35%	120
1962	Truman	Mild Ale	17	1033.3	1011.3	2.84	66.07%	110
1962	Watney	Mild Ale	14	1032.3	1012	2.62	62.85%	120
1962	Whitbread	Best Ale	14	1034				
1963	Friary Meux	Keg Mild Ale	20	1030.1	1008.8	2.66	70.76%	110
1964	Whitbread	Best Ale		1030.6	1007.5	3.06	75.49%	100
1965	Whitbread	Best Ale		1030.0	1008.3	2.87	72.33%	105
	Average		***13.8***	***1031.7***	***1009.7***	***2.83***	***69.49%***	***108.9***

Sources:
Whitbread Gravity book held at the London Metropolitan Archives, document number LMA/4453/D/02/002.
Whitbread brewing records.
Which Beer Report, 1960, pages 171 - 173.

Friary Meux Keg Mild is 3d per pint more expensive than the next dearest beer and 6d more than the average. While it's also one of the weakest examples. More proof of what poor value keg beer was.

The colour remains very dark and the attenuation poor. You'll see in the next section that elsewhere in the country Attenuation was around 80%.

This is around the time when Mild started to entre a steep decline in the capital. By the end of the 1970s it had been all but wiped out, save for the occasional keg example.

Provincial Mild

There was a surprisingly large variation in Mild Ale between different regions of the UK. Mild in the capital was quite different to that elsewhere.

1940s

Provincial Mild Ale 1946 - 1949								
Year	**Brewer**	**Beer**	**Price per pint d**	**OG**	**FG**	**ABV**	**App. Atten-uation**	**colour**
1946	Lees	K		1028.0				
1946	Lees	Bot. B		1030.0				
1946	Lees	BM		1033.0				
1948	Lees	K		1028.0				
1948	Lees	BM		1032.0				
1948	Lees	Bot. B		1030.0				
1949	Ansell	Mild Ale	13	1035.4	1007.4	3.64	79.10%	50
1949	Atkinsons	Mild Ale	13	1034.6	1004.8	3.88	86.13%	50
1949	Brickwoods	Mild Ale	13	1033.2	1004.8	3.70	85.54%	20.5
1949	Burtonwood	Mild Ale	13	1027.5	1003.5	3.12	87.27%	80
1949	City Brewery	Mild Ale	13	1032.6	1006.8	3.35	79.14%	21
1949	Dare	Mild Ale	13	1034.6	1006.9	3.60	80.06%	58
1949	Davenport	Mild Ale	13	1032	1007.9	3.12	75.31%	58
1949	Frederick Smith	Mild Ale	13	1035	1008.6	3.42	75.43%	58
1949	Mitchell & Butler	XX	18	1034.6	1003.9	4.00	88.73%	35
1949	Morgans	Mild Ale	11	1027.7	1002.8	3.24	89.89%	50
1949	Portsmouth United	Mild Ale	13	1029.3	1003.1	3.41	89.42%	19
1949	St. Annes Brewery	Mild Ale	13	1034.9	1003	4.16	91.40%	20
1949	Steward & Patteson	Mild Ale	11	1027.7	1004.5	3.01	83.75%	50
	Average		***13.1***	***1032.2***	***1005.2***	***3.51***	***83.94%***	***43.8***

Sources:
Lees brewing records held at the brewery.
Whitbread Gravity book held at the London Metropolitan Archives, document number LMA/4453/D/02/002.

A note about where the breweries above were located. Six were from Birmingham: Ansell, Atkinson, Dare, Davenport, Frederick Smith and Mitchell & Butler. Two from Exeter: City Brewery and St. Annes. Two from Norwich: Morgans and Steward and Patteson. Two from Portsmouth: Brickwood and Portsmouth United. And finally Burtonwood of Warrington.

The Birmingham Milds all have relatively high gravities. Coupled my decent attenuation, it means they're mostly over 3.5% ABV. Which is very high for the period. If you remember, most of the London Milds were under 3% ABV. I'm not surprised that the Norwich Milds have some of the lowest gravities. Beers from rural areas tended to be weaker, for some reason.

Most interesting of all is the colour. Or rather lack of it. Because there's only one of this set – Burtonwood – that's properly dark. Three examples – City, Brickwood, Portsmouth United and St. Annes are pale. That is, all the ones from Exeter and Portsmouth. The Birmingham beers are all semi-dark, as are those from Norwich.

The real fun comes when you compare the colours of the London and provincial Milds. Only one London example was pale and one semi-dark. All the rest were properly dark. Here's a comparison of the London and provincial analyses:

London vs. provincial Mild Ale 1946 - 1949						
region	Price per pint d	OG	FG	ABV	App. Atten-uation	colour
London	12.5	1030.6	1008.7	2.84	71.64%	100.9
Provinces	13.1	1032.2	1005.2	3.51	83.94%	43.81

Provincial beers were a halfpenny a pint dearer, slightly higher in gravity, considerably higher in ABV and much paler in colour than their London counterparts. The difference is much greater than I would have imagined. Given the higher FG and lower attenuation, my guess is that London Milds were sweeter.

1950s

Midlands Mild Ale 1950 - 1951								
Year	Brewer	Beer	Price per pint d	OG	FG	ABV	App. Atten-uation	colour
1950	Ansell	Mild Ale	13	1034.8	1005.2	3.85	85.06%	50
1950	Bass, Burton	Mild Ale	15	1041.4	1008	4.34	80.68%	40.1
1950	Mitchell & Butler	Mild Ale	13	1034.6	1005.4	3.80	84.39%	37
1950	Mitchell & Butler	Mild Ale	17	1034.5	1003.8	4.00	88.99%	38
1950	Mitchell & Butler	X	15	1038.4				41
1950	Offilers	Mild Ale	13	1031.2	1004.7	3.45	84.94%	70
1951	Ansell	Mild Ale	15	1038.3	1005.7	4.25	85.12%	45
	Average		***14.4***	***1036.2***	***1005.5***	***3.95***	***84.86%***	***45.9***

Sources:
Whitbread Gravity book held at the London Metropolitan Archives, document number LMA/4453/D/02/002.
Truman Gravity Book held at the London Metropolitan Archives, document number B/THB/C/252

Moving on to the 1950s, I've far too many analyses to make a single manageable table. Splitting them up makes sense. And it also highlights regional variations.

Kicking off with the middle bit of the England. Which I've divided into the Midlands and East Anglia. For no particular reason, other than convenience. I have to draw the lines somewhere. What's fascinating about these two sets is how different they are. It illustrates the considerable regional variations in Mild.

East Anglia Mild Ale 1950 - 1953								
Year	**Brewer**	**Beer**	**Price per pint d**	**OG**	**FG**	**ABV**	**App. Atten-uation**	**colour**
1950	Grays	X	11	1029.1				56
1950	Lacons	X	12	1032.7				100
1951	Lacons	Mild Ale	14	1031.4	1006.9	3.18	78.03%	65
1951	Lacons	X	13	1034.4				88
1951	Morgans	Mild Ale	14	1032.4	1007.2	3.27	77.78%	65
1951	Ridley	Mild Ale	13	1030.3	1004.9	3.30	83.83%	70
1951	Tollemache	Mild Ale	14	1028.7	1005.6	3.00	80.49%	60
1951	Wells & Winch	Mild Ale	14	1029.3	1008.6	2.68	70.65%	80
1951	Young Crawshay	Mild Ale	14	1031.2	1003.7	3.58	88.14%	70
1952	Lacons	X	14	1031.9				92
1953	Tollemache	X	16	1037.7				144
	Average		***13.5***	***1031.7***	***1006.2***	***3.17***	***79.82%***	***80.9***

Sources:
Whitbread Gravity book held at the London Metropolitan Archives, document number LMA/4453/D/02/002.
Truman Gravity Book held at the London Metropolitan Archives, document number B/THB/C/252

Starting with the colour. All the East Anglian Milds are dark, with the exception of the one from Grays. The average, just over 80, is well in dark brown territory. While the Midlands Milds are, except for Offiler's, in the twilight zone between pale and dark. Significantly, that's the only example from the East Midlands. The average of 45.9 is well short of dark brown.

There's a big difference between the gravities, too. Remove Tollemache from the East Anglian set and the remainders are weaker than every Midlands Mild, except Offiler's. The average ABV of the Midlands set it 0.75% higher than the East Anglian ones.

Both sets have high rates of attenuation, but it's particularly high for the Midlands. Note that the FG's are very similar for the two sets, despite the much higher average OG for the Midlands.

It seems that in the West Midlands they liked their Mild strong but quite pale. While in East Anglia they preferred it weaker and darker.

Now we head further North. There, unlike London where all Mild was dark, breweries had a habit of brewing two Milds, one pale and one dark. At least ones in Yorkshire and Lancashire did. You can see the practice a little in the table. Through Lees. They had a pale Ordinary Mild and a dark Best Mild. Which in itself is a bit unusual. They were usually the other way around, the stronger Mild being the paler one. No idea why that was different at Lees.

It's a shame that I don't have the FG for most examples. Because for those where I do, it's exceptionally low, leaving a couple of beer over 4% ABV. I'm looking at Vaux in particular. Speaking of Vaux, I can remember their Mild. It was a pretty rare beer in its final days, the

Northeast not being a great mild-drinking area. And, unlike the one in the table, was very dark as I recall.

Mild wasn't very common by this period in Scotland. My suspicion is that these samples were taken south of the border. Probably in London, as they were performed by Truman. Younger had pubs selling their beer in the capital, both free houses and tied houses. These would have needed to have a Mild Ale to satisfy the demands of English drinkers. Which would explain why all the samples are dark in colour.

Northern and Scottish Mild Ale 1950 - 1953

Year	Brewer	Beer	Price per pint d	OG	FG	ABV	App. Atten-uation	colour
1951	Groves & Whitnall	Mild Ale	14	1030.6	1004.1	3.45	86.60%	50
1951	Mitchell	Mild Ale	15	1037.2	1004.8	4.22	87.10%	60
1951	Vaux	Mild Ale	15	1035.6	1002.9	4.27	91.85%	24.5
1951	Wilsons	Mild Ale	14	1034.8	1005.3	3.84	84.77%	50
1952	Hull Brewery	Mild Ale	16	1032.1	1005.6	3.44	82.55%	85
1952	Lees	Bot. B		1035.0				35
1952	Lees	K		1031.0				34
1952	Lees	Best Mild		1034.0				100
1952	Tetley	X	13	1031.3				58
1953	Tetley	X	13	1031.4				58
	Average		***14.3***	***1033.3***	***1004.5***	***3.8***	***86.6%***	***55.5***
1951	Wm. Younger	X	13	1030.0				72
1952	Wm. Younger	X	14	1031.2				80
1952	Wm. Younger	X	14	1033.5				92
1953	Wm. Younger	X	14	1033.3				82
	Average		***13.8***	***1032.0***				***81.5***

Sources:
Lees brewing records held at the brewery.
Whitbread Gravity book held at the London Metropolitan Archives, document number LMA/4453/D/02/002.
Truman Gravity Book held at the London Metropolitan Archives, document number B/THB/C/252

The Southeast next. Using London Milds as my baseline, this lot have a slightly lower average gravity. Buy a higher rate of attenuation leaving the ABV a little higher. There's very little variation in gravity, all the beers lying 1 or 2 points above or below 1030°. London Milds, with their higher FGs, probably tasted sweeter and fuller.

There are two out-and-out pale examples, from Shepherd Neame and Fremlins. But both also brewed a dark version. As the two beers have very similar gravities in both cases, I assume they are versions of the same basic beer. Those aside, everything else is reasonably dark, though a bit paler than in London.

Southeastern Mild Ale 1950 - 1953								
Year	**Brewer**	**Beer**	**Price per pint d**	**OG**	**FG**	**ABV**	**App. Atten-uation**	**colour**
1950	Cobb & Co.	X		1030.7				72
1950	Daniells	X	11	1031.2				56
1950	Gardner	X	12	1030.0				96
1950	Shepherd Neame	X		1030.1				63
1950	Simonds	Ale	12	1030.4				56
1950	Tomson & Wotton	X		1026.8				76
1950	Wells	X	12	1030.4				104
1951	Cobb & Co.	X	12	1028.4				88
1951	Daniells	Mild Ale	14	1029.9	1003.9	3.38	86.96%	110
1951	Daniells	X	12	1032.1				72
1951	Daniels	Ale	13	1032.9				86
1951	Fremlin	XXL	12	1029.4				22
1951	Fremlin	XX	12	1030.6				60
1951	JJ Young	Mild Ale	14	1030.6	1004.8	3.35	84.31%	65
1951	Morrell	Mild Ale	14	1029.7	1003.7	3.38	87.54%	80
1951	Portsmouth United	Mild Ale	14	1029.3	1005.1	3.14	82.59%	75
1951	Shepherd Neame	X	12	1031.4				24
1951	Simonds	Mild Ale	14	1032.0	1005.5	3.44	82.81%	80
1951	Simonds	Mild Dark Sweet	14	1031.5	1005.7	3.35	81.90%	80
1951	Tamplin	Mild Ale	14	1029.9	1005.2	3.21	82.61%	70
1951	Tomson & Wotton	X	12	1029.2				80
1951	Wells	Mild Ale	14	1028.6	1005	3.07	82.52%	75
1953	Benskins	X	13	1031.5				84
	Average		***12.9***	***1030.3***	***1004.9***	***3.29***	***83.9%***	***72.8***

Sources:
Whitbread Gravity book held at the London Metropolitan Archives, document number LMA/4453/D/02/002.
Truman Gravity Book held at the London Metropolitan Archives, document number B/THB/C/252

The finally set is from the Southwest of England and Wales.

It's surprising how strong the Southwestern Milds are, averaging almost 4% ABV. I'd have expected the opposite. Especially remembering St. Austell and Devenish beers from the 1970's which were pretty weak. Though you paid a price. Literally. Rather than 13d or 14d a pint, these were 17d or 18d. Other than the Starkey, Knight & Ford beer which looks excellent value.

You'll note that the real Southwestern beers are quite pale and fairly highly, but not ridiculously so, attenuated. Odd thing is, I remember Plymouth Heavy, which is what Plymouth Breweries Mild was called when I drank it. I recall it being very dark. And very nice. It was a real shame when Courage closed the brewery and it disappeared.

It's hard to draw many conclusions based on just two beer. So I don't really know what to say about the Welsh Milds. Other than that I would have expected them to be darker.

Southwestern and Welsh Mild Ale 1950 - 1951								
Year	Brewer	Beer	Price per pint d	OG	FG	ABV	App. Atten-uation	colour
1950	Plymouth Breweries	Mild Ale	17	1038.1	1006.9	4.06	81.89%	43
1950	Starkey, Knight & Ford	Mild Ale	14	1037.8	1008.5	3.80	77.51%	50
1951	Flowers	Mild Ale	15	1030.7	1003.9	3.49	87.30%	120
1951	Plymouth Breweries	Mild Ale	18	1040.3	1009.5	4.00	76.43%	42
	Average		***16***	***1036.7***	***1007.2***	***3.84***	***80.78%***	***63.8***
1950	Clubs Brewery Ltd	Mild Ale	13	1030	1007.5	2.92	75.00%	55
1951	Brains	Mild Ale	15	1033.9	1004.3	3.85	87.32%	85
	Average		***14***	***1032.0***	***1005.9***	***3.39***	***81.16%***	***70***

Source:
Whitbread Gravity book held at the London Metropolitan Archives, document number LMA/4453/D/02/002.

I have a limited number of analyses for the remainder of the 1950s, so there just a single table for everywhere outside London.

Though it's more like Northern Mild Ale rather than provincial. Only four of the breweries aren't in the North: Hancock (Cardiff), Home (Nottingham), William Younger (Edinburgh) and Worthington (Burton).

Provincial Ordinary Mild 1955 - 1959								
Year	Brewer	Beer	Price per pint d	OG	FG	ABV	App. Atten-uation	colour
1955	Hancock	Dark Malt		1032				
1955	Hancock	XXXX		1031				
1955	Lees	K		1030.0				
1955	Thwaites	Mild Ale	16	1032.2	1006.1	3.39	81.06%	40
1955	Younger, Wm.	X	14	1030.2				96
1957	Lees	Mild		1032.0				
1958	Home Brewery	Mild Ale		1034.5	1007.6	3.49	77.97%	60
1958	Scarsdale	Mild Ale		1035.4	1006.6	3.74	81.36%	130
1958	Vaux & Co	Mild Ale	15	1030.3	1005.8	3.18	80.86%	27
1959	Bentleys	Mild	13	1032.9	1005.4	3.44	83.59%	30
1959	Bents	Mild Ale	12	1033.2	1003.6	3.86	89.16%	55
1959	Chester Northgate Brewery	Mild Ale	14	1030.6	1005.6	3.25	81.70%	95
1959	Greenall Whitley	Mild Ale	12	1030.4	1005.5	3.23	81.91%	80
1959	Lees	Mild		1032.0				
1959	Ramsdens	Mild	12	1029.2	1004.7	3.06	83.90%	45
1959	Threlfalls	Mild Ale	12	1032.8	1004.3	3.71	86.89%	50
1959	Websters	Mild	12	1031.6	1004.8	3.35	84.81%	55
	average		***13.2***	***1031.8***	***1005.5***	***3.43***	***83.02%***	***63.6***

Sources:
Lees brewing records held at the brewery.
"Cardiff Pubs and Breweries" by Brian Glover, 2005. pages 97-101
Truman Gravity Book held at the London Metropolitan Archives, document number B/THB/C/252
Whitbread Gravity book held at the London Metropolitan Archives, document number LMA/4453/D/02/002.

It's nice having both the Ordinary Mild and Best Milds from a couple of breweries. Dead handy, because it helps show the relationship between the two at a brewery. It's clear that Ordinary Mild was around 1032° while Best Mild was 1035°. And that Best Mild cost 1d per pint more. The difference in gravity is probably based around that price differential. Expecting consumers to be prepared to pay a penny a pint more for "Best".

The colours differed, too. Ordinary Mild was usually darker, though in the case Ramsdens and Websters – both Yorkshire breweries – the colour wasn't that dark. I know from earlier Lees records that they had it the other way around, Ordinary Mild being pale and Best Mild dark. I think that was unusual. "The Pub and the People", based on an investigation into Bolton puns in the late 1930's, states that Ordinary Mild was dark and Best Mild pale. I tend to believe that was the usual relationship.

Having said that, about the only example of a brewery I personally experienced selling both Mild and Best Mild, Thwaites, had two dark beers.

Not much else to say, other than that Worthington's Mild was pretty bad value. Mind you, beer from the famous Burton breweries sold at a premium price. Even their Mild. Oh, and there are very few really properly brown examples. I count that as 80 plus and only five examples hit that.

Provincial Best Mild 1955 - 1959

Year	Brewer	Beer	Price per pint d	OG	FG	ABV	App. Atten-uation	colour
1955	Lees	Best Mild		1035.0				
1955	Lees	Bot. B		1035.0				
1955	Worthington	Special Mild Ale	19	1036.9	1007.9	3.77	78.59%	85
1956	Lees	Best Mild		1035.0				
1956	Lees	Bottling Beer		1035.0				
1959	Lees	Best Mild		1035.0				
1959	Ramsdens	Best Mild	13	1035.5	1006.5	3.63	81.69%	35
1959	Websters	Best Mild	13	1035	1005.9	3.64	83.14%	20
1959	Whitaker	Best Mild	13	1033.1	1010.2	2.86	69.18%	45
	average		***14.5***	***1035.1***	***1007.6***	***3.47***	***78.15%***	***46.3***

Sources:
Lees brewing records held at the brewery.
Whitbread Gravity book held at the London Metropolitan Archives, document number LMA/4453/D/02/002.

1960s

Finally, for the 1960s, I've split the analyses into three tables: North, Midlands and South (other than London).

The Northern breweries straddle the Pennines and stretch over into Scotland with William Younger.

Northern Mild 1960 - 1965								
Year	**Brewer**	**Beer**	**Price per pint d**	**OG**	**FG**	**ABV**	**App. Atten-uation**	**colour**
1964	John Smith	Mild Ale	15	1030.9	1008.5	2.80	72.49%	30
1960	Carlisle State Management	Mild	11	1031.2	1008.8	2.90	71.79%	
1960	Greenall Whitley	Mild	12	1030.8	1004.7	3.40	84.90%	
1960	John Smiths	Mild	12	1033.6	1009.7	3.10	71.28%	
1960	Tetley	Mild Ale	12	1031.9	1003.6	3.54	88.71%	60
1960	Thwaites	Mild	12	1031.1	1005	3.40	84.08%	
1960	Wilson	Mild	12	1031.2	1005.8	3.30	81.41%	
1961	Cornbrook	Keg Mild	17	1035	1002.3	4.09	93.43%	20
1961	Threllfalls	Keg Mild	16	1034	1003.2	3.85	90.59%	75
1961	Workington	Mild	14	1029.6	1004.7	3.11	84.12%	105
1961	Younger, Wm.	Mild	15	1029.2	1004.5	3.21	84.59%	75
1960	Hammond United	Best Mild KB	12	1032.7	1005	3.60	84.71%	
	Average		***13.3***	***1031.8***	***1005.5***	***3.36***	***82.68%***	***60.8***

Sources:
Whitbread Gravity book held at the London Metropolitan Archives, document number LMA/4453/D/02/002.
Which Beer Report, 1960, pages 171 - 173.

No surprise that the cheapest beer is from the nationalised Carlisle State Management Scheme. They generally sold their beer 1d per pint cheaper than their rivals. The two keg Milds are noticeably more expensive than the other examples. Though do also have the highest gravities and ABVs.

The common feature most have is a very high degree of attenuation: the average is almost 83% and the highest are over 90%. There's a great degree of variation in colour from 20, which is pale even for a Bitter, to 105 which is a very dark brown.

There are fewer analyses of Midland Milds, from just two breweries: Ansells and Mitchells & Butlers. Who were, undoubtedly, two of the largest breweries in the region.

Midlands Mild 1960 - 1965								
Year	**Brewer**	**Beer**	**Price per pint d**	**OG**	**FG**	**ABV**	**App. Atten-uation**	**colour**
1960	Ansell	Mild Ale	13	1038				
1960	Ansell	Mild	12	1036.5	1009.5	3.50	73.97%	
1961	Ansell	King Pin Mild	19	1037.6	1006.7	3.86	82.18%	45
1961	M & B	Keg Mild	19	1038.5	1009.9	3.58	74.29%	45
1962	Ansell	King Pin Mild	22	1035.9	1007.4	3.56	79.39%	50
1963	M & B	Keg Mild	20	1037.9	1010.2	3.46	73.09%	50
	Average		***17.5***	***1037.4***	***1008.7***	***3.59***	***76.58%***	***47.5***

Sources:
Whitbread Gravity book held at the London Metropolitan Archives, document number LMA/4453/D/02/002.
Which Beer Report, 1960, pages 171 - 173.

The gravities are significantly higher than elsewhere. Though lower degree of attenuation leaves the ABV barely higher than in the North. The colour is firmly in the no man's land between pale and dark.

Finally we have Southern Milds (excluding London).

Southern Mild 1960 - 1965								
Year	**Brewer**	**Beer**	**Price per pint d**	**OG**	**FG**	**ABV**	**App. Atten-uation**	**colour**
1960	Greene King	Mild	12	1030.7	1006.1	3.20	80.29%	
1960	Fremlins	Mild	12	1033.3	1005.6	3.60	83.18%	
1960	Ind Coope	XXX	12	1034.3	1009.6	3.20	72.01%	
1962	Flowers	Mild Ale	14	1031.2	1005.2	3.25	83.33%	75
1962	Ind Coope	Mild Ale	14	1033.7	1009.5	3.13	71.81%	20
1962	McMullen	Mild Ale	14	1034	1006.3	3.46	81.47%	20
	Average		***14.4***	***1033.5***	***1006.6***	***3.40***	***80.26%***	***51.9***
Sources: Whitbread Gravity book held at the London Metropolitan Archives, document number LMA/4453/D/02/002. Which Beer Report, 1960, pages 171 - 173.								

The OG is between that of the Northern and Midlands Milds. Again the average rate of attenuation is high at over 80%, leaving an average ABV not much different from the other two sets.

Mild Grists

We've already seen how diverse Mild was in terms of strength and colour. It should come as no surprise that the ingredients used to brew Mild were also diverse. Once again, I've divided them up by region.

Starting with the South (excluding London).

Southern Mild grists 1947 - 1964: malts									
Year	Brewer	Beer	OG	mild malt	pale malt	black malt	amber malt	crystal malt	enzymic malt
1947	Adnams	XX	1027.1	71.32%			5.09%	5.09%	
1951	Adnams	XXX	1031.0	80.68%			5.93%	5.93%	
1965	Adnams	XXX	1031.0	74.65%				8.78%	2.90%
1947	Shepherd Neame	MB	1027.1		68.70%				
1954	Shepherd Neame	SM	1030.2		88.11%				
1952	Strong	XXX	1033.5	56.60%	28.30%				
1955	Flowers	XXX	1032.4		81.82%				
1959	Ushers	X	1030.7		79.16%	2.29%		9.18%	
1949	Elgood	XK	1026.5	80.49%				7.32%	
1953	Elgood	X	1026.0	80.00%					
1964	Eldridge Pope	SM	1026.3		70.13%			11.69%	

Sources:
Adnams brewing record Book 34 held at the brewery
Adnams brewing record Book 38 held at the brewery
Adnams brewing record held at the brewery
Shepherd Neame 1947 brewing book held at the brewery
Shepherd Neame 1954 brewing book H/500 held at the brewery
79A01-A3-3-27
Ref Shakespeare Birthplace Trust DR227/215 Brewing Record Book No2
1075-275-6 Wiltshire archives at Chippenham
Elgood brewing record held at the brewery

There's not a single malt they all have in common. The most popular are mild, pale and crystal malt, which all appear in six of the eleven examples.

There are just two roasted malts: black and amber. They appear in a mere three of the beers. It was quite unusual for Dark Mild to be coloured with malt.

Next we'll take a look at the adjuncts in these same beers.

Southern Mild grists 1947 - 1964: adjuncts						
Year	Brewer	Beer	OG	flaked rice	flaked barley	wheat flour
1947	Adnams	XX	1027.1		10.19%	
1951	Adnams	XXX	1031.0			
1965	Adnams	XXX	1031.0			
1947	Shepherd Neame	MB	1027.1		9.16%	
1954	Shepherd Neame	SM	1030.2			
1952	Strong	XXX	1033.5			
1955	Flowers	XXX	1032.4			
1959	Ushers	X	1030.7			
1949	Elgood	XK	1026.5			
1953	Elgood	X	1026.0	3.30%	6.70%	
1964	Eldridge Pope	SM	1026.3			3.80%

Surprisingly, very few adjuncts were used. That's not particularly typical. The flaked barley is a hangover from wartime restrictions. I've no idea why Elgood used wheat flour. It's a bit odd.

Southern Mild grists 1947 - 1964: sugars									
Year	Brewer	Beer	OG	no. 3 sugar	invert	lactose	caramel	malt extract	other sugar
1947	Adnams	XX	1027.1	6.79%			1.52%		
1951	Adnams	XXX	1031.0	6.33%			1.13%		
1965	Adnams	XXX	1031.0	8.78%					4.89%
1947	Shepherd Neame	MB	1027.1	9.16%				9.92%	3.05%
1954	Shepherd Neame	SM	1030.2	5.59%				0.70%	5.59%
1952	Strong	XXX	1033.5	3.77%				3.77%	7.55%
1955	Flowers	XXX	1032.4			6.55%		4.36%	7.27%
1959	Ushers	X	1030.7		5.35%		2.49%	1.53%	
1949	Elgood	XK	1026.5		4.88%			4.88%	2.44%
1953	Elgood	X	1026.0		3.33%			3.33%	3.33%
1964	Eldridge Pope	SM	1026.3					3.80%	5.48%

No surprise that No. 3 invert sugar was popular in Mild. It's quite possible that what's listed as simply "invert" was also No. 3. Some breweries weren't very specific about the type of invert sugar they used. Along with caramel. No. 3 invert was the main colorant in many Dark Milds.

That so many contained malt extract might seem strange, but many breweries threw it into all their beers. The other sugar column mostly consists of proprietary sugars of various types.

Lactose occasionally shows up in beers other than Milk Stout. Including Mild. Though it's by no means a common occurrence.

In the other sugar column a wide variety of products are represented, most of them proprietary sugar, but sometimes candy or cane sugar.

Now it's time to move North to look at its Milds.

Northern Mild grists 1947 - 1964: malts								
Year	Brewer	Beer	OG	pale malt	black malt	crystal malt	high dried malt	enzymic malt
1947	Boddington	XX	1028.0	61.48%	0.91%	9.22%		2.27%
1951	Boddington	XX	1032.0	65.05%	0.70%	20.70%		2.22%
1966	Boddington	BM	1033.5	68.52%		10.28%		2.57%
1953	Truman (Burton)	XX	1030.7	83.54%			14.53%	
1964	Truman (Burton)	XX	1030.7	76.53%		10.20%		
1956	Tennant	Rock Ale	1032.9	76.68%				2.69%
1946	Tetley	M	1033.0	64.99%				
1961	Clarke	1/2 MB	1032.9	78.42%				1.40%

Sources:
Boddington brewing record held at Manchester Central Library, document number M693/405/130.
Boddington brewing record held at Manchester Central Library, document number M693/405/133.
Truman brewing record held at the London Metropolitan Archives, document number B/THB/C/355.
Truman brewing record held at the London Metropolitan Archives, document number B/THB/C/374.
Tennant brewing record held at Sheffield City Archive, document number MD7518/38/34.
Tetley brewing record held at the West Yorkshire Archives, document number WYL756/ACC3349/565
Clarke brewing record held at Manchester Central Library, document number M693/405/137.

The biggest difference with the malts used in Southern Milds is the absence of mild malt as base. All five breweries used pale malt as their base. Surprisingly, only two breweries included crystal malt. While three used the 1950s favourite, enzymic malt.

As a ta Boddington, small quantities of black malt were sometimes employed for colour. From the way it's listed in the brewing record, it looks as if in this case it was added in the copper.

Looking at the adjuncts, I'm starting to realise that the use of flaked maize wasn't quite as extensive as I had thought:

Northern Mild grists 1947 - 1964: adjuncts						
Year	Brewer	Beer	OG	flaked maize	flaked barley	wheat
1947	Boddington	XX	1028.0		14.32%	
1951	Boddington	XX	1032.0			
1966	Boddington	BM	1033.5			3.43%
1953	Truman (Burton)	XX	1030.7			
1964	Truman (Burton)	XX	1030.7	5.10%		
1956	Tennant	Rock Ale	1032.9			
1946	Tetley	M	1033.0		13.84%	
1961	Clarke	1/2 MB	1032.9	3.74%		

I'm not sure what form the wheat was in as it'd listed as simply "wheat" in the brewing record.

Northern Mild grists 1947 - 1964: sugars										
Year	**Brewer**	**Beer**	**OG**	**no. 2 sugar**	**no. 3 sugar**	**invert**	**caramel**	**glucose**	**malt extract**	**other sugar**
1947	Boddington	XX	1028.0			6.15%	0.51%		3.07%	2.05%
1951	Boddington	XX	1032.0			3.94%	0.49%		3.94%	2.96%
1966	Boddington	BM	1033.5			6.85%	0.36%		4.57%	3.43%
1953	Truman	XX	1030.7		1.94%					
1964	Truman	XX	1030.7		6.80%					1.36%
1956	Tennant	Rock Ale	1032.9	1.79%			2.69%		1.79%	14.35%
1946	Tetley	M	1033.0							21.17%
1961	Clarke	1/2 MB	1032.9			3.73%	1.50%	3.73%	3.73%	3.73%

There's not much of a recognisable pattern in the sugar usage. Other than that some sort of invert and malt extract were popular. There's also quite a lot of caramel for colouring purposes.

We finish with London Mild grists.

London Mild grists 1947 - 1965: malts								
Year	**Brewer**	**Beer**	**OG**	**pale malt**	**mild malt**	**SA malt**	**amber malt**	**crystal malt**
1948	Whitbread	XX	1027.7	20.79%	63.48%			7.87%
1955	Whitbread	MA	1030.9		79.44%			6.27%
1965	Whitbread	Best Ale	1030.7		80.00%			5.88%
1946	Fullers	X	1030.7	78.50%				
1958	Fullers	X	1031.3	81.06%				
1947	Barclay Perkins	XX	1030.4		25.48%	46.33%	4.63%	6.95%

Sources:
Whitbread brewing record held at the London Metropolitan Archives, document number LMA/4453/D/01/116.
Whitbread brewing record held at the London Metropolitan Archives, document number LMA/4453/D/01/122.
Whitbread brewing record held at the London Metropolitan Archives, document number LMA/4453/D/01/132.
Fullers brewing records held at the brewery.
Barclay Perkins brewing record held at the London Metropolitan Archives, document number ACC/2305/01/627.

As with Southern Milds, there's a mixture of pale and mild malt as the base. Except at Barclay Perkins where SA malt – a malt that produces a less readily fermentable wort – makes an appearance. Along with amber malt, which isn't very common in Mild, and crystal malt.

Once again, there aren't a great number of adjuncts in play.

London Mild grists 1947 - 1965: adjuncts					
Year	Brewer	Beer	OG	flaked maize	flaked barley
1948	Whitbread	XX	1027.7		
1955	Whitbread	MA	1030.9		
1965	Whitbread	Best Ale	1030.7		
1946	Fullers	X	1030.7		14.54%
1958	Fullers	X	1031.3	9.01%	
1947	Barclay Perkins	XX	1030.4		4.63%

Flaked barley was a wartime substitution for flaked maize that quickly lost favour when it was no longer compulsory.

London Mild grists 1947 - 1965: sugars								
Year	Brewer	Beer	OG	no. 2 sugar	no. 3 sugar	caramel	glucose	other sugar
1948	Whitbread	XX	1027.7		5.99%			1.87%
1955	Whitbread	MA	1030.9		11.15%			3.14%
1965	Whitbread	Best Ale	1030.7		10.98%			3.14%
1946	Fullers	X	1030.7			1.53%	3.49%	1.94%
1958	Fullers	X	1031.3	4.80%				5.14%
1947	Barclay Perkins	XX	1030.4		10.81%	1.16%		

Invert sugars were popular in London, too. Glucose was another wartime thing, turning up in many 1940s recipes when many other types of sugar weren't available.

Pale Ale

I'm not going to try to split apart Pale Ale and IPA because it's pointless. Beers were fairly randomly labelled as either the one or the other. In this category I'm going to lump together both types, just for my own convenience, really.

Pale Ale colour in 1952							
Year	Brewer	Beer	Price	size	package	OG	colour
1952	Ansell	Spotlight	10d	half pint	bottled	1038.3	19
1952	Cobbs Brewery	Pale Ale	10d	half pint	bottled	1031.5	26
1952	Barclay Perkins	Pale Ale	15d	pint	draught	1034.6	19
1952	Barclay Perkins	Pale Ale	16d	pint	draught	1033.22	24
1952	Barclay Perkins	Pale Ale	16d	pint	draught	1032.78	23
1952	Bass	H & O Pale Ale		half pint	bottled	1036.7	20
1952	Bass	Pale Ale	19d	pint	draught	1044.81	22
1952	Bass	Pale Ale	19d	pint	draught	1046.44	24
1952	Beasley	Pale Ale	17d	pint	draught	1037.18	30
1952	Benskins	Pale Ale	18d	pint	draught	1038.98	23
1952	Charrington	Pale Ale	15d	pint	draught	1034.06	18
1952	Courage	Pale Ale	16d	pint	draught	1037.47	24
1952	Courage	Pale Ale	19d	pint	draught	1039.99	26
1952	Courage	Pale Ale	18d	pint	draught	1039.04	32

Pale Ale colour in 1952							
Year	**Brewer**	**Beer**	**Price**	**size**	**package**	**OG**	**colour**
1952	Ind Coope	Pale Ale	19d	pint	draught	1044.08	26
1952	Ind Coope	Pale Ale	19d	pint	draught	1043.7	23
1952	Ind Coope	Pale Ale	19d	pint	draught	1044.86	23
1952	Ind Coope	Coronet Pale Ale	11d	half pint	bottled	1035.6	22
1952	Lacons	Pale Ale	17d	pint	draught	1037.98	30
1952	Lacons	Pale Ale	18d	pint	draught	1037.93	25
1952	Lacons	Pale Ale	17d	pint	draught	1037.36	28
1952	Lees	Bitter				1040.0	20
1952	Lees	Bitter				1040.0	20
1952	Mann Crossman	Pale Ale	20d	pint	draught	1044.91	20
1952	McMullen	Macs No.1 Pale Ale	10.5d	half pint	bottled	1038.2	30
1952	Meux	Pale Ale	17d	pint	draught	1036.04	20
1952	Taylor Walker	Pale Ale	17d	pint	draught	1037.65	24
1952	Tetley	Pale Ale	16d	pint	draught	1036.27	20
1952	Tollemache	Pale Ale	18d	pint	draught	1035.96	23
1952	Tooth & Co	Resch's Bitter Ale		half pint	bottled	1043.1	13
1952	Truman	Pale Ale	17d	pint	draught	1037.15	20
1952	Truman	Pale Ale	17d	pint	draught	1037.14	24
1952	Truman	Pale Ale	17d	pint	draught	1036.72	20
1952	Truman	Pale Ale	17d	pint	draught	1036.52	24
1952	Watney	Pale Ale	17d	pint	draught	1037.42	24
1952	Watney	Pale Ale	17d	pint	draught	1035.72	26
1952	Wenlock	Pale Ale	17d	pint	draught	1036.09	32
1952	Wenlock	Pale Ale	16d	pint	draught	1036.69	27
1952	Whitbread	Pale Ale	17d	pint	draught	1038.12	28
1952	Younger	Pale Ale	17d	pint	draught	1035.92	26
1952	Wm.Younger	"Monk" Export	1/1d	half pint	bottled	1046.9	24
	Average					***1038.4***	***23.7***

Sources:
Truman Gravity Book held at the London Metropolitan Archives, document number B/THB/C/252.
Whitbread Gravity book held at the London Metropolitan Archives, document number LMA/4453/D/02/002.
Lees brewing records

Draught Pale Ale

After WW II, the vast majority of Pale Ale was consumed in the form of draught Bitter. Mostly fairly puny Ordinary Bitter of around 3.5 % ABV. Though as the 1950s went on, more breweries reintroduced a stronger Bitter for those with a few more bob in their pocket. Fullers London Pride and Youngs Special are good examples.

Draught Bass Pale Ale was still a respectable strength and one of the few draught beers allowed onto the bar of other brewers' tied houses. Still run through union sets, it was a distinctive beer with an air of class that drinkers were willing to pay that little bit extra for.

Boys Bitter

The name is one which was later – I think in the 1970s – was given to a type of low-gravity draught Bitter found in the Southwest of England. By the 1970s these beers often played the role of draught Mild, which by then had mostly disappeared from the region.

I'm using the term to refer to any draught Bitter under 1036°. It's a pretty arbitrary distinction, but it stops the tables getting too big.

Boys Bitter 1953 to 1959								
Year	**Brewer**	**Beer**	**Price per pint (d)**	**OG**	**FG**	**ABV**	**App. Atten-uation**	**colour**
1959	Fuller	Bitter	14	1031.6	1004.1	3.58	87.03%	23
1959	Charrington	BBB	17	1032.8	1007.8	3.24	76.22%	14
1954	Barclay Perkins	XLK	15	1032.9	1004.5	3.70	86.32%	
1954	Meux	PA	17	1033.7	1007.3	3.43	78.34%	24
1954	Barclay Perkins	XLK	15	1033.8	1006.9	3.49	79.59%	19
1954	Taylor Walker	EPA	17	1034	1008.6	3.29	74.71%	23
1958	Vaux & Co	Bitter Ale	17	1034.2	1007.8	3.43	77.19%	26
1953	Whitbread	Pale Ale	16	1035.1				22
1957	Ind Coope	Best Bitter	17	1035.2	1008	3.53	77.27%	19
1954	Mann Crossman	KK	17	1035.3	1007.7	3.58	78.19%	19
1957	Charrington	PA	15	1035.5	1004.9	3.98	86.20%	23
1959	Whitaker	Bitter	14	1035.6	1010.2	3.17	71.35%	22
	Average		***15.9***	***1034.1***	***1007.1***	***3.49***	***79.3%***	***21.5***
Sources:								
Truman Gravity Book held at the London Metropolitan Archives, document number B/THB/C/252.								
Whitbread Gravity book held at the London Metropolitan Archives, document number LMA/4453/D/02/002.								
document from the Steel Coulson archive held at the Scottish Brewing Archives								
T & J Bernard's brewing records held at the Scottish Brewing Archive								

The rate of attenuation – which is just under 80% - is pretty high. Presumably that's an attempt to compensate for the low gravity. It leaves the average ABV a respectable 3.5%.

The 1960s didn't bring about any huge changes to this type of beer, as you can see in the next table.

Boys Bitter 1960 - 1964								
Year	**Brewer**	**Beer**	**Price per pint d**	**OG**	**FG**	**ABV**	**App. Atten-uation**	**colour**
1960	Beasley	Bitter	15	1034.3	1004.5	3.72	86.88%	35
1960	Blatch Brewery	Bitter	14	1031.8	1003.9	3.49	87.74%	20
1960	Burt & Co.	Best Bitter	13	1032.6	1004.5	3.51	86.20%	20
1964	Camerons	Ordinary Bitter	15	1031.3	1006.7	3.07	78.59%	30
1960	Charles Wells	Bitter	18	1034.4	1006.6	3.48	80.81%	18
1960	Charrington	Ordinary Bitter	14	1033.8	1008	3.35	76.33%	18
1960	Clinch	Bitter	13	1034	1006.1	3.49	82.06%	20

Boys Bitter 1960 - 1964								
Year	Brewer	Beer	Price per pint d	OG	FG	ABV	App. Atten-uation	colour
1960	Dunmow Brewery	Bitter	14	1033.6	1006.6	3.37	80.36%	25
1960	Fremlin	XXX Bitter	14	1035.5	1005.7	3.72	83.94%	26
1960	Friary	Bitter	14	1033.8	1005.2	3.57	84.62%	20
1960	Fullers	Ordinary Bitter	16	1032.2	1005.3	3.50	83.54%	24
1960	Garne & Sons	Bitter	13	1031.2	1004.3	3.36	86.22%	21
1960	Georges	Bitter	13	1030.9	1004.75	3.40	84.63%	
1960	Gray's	Bitter	13	1033.6	1006.1	3.44	81.85%	21
1960	Greenall Whitley	Bitter	14	1034.4	1005.95	3.70	82.70%	
1960	Greene King	Ordinary Bitter	13	1033.9	1005.7	3.53	83.19%	26
1964	Hammond	Caledonian Scotch	15	1031.2	1008.7	2.81	72.12%	30
1960	Hammond	Best Bitter	16	1035.5	1004.05	4.10	88.59%	
1960	Harvey's	Bitter	14	1033.8	1006.1	3.46	81.95%	22
1960	Kemp Town	Bitter	12	1031.5	1004	3.44	87.30%	16
1960	Morland	Bitter	14	1035.6	1006.1	3.69	82.87%	18
1960	Morrell	Light Bitter	12	1030.7	1005	3.21	83.71%	17
1960	Morrell	Best Bitter	15	1035.3	1005.3	3.75	84.99%	23
1964	Newcastle Breweries	Scotch Ale	15	1032.3	1005.4	3.36	83.28%	30
1964	Northern Clubs Federation	Ordinary Bitter	13	1033.1	1004.5	3.57	86.40%	25
1960	Rayments	Bitter	12	1030.3	1004.1	3.27	86.47%	18
1960	Rayments	Best Bitter	14	1035.7	1006.4	3.66	82.07%	22
1961	Rhymney	Silver Drum	18	1035.1	1007.1	3.50	79.77%	17
1960	Ridley	Ordinary Bitter	14	1034.2	1009.8	3.05	71.35%	19
1960	Star Brewery, Eastbourne	Bitter	12	1029.5	1003.3	3.28	88.81%	20
1960	Tamplin	Bitter	14	1034.3	1006	3.54	82.51%	24
1960	Thwaites	Bitter	16	1035.8	1006.6	3.80	81.56%	
1960	Tollemache	Bitter	16	1033.3	1003.4	3.74	89.79%	20
1960	Usher	Ordinary Bitter	13	1032.5	1007.3	3.15	77.54%	18
1960	Ushers	Bitter	13	1031.9	1008.75	3.00	72.57%	
1960	Vaux	Best Bitter	15	1034.8	1005.6	3.80	83.91%	
1960	Wenlock	Bitter	16	1035	1008.7	3.41	75.14%	26
	Average		***14.2***	***1033.3***	***1005.8***	***3.47***	***82.50%***	***22.2***

Sources:
Whitbread Gravity book held at the London Metropolitan Archives, document number LMA/4453/D/02/002.
Which Beer Report, 1960, pages 171 - 173.

The average rate of attenuation is even higher than in the 1950s, over 80%. And, surprisingly, the average price per pint is lower, just over 14d rather than almost 16d.

Ordinary Bitter

For simplicity's sake, I'm classing anything between 1036° and 1037.9° as Ordinary Bitter.

Ordinary Bitter in the 1953 to 1959								
Year	**Brewer**	**Beer**	**Price per pint (d)**	**OG**	**FG**	**ABV**	**App. Atten-uation**	**colour**
1953	Benskins	Pale Ale	16	1037.2				18
1954	Charrington	BBB	15	1036.8	1008.9	3.62	75.82%	26
1954	Courage	Alton PA	18	1037.7	1008.1	3.84	78.51%	24
1957	Ind Coope	PA	17	1036.3	1006.5	3.88	82.09%	19
1959	Ind Coope	Red Hand	22	1037.5	1011.5	3.37	69.33%	18
1953	Mann	Pale Ale	17	1037.5				25
1953	Meux	Pale Ale	17	1036.8				27
1953	Taylor Walker	Pale Ale	18	1036.3				27
1953	Tetley	Pale Ale	16	1037.3				20
1954	Truman	PA	17	1036.7	1006.4	3.94	82.56%	18
1955	Truman	PA Burton Brewed	17	1037.7	1005.9	4.14	84.35%	17
1957	Truman	PA	17	1037.2	1007.1	3.91	80.91%	18
1954	Watney	IPA	17	1036.7	1008.4	3.67	77.11%	23
1957	Watney	PA	17	1036.8	1006.9	3.89	81.25%	26
1959	Websters	Bitter	15	1037	1005.4	3.95	85.41%	20
1953	Wenlock	Pale Ale	16	1037				24
1954	Whitbread	PA	17	1037.9	1004.8	4.31	87.34%	24
1953	Young & Co	Pale Ale	16	1036.8				20
	Average		***16.9***	***1037.1***	***1007.3***	***3.87***	***80.4%***	***21.9***

Sources:
Truman Gravity Book held at the London Metropolitan Archives, document number B/THB/C/252.
Whitbread Gravity book held at the London Metropolitan Archives, document number LMA/4453/D/02/002.

The rate of attenuation is similar to Boys Bitter at around 80%, leaving average ABV not far short of 4%. The list is very London dominated. Only Websters and Benskins are from outside the capital.

Ordinary Bitter 1960 - 1965								
Year	**Brewer**	**Beer**	**Price per pint d**	**OG**	**FG**	**ABV**	**App. Atten-uation**	**colour**
1964	Camerons	Special Scotch	17	1037.3	1007.7	3.70	79.36%	40
1965	Charrington	Plus Four	17	1036.4	1008.5	3.62	76.65%	22
1961	Dares	Drum Treble Gold	22	1037	1007.7	3.66	79.19%	10
1961	Evan Evans Bevan	Crown Bitter	20	1036.7	1004	4.09	89.10%	20
1961	Everards	Golden Bitter	20	1037.6	1003.7	4.24	90.16%	14
1960	Greene King	Bitter	15	1037.0	1006.25	4.00	83.11%	
1960	Ind Coope	Bitter (BB)	15	1037.7	1008.4	3.80	77.72%	
1961	Ind Coope	Red Hand	21	1036.7	1011	3.33	70.03%	18
1960	John Smiths	Best Bitter	16	1036.8	1010.55	3.40	71.33%	
1960	McMullen	Ordinary Bitter	15	1037	1008	3.63	78.38%	22
1960	Mew Langton	Best Bitter	18	1037	1008.6	3.55	76.76%	19
1964	Newcastle	Four Star	17	1037.6	1008.7	3.61	76.86%	30

Ordinary Bitter 1960 - 1965								
Year	**Brewer**	**Beer**	**Price per pint d**	**OG**	**FG**	**ABV**	**App. Atten-uation**	**colour**
	Breweries							
1965	Nimmo	Durham Ale	18	1036.7	1006.2	3.81	83.11%	40
1961	Rhymney	Hobby Horse	20	1036.4	1007.3	3.64	79.95%	13
1960	Simpson & Co.	Bitter	15	1036.2	1008	3.53	77.90%	24
1961	Strongs	Barley Corn Bitter	24	1037.6	1006.3	3.91	83.24%	23
1960	Tetley	Bitter	16	1037.9	1003.7	4.28	90.24%	20
1961	Tomson & Wotton	Bitter	24	1037.7	1004.1	4.20	89.12%	20
1960	Truman	Ordinary Burton Bitter	16	1037.4	1007.6	3.87	79.68%	20
1961	Walkers	Goblet Pale Ale	19	1037.9	1006.4	3.94	83.11%	17
1960	Wells & Winch	Bitter	16	1036	1010.3	3.21	71.39%	12
1960	Wilson	Bitter	15	1036.1	1006.1	3.90	83.10%	
1960	Young & Co	Ordinary Bitter	15	1037.5	1006.6	3.86	82.40%	19
	Average		***18.0***	***1037.1***	***1007.1***	***3.8***	***80.82%***	***21.4***

Sources:
Whitbread Gravity book held at the London Metropolitan Archives, document number LMA/4453/D/02/002.
Which Beer Report, 1960, pages 171 - 173.

Best Bitter

Continuing my arbitrary classifications, I'm calling anything with an OG 1038° to 1044.9° Best Bitter.

Best Bitter in the 1953 to 1959								
Year	**Brewer**	**Beer**	**Price per pint (d)**	**OG**	**FG**	**ABV**	**App. Atten-uation**	**colour**
1954	Taylor Walker	PA	17	1038	1009.9	3.64	73.95%	23
1959	Websters	Bitter	16	1038	1004.7	4.16	87.63%	22
1954	Courage	PA	18	1038.4	1006.4	4.16	83.33%	28
1954	Charrington	PA	15	1038.6	1008.1	3.96	79.02%	20
1957	Whitbread	PA	19	1038.6	1010	3.71	74.09%	20
1957	Whitbread	PA	19	1038.6	1010	3.71	74.09%	20
1957	Taylor Walker	PA	17	1038.8	1009.3	3.83	76.03%	19
1959	Ramsdens	Bitter	16	1038.9	1006	4.28	84.58%	16
1955	Hancock	HB		1039				
1957	Barclay Perkins	PA	18	1039.5	1005.9	4.38	85.06%	26
1959	Bentleys	Bitter	16	1039.5	1010.2	3.66	74.18%	19
1954	Whitbread	PA	17	1039.5				
1957	Courage	PA	18	1039.8	1005.4	4.48	86.43%	27
1954	Barclay Perkins	Best Bitter	18	1040.4	1007.5	4.28	81.44%	22
1959	Ramsdens	Bitter	16	1040.7	1006.2	4.31	84.77%	18
1959	Courage & Barclay	Bitter	22	1040.9	1009.8	4.04	76.04%	23

Best Bitter in the 1953 to 1959								
Year	Brewer	Beer	Price per pint (d)	OG	FG	ABV	App. Atten-uation	colour
1959	Fuller	Best Bitter	19	1041.4	1006.1	4.60	85.27%	32
1953	Watney	Pale Ale	19	1042.8				27
1957	Ind Coope	Double Diamond	20	1043.8	1008.1	4.65	81.51%	20
1957	Watney	Best PA	21	1044	1014.2	3.86	67.73%	20
1957	Bass, Burton	Pale Ale	21	1044.6	1005.4	5.12	87.89%	21
1953	Bass, Burton	Pale Ale	19	1044.7				26
1953	Watney	Special Bitter	20	1044.9	1009.6	4.59	78.62%	28
	Average		***18.2***	***1040.6***	***1008.0***	***4.18***	***80.09%***	***22.6***

Sources:
Truman Gravity Book held at the London Metropolitan Archives, document number B/THB/C/252.
Whitbread Gravity book held at the London Metropolitan Archives, document number LMA/4453/D/02/002.
"Cardiff Pubs and Breweries" by Brian Glover, 2005. pages 97-101

I'm slightly surprised that Draught Bass was one of the paler examples. I always thought that was on the dark side. Though it's also one of the strongest, at around 5% ABV. As a relatively expensive beer, it was able to maintain its gravity better than most. The

There's quite a big variation in colour, from 16 to 32. Somewhere between 20 and 25 is the colour I would expect for this type of beer.

The attenuation is all over the place – 68% to 88% - but averages only a little lower than the previous two sets.

Best Bitter 1960 - 1964								
Year	Brewer	Beer	Price per pint (d)	OG	FG	ABV	App. Atten-uation	colour
1961	Ansell	King Pin Bitter	23	1044.8	1004.4	5.05	90.18%	17
1960	Bass	Bitter	21	1044	1009.8	4.45	77.73%	19
1964	Camerons	Strong Arm	20	1044	1010.3	4.21	76.59%	35
1960	Carlisle State Management	Bitter	14	1038.2	1008.2	3.90	78.53%	
1960	Charrington	Best Bitter	19	1044.5	1012.9	4.10	71.01%	24
1960	Courage & Barclay	Alton Pale Ale	17	1040.4	1009.4	4.03	76.73%	25
1961	Devenish	High Life	21	1038.9	1007.1	3.98	81.75%	24
1960	Flowers	Bitter	19	1040.6	1008.8	3.97	78.33%	24
1960	Fremlins	Best Bitter	21	1044.7	1009.3	4.60	79.19%	
1960	Friary Meux	Treble Gold	18	1042.3	1008.9	4.18	78.96%	23
1960	Fullers	London Pride	20	1042.3	1010.5	4.13	75.18%	24
1960	Garne & Sons	Best Bitter	17	1042.9	1009.5	4.18	77.86%	30
1960	Greene King	Best Bitter	15	1038.4	1007.4	3.88	80.73%	20
1964	Hammond	Caledonian Special	20	1041.7	1011.5	3.78	72.42%	17
1961	Hancock	Barley Brite	24	1038.5	1006.7	3.97	82.60%	17
1960	Ind Coope	Double Diamond	19	1040.2	1010	3.92	75.12%	22

Best Bitter 1960 - 1964								
Year	Brewer	Beer	Price per pint (d)	OG	FG	ABV	App. Atten-uation	colour
1964	John Smith	Bitter	18	1038.3	1007.6	3.84	80.16%	23
1964	John Smith	Draught Magnet	20	1043	1007.4	4.45	82.79%	35
1961	Matthew & Co.	Buffalo Ale	21	1044.6	1013.7	3.86	69.28%	27
1960	McMullen	Best Bitter	16	1041.1	1010.8	3.79	73.72%	25
1961	Mitchell & Butler	Anker	23	1043.4	1010.9	4.06	74.88%	16
1964	Newcastle Breweries	Exhibition Ale	20	1043.2	1008.8	4.30	79.63%	18
1961	Norman & Pring	Tan Bitter	24	1038.4	1005.2	4.15	86.46%	18
1964	Northern Clubs Federation	Special	17	1040.9	1011.5	3.68	71.88%	17
1960	Simonds	Best Bitter	19	1042.3	1007.5	4.35	82.27%	17
1961	St. Austell	Extra	20	1039.9	1005.6	4.29	85.96%	25
1960	Star Brewery, Eastbourne	SPA	17	1039.5	1005.8	4.21	85.32%	22
1960	Tennant	Queen's Ale	18	1041.7	1008.6	4.30	79.38%	
1960	Truman	Best Burton Bitter	18	1042.7	1009.7	4.29	77.28%	19
1960	Usher, Trowbridge	Best Bitter	18	1043.6	1010	4.20	77.06%	21
1964	Vaux	Samson	20	1043.1	1011.1	4.00	74.25%	25
1961	Warwick & Richardson	Crystal Bitter	18	1038	1009.1	3.61	76.05%	20
1960	Watney	Special Bitter	19	1044.2	1009.6	4.50	78.28%	26
1961	Watney	Red Barrel	23	1038.6	1006.6	4.16	82.90%	26
1960	Whitbread	Bitter	17	1038.5	1011	3.56	71.43%	20
1961	Workington Brewery	Golden Bitter	21	1044.7	1008.1	4.58	81.88%	26
	Average		***19.3***	***1041.6***	***1009.0***	***4.12***	***78.44%***	***22.6***

Sources:
Whitbread Gravity book held at the London Metropolitan Archives, document number LMA/4453/D/02/002.
Which Beer Report, 1960, pages 171 - 173.

Little has changes with this 1960s set. The average attenuation has declined a little, as has the ABV. While the average OG has increased a little.

Strong Bitter

According to my classification, Strong Bitter is anything above 1045°. Beers of this type pretty much disappeared in the 1940s. As restrictions on brewing were lifted in the early 1050s, breweries started to introduce stronger Bitters, similar in strength to pre-war Best Bitter.

About the only exception to this was Draught Bass, which even during the war remained over 1045°.

Beers of this strength didn't sell in enormous quantities, but were profitable enough to be worth a brewery's while. Often they were parti-gyled with standard Bitter, an economical way of producing a small batch beer. Which is still the way Fullers produce ESB.

Strong Bitter 1953 - 1964								
Year	Brewer	Beer	Price per pint d	OG	FG	ABV	App. Atten-uation	colour
1960	Ansells	Bitter	17	1045.3	1010.7	4.50	76.38%	
1954	Bass	Pale Ale	19	1046	1008.7	4.86	81.09%	20
1965	Bass	Draught PA		1050.5	1009.4	5.36	81.39%	16
1964	Camerons	Strong Arm	25	1045.2	1013.1	4.01	71.02%	45
1953	Charrington	Pale Ale	17	1046.4				29
1959	Charrington	Toby Ale	15	1046.6	1009.4	4.84	79.83%	20
1963	Charrington	Toby Ale	33	1048.1	1008.3	5.19	82.74%	18
1960	Courage & Barclay	Directors' Bitter	24	1048.8	1008.4	5.27	82.79%	26
1960	Greene King	Abbot Ale	22	1051.3	1007.9	5.43	84.60%	20
1960	Ridley	Best Bitter	21	1047	1007.8	4.90	83.40%	22
1961	Southams	Pressure PA	24	1045.8	1007.1	4.84	84.50%	17
1954	Watney	Special Bitter	20	1045.5	1013.7	4.12	69.89%	23
1963	Watney	Red Barrel Ex. PA	31	1047.7	1012.9	4.52	72.96%	20
1965	Watney	PA		1050.3	1011.5	5.05	77.14%	23
1960	Young & Co	Best Bitter	20	1048.4	1011.5	4.61	76.24%	24
	Average		***21.4***	***1047.5***	***1010.0***	***4.82***	***76.24%***	***23.1***

Sources:
Whitbread Gravity book held at the London Metropolitan Archives, document number LMA/4453/D/02/002.
Which Beer Report, 1960, pages 171 - 173.

Keg Bitter

At a time when the quality of cask beer was often questionable, but bottled beer was rather expensive for the average drinker, Keg Bitter was an attractive proposition Brewers often described it as being bulk bottled beer.

Crystal clear and sparkling, it had the visual characteristics associated with good-quality beer. And, being pasteurised, there was little chance of it turning sour before the keg ran dry.

Keg Bitter in the 1957 to 1959								
Year	Brewer	Beer	Price per pint (d)	OG	FG	ABV	App. Atten-uation	colour
1959	Simonds	Keg Bitter	22	1037.4	1007.3	3.76	80.48%	19
1959	South London Brewery	Golden Keg	18	1037.9	1005.7	4.03	84.96%	19
1959	Watney	Red Barrel	22	1038.5	1010	3.70	74.03%	24
1959	Flowers	Keg Bitter	22	1039	1010.7	3.54	72.56%	23
1959	Whitbread	Tankard Bitter	22	1039.1	1011.9	3.52	69.57%	22
1957	Watney	Keg Bitter	24	1039.4	1007.6	4.14	80.71%	23
1959	Truman	Keg Bitter	22	1040.5	1008.8	4.12	78.27%	22
1957	Courage & Barclay	Keg Bitter	22	1042.8	1006.6	4.72	84.58%	22

Keg Bitter in the 1957 to 1959								
Year	**Brewer**	**Beer**	**Price per pint (d)**	**OG**	**FG**	**ABV**	**App. Atten-uation**	**colour**
1959	Wm. Younger	Keg Bitter	19	1043.7	1007.8	4.68	82.15%	55
	Average		***21.4***	***1039.8***	***1008.5***	***4.02***	***78.6%***	***25.4***
	Without Younger							***21.75***
Sources: Whitbread Gravity book held at the London Metropolitan Archives, document number LMA/4453/D/02/002.								

The first Keg Bitters of the 1950s were promoted as high-class Pale Ales. And that's where the origin of some truly lay. Double Diamond was a version of Allsopp's IPA and Ben Truman was the descendent of a 19th-century bottled IPA. These beers were priced according to their perceived prestige. Keg Bitter was, on average, 3d per pint more expensive than an equivalent cask beer.

As brewers moved away from cask-conditioning, mostly for reasons of consistency and convenience, standard Bitters were also presented in keg form. Though still generally at a higher price than the cask version. It's a trend that continues today: cask is generally cheaper than keg.

As keg began to spread to smaller breweries, more lower-gravity Keg Bitters were brewed. More like Ordinary Bitter than Best Bitter. For the most part, however, they still weren't cheap.

Keg Bitter 1960 - 1965								
Year	**Brewer**	**Beer**	**Price per pint (d)**	**OG**	**FG**	**ABV**	**App. Atten-uation**	**colour**
1960	Bass	Worthington "E"	18	1041.8	1006.5	4.60	84.45%	
1960	Gibbs Mew	Blue Keg Bitter	18	1036	1007.6	3.55	78.89%	25
1960	Ind Coope	Double Diamond	19	1040.2	1010	3.92	75.12%	22
1960	Marston	Burton Keg	21	1036	1006.8	3.65	81.11%	20
1961	Arkells	King Keg	24	1040.5	1007.2	4.16	82.22%	20
1961	Birkenhead Brewery	Keg Gold	20	1043.1	1006.5	4.57	84.92%	23
1961	Brickwoods	Sunshine Keg Bitter	21	1035	1008.4	3.33	76.00%	28
1961	Dryborough	Keg	19	1037.6	1006.8	3.85	81.91%	10
1961	Flowers	Keg	24	1039.3	1012.5	3.35	68.19%	27
1961	Fremlin	Keg	24	1040.4	1005.8	4.33	85.64%	23
1961	Gibbs Mew	Red Keg	22	1040.4	1003.7	4.59	90.84%	21
1961	Gibbs Mew	Blue Keg	18	1034.7	1002.8	3.99	91.93%	24
1961	Home Brewery	5 Star	22	1047.5	1007.7	4.97	83.79%	18
1961	Howcrofts	Silver Keg	15	1037.3	1006.9	3.80	81.50%	20
1961	Lacon	Keg Bitter	24	1040.1	1007.1	4.12	82.29%	17
1961	Starkey, Knight & Ford	Star Keg	23	1042.3	1008	4.29	81.09%	27

Keg Bitter 1960 - 1965								
Year	**Brewer**	**Beer**	**Price per pint (d)**	**OG**	**FG**	**ABV**	**App. Atten-uation**	**colour**
1961	Tennant Bros.	Keg Bitter	21	1036.8	1005	3.97	86.41%	15
1961	Threllfalls	Keg Bitter	18	1038.5	1004.9	4.20	87.27%	17
1961	Truman	Keg Bitter	21	1039	1006.2	4.27	84.10%	16
1961	Vaux	Keg Beer	20	1034.8	1002.2	4.07	93.68%	14
1961	West Country Breweries	Star Bright Keg	16	1029.8	1004.6	3.15	84.56%	22
1961	Whitbread	Tankard Bitter	24	1038.6	1011	3.58	71.50%	18
1961	Yates's Castle Brewery	Keg	20	1037.8	1006.8	3.88	82.01%	16
1963	Watney	Red Barrel Ex. PA	31	1047.7	1012.9	4.52	72.96%	20
1964	John Smith	Golden Keg	24	1039.1	1009.4	3.71	75.96%	23
	Average		***24***	***1039.1***	***1009.4***	***3.71***	***75.96%***	***23***

Sources:
Whitbread Gravity book held at the London Metropolitan Archives, document number LMA/4453/D/02/002.
Which Beer Report, 1960, pages 171 - 173.

It's interesting to note the date when smaller, regional breweries started brewing Keg Bitter: around 1960. Also when they started brewing Lager. That's probably not a coincidence. There's overlap in the equipment used to make the two

Bottled Pale Ale

There was a huge variation in strength amongst bottled Pale Ales. The weakest – which, to be honest, are hard to differentiate from Light Ale – were under 1030°.

Once again, to make it more manageable, I've split them by strength. The groups are <1034°, 1034° to 1038°, 1038° to 1045°, 1045° to 1055° and >1055°.

Immediately after WW II there were a lot of very weedy Pale Ales. But what would you expect when average OG was only 1033°?

London bottled Pale Ale below 1034° 1946 - 1951								
Year	**Brewer**	**Beer**	**Price per pint d**	**OG**	**FG**	**ABV**	**App. Atten-uation**	**colour**
1947	Barclay Perkins	PA	13	1031.2	1007.5	3.07	75.96%	19
1950	Barclay Perkins	PA	15	1029.6	1007.1	2.92	76.01%	20
1946	Beasley	Pale Ale	12	1030.3	1005.6	3.21	81.52%	19
1946	Benskin	Light Sparkling Ale	13	1028.9	1004.9	3.12	83.04%	20.5
1951	Benskin	Light Sparkling Ale	16	1032.6	1008.1	3.18	75.15%	18
1947	Charrington	Toby Ale	13	1031.4	1005.7	3.34	81.85%	17.5
1950	Charrington	Pale Ale	15	1033.3	1010.8	2.91	67.57%	21
1948	Courage	Pale Ale	15	1027.8	1006.1	2.81	78.06%	25
1951	Courage	Pale Ale	14	1033.1	1005.5	3.59	83.38%	

London bottled Pale Ale below 1034° 1946 - 1951								
Year	Brewer	Beer	Price per pint d	OG	FG	ABV	App. Atten-uation	colour
1950	Hammerton	Light VC	15	1031.6	1004.7	3.50	85.13%	27
1947	Hodgson's Kingston Brewery	Pale Ale	13	1030.4	1005.3	3.26	82.57%	20
1951	Ind Coope	Sparkling Ale	18	1032.6	1007.6	3.24	76.69%	21
1946	Isleworth	Pale Ale	12	1029.6	1007.3	2.89	75.34%	21
1946	Mann Crossman	PA	13	1033.4	1006.3	3.52	81.14%	18.5
1950	Mann Crossman	Pale Ale	17	1032.6	1007.6	3.24	76.69%	19
1950	Meux	London Pale Ale	17	1029	1005	3.12	82.76%	26
1948	South London Brewer	SLB Pale Ale	16	1027.4	1008.1	2.50	70.44%	22.5
1946	Taylor Walker	PA	17	1029.8	1010.4	2.51	65.10%	22
1951	Taylor Walker	Pale Ale	17	1031.8	1007	3.22	77.99%	25
1946	Truman	Eagle Ale	13	1030.8	1008.7	2.86	71.75%	25
1951	Truman	Eagle Ale	17	1031.6	1005.4	3.41	82.91%	20
1946	Watney	PA	12.5	1031.1	1007	3.13	77.49%	21
1951	Watney	Pale Ale	17	1030	1009.5	2.65	68.33%	27
1950	Wenlock	Pale Ale	15	1029.6	1009.6	2.59	67.57%	24
	Average		***14.8***	***1030.8***	***1007.1***	***3.07***	***76.85%***	***21.7***
Source: Whitbread Gravity book held at the London Metropolitan Archives, document number LMA/4453/D/02/002.								

There are some pretty weak beers in that set, plenty are under 3% ABV and some just 2.5% ABV. The average price is quite low. Not that much more than draught Pale Ale of a similar strength.

Next, bottled Pale Ale from other parts of the country. Though, with the exception of Hancocks, which was in Cardiff, all the others are from the South.

Other bottled Pale Ale below 1034° 1946 - 1951								
Year	Brewer	Beer	Price per pint d	OG	FG	ABV	App. Atten-uation	colour
1949	Davenport	Best Bitter	14	1032.8	1006.5	3.42	80.18%	19
1946	Fremlin	Dinner Ale	11.5	1028.8	1006	2.96	79.17%	18.5
1946	Fremlin	Elephant Brand Ale	13	1033.1	1006.1	3.51	81.57%	19
1948	Fremlin	Elephant Brand Ale	15	1031.8	1006.5	3.28	79.56%	19
1950	Fremlin	Dinner Ale	13	1028.4	1006.1	2.89	78.52%	24
1950	Gale	Horndean Pale Ale	14	1027	1005.6	2.78	79.26%	21
1951	Hancocks	Bitter Ale	13	1031.2	1010.3	2.70	66.99%	19
1946	Simonds	SB Pale Ale	13	1029.4	1005.1	3.16	82.65%	25
1950	Simonds	SB Pale Ale	18	1032.5	1008.5	3.11	73.85%	26
1949	Style & Winch	Farmer Ale	16	1031	1006.3	3.21	79.68%	18
1951	Style & Winch	Farmer Ale	20	1030.5	1007.8	2.94	74.43%	20
1946	Tollemache	Light Bitter	13	1031.1	1006.1	3.25	80.39%	17
	Average		***14.5***	***1030.6***	***1006.7***	***3.10***	***78.02%***	***20.5***
Source: Whitbread Gravity book held at the London Metropolitan Archives, document number LMA/4453/D/02/002.								

There's not a huge amount of difference with the London beers, other than a slightly higher rate of attenuation.

In the 1950s and 1960s, not a great deal had changed.

London bottled Pale Ale below 1034° 1953 - 1965

Year	Brewer	Beer	Price per pint d	OG	FG	ABV	App. Atten-uation	colour
1959	Beasley	Pale Ale	20	1031.1	1006.8	3.15	78.14%	26
1956	Benskin	Light Ale	19	1031.4	1009.8	2.79	68.79%	25
1959	Charrington	Pale Ale	20	1033.1	1006.9	3.40	79.15%	16
1955	Courage	Pale Ale	24	1033.7	1007.2	3.44	78.64%	25
1965	Courage	Jack Pot	21.25	1032.4	1009.3	2.99	71.30%	22
1959	Friary Meux	Friary Ale	20	1031.5	1007.9	3.06	74.92%	18
1965	Friary Meux	Pipkin 4	23	1029.5	1007.6	2.84	74.24%	16
1956	Fullers	PA	20	1032.1	1008.5	3.06	73.52%	27
1956	Harman's Uxbridge Brewery	Pale Ale	22	1032.1	1008.4	3.07	73.83%	27
1956	Ind Coope	Light Ale	20	1031	1010.5	2.65	66.13%	22
1957	John Egan & Sons	Pale Ale	20	1032.1	1006.3	3.35	80.37%	25
1956	Lovibond	Yeoman Ale	20	1031.6	1005.5	3.39	82.59%	25
1959	Mann Crossman	Pale Ale	20	1029.7	1007.8	2.84	73.74%	
1956	Meux	London Pale Ale	22	1030.4	1009.3	2.73	69.41%	22
1956	South London Brewery	PA	20	1030.3	1007.1	3.01	76.57%	23
1956	Taylor Walker	Pale Ale	20	1032.1	1007.3	3.22	77.26%	23
1954	Truman	Eagle Light Ale	19	1031.3	1005.3	3.38	83.07%	22
1963	Truman	Light Ale	22	1031.8	1008.3	3.05	73.90%	21
1954	Watney	Pale Ale	19	1033.1	1009.7	3.03	70.69%	22
1959	Watney	Pale Ale	20	1033.2	1010.1	2.99	69.58%	23
1956	Wenlock	Light Ale	22	1033.1	1009.3	3.08	71.90%	22
1959	Young	Pale Ale	20	1032.4	1008.9	3.04	72.53%	23
	Average		***20.6***	***1031.8***	***1008.1***	***3.07***	***74.56%***	***22.6***

Source:
Whitbread Gravity book held at the London Metropolitan Archives, document number LMA/4453/D/02/002.

There are still plenty of beers under 3% ABV. Though there's one thing that has gone up: the price. It averages 6d per pint more than the first set.

Southern bottled Pale Ale below 1034° 1953 - 1965

Year	Brewer	Beer	Price per pint d	OG	FG	ABV	App. Atten-uation	colour
1959	Brickwoods	Light Bitter Ale	20	1031.8	1007.4	3.16	76.73%	21
1960	Cheltenham & Hereford Brewery	Cheltenham Ale	18	1032.1	1007.6	3.06	76.32%	25
1953	Ely Brewery Co Ltd	Davids Ale	18	1033.1	1003.7	3.83	88.82%	23
1953	Fremlin	Elephant Light Ale	20	1031.6	1006.9	3.21	78.16%	20
1965	Fremlin	Jumbo	21.25	1029.9	1006.9	2.88	76.92%	20

Southern bottled Pale Ale below 1034° 1953 - 1965								
Year	Brewer	Beer	Price per pint d	OG	FG	ABV	App. Atten-uation	colour
1960	Norman & Pring	Pale Ale	20	1031	1003.8	3.40	87.74%	15
1959	Shepherd Neame	India Pale Ale	20	1031.2	1005.4	3.35	82.69%	21
1955	Simonds	SB Pale Ale	18	1033	1009	3.11	72.73%	21
1960	Starkey, Knight & Ford	Tivvy Pale Ale	20	1030.5	1005.1	3.18	83.28%	28
1959	Strong	Golden Ale	22	1032	1006.3	3.34	80.31%	18
1960	Stroud Brewery	Allbright Ale	18	1030.9	1008	2.86	74.11%	25
1953	Tamplin	Baby Tamp	22.5	1031.8	1005.6	3.40	82.39%	20
1959	Timothy Taylor	Special Pale Ale	19	1032.5	1006.5	3.25	80.00%	23
1956	Tollemache	Light Bitter	20	1030.4	1006.7	3.07	77.96%	19
1960	Tomson & Wotton	Allbright Pale Ale	20	1029.9	1005.8	3.01	80.60%	18
1959	Wethered	Amber Ale	22	1031.7	1006	3.34	81.07%	25
	Average		***19.9***	***1031.5***	***1006.3***	***3.22***	***79.99%***	***21.4***
Source: Whitbread Gravity book held at the London Metropolitan Archives, document number LMA/4453/D/02/002.								

The Southern set averages out a little cheaper. The rate of attenuation is a good bit higher at just about 80%.

The next strength band up is roughly equivalent to Ordinary Bitter.

Bottled Pale Ale 1034° to 1038° 1947 - 1952								
Year	Brewer	Beer	Price per pint d	OG	FG	ABV	App. Atten-uation	colour
1947	Barclay Perkins	PA	12	1037.8	1006.3	4.10	83.33%	20.5
1952	Bass	H & O Pale Ale		1036.7	1007	3.86	80.93%	20
1948	Carlisle State Brewery	Pale Ale	20	1037.5	1006.5	4.03	82.67%	17.5
1950	Charrington	Pale Ale	17	1035.7	1006.5	3.80	81.79%	20
1952	Ind Coope	Coronet Pale Ale	22	1035.6	1008.6	3.50	75.84%	22
1948	Jenners	Pale Ale (Export)		1035.6	1009.7	3.36	72.75%	22
1950	Northampton Brewery	PA		1035.2	1007.8	3.56	77.84%	32
1951	Peter Walker	SB Ale	19	1035.1	1005.7	3.82	83.76%	28
1950	Timothy Taylor	Special Pale Ale	28	1034.7	1008.3	3.42	76.08%	24
1947	Tollemache	Light Ale	17	1037.7	1005.3	4.22	85.94%	18
1952	Tollemache	Light Tolly	24	1037	1004.1	4.29	88.92%	
1947	Watney	Pale Ale	12	1037.2	1004.4	4.28	88.17%	20.5
	Average		***19***	***1036.3***	***1006.7***	***3.85***	***81.50%***	***22.7***
Source: Whitbread Gravity book held at the London Metropolitan Archives, document number LMA/4453/D/02/002.								

It's quite a small, which implies not that many beers of this strength were being brewed. The small number of samples is why I haven't split this set geographically. The rate of attenuation is high, averaging over 80%.

Moving slightly forward in time, I've a small London set.

London bottled Pale Ale 1034° to 1038° 1953 - 1963								
Year	Brewer	Beer	Price per pint d	OG	FG	ABV	App. Atten-uation	colour
1956	Charrington	Pale Ale	20	1036.1	1008.8	3.54	75.62%	19
1963	Charrington	Pale Ale	22	1034	1007.2	3.48	78.82%	18
1954	Courage	Pale Ale	19	1034	1007.2	3.48	78.82%	28
1953	Truman	Eagle Light Ale	19	1034	1004.6	3.83	86.47%	21
1961	Watney	Pale Ale	22	1035.9	1007.4	3.70	79.39%	23
	Average		***20.4***	***1034.8***	***1007.0***	***3.61***	***79.83%***	***21.8***
Source: Whitbread Gravity book held at the London Metropolitan Archives, document number LMA/4453/D/02/002.								

There's a slightly larger Southern set.

Southern bottled Pale Ale 1034° to 1038° 1955 - 1960								
Year	Brewer	Beer	Price per pint d	OG	FG	ABV	App. Atten-uation	colour
1956	Lacons	Pale Ale	20	1035.9	1009.4	3.44	73.82%	23
1956	McMullen	Mac's No 1. PA	22	1036.4	1005.6	4.01	84.62%	26
1955	Morgans	Light Bitter Ale	22	1034.5	1005.7	3.75	83.48%	18
1959	Simonds	SB Light Ale	20	1034.2	1010.3	3.09	69.88%	19
1955	St Austell	Light Bitter Ale	22	1034.4	1008	3.43	76.74%	22
1955	Steward & Patteson	Pale Ale	21	1036.4	1010.6	3.34	70.88%	20
1960	Stroud Brewery	Cotswold Ale	24	1034.8	1004.3	3.81	87.64%	45
1955	Tollemache	Light Bitter Pale Ale	22	1037.9	1009	3.75	76.25%	17
	Average		***21.6***	***1035.6***	***1007.9***	***3.6***	***77.91%***	***23.8***
Source: Whitbread Gravity book held at the London Metropolitan Archives, document number LMA/4453/D/02/002.								

I've rather more Northern beers. Whitbread seems to have had an unhealthy interest in the breweries from some regions.

Northern bottled Pale Ale 1034° to 1038° 1955 - 1964								
Year	Brewer	Beer	Price per pint d	OG	FG	ABV	App. Atten-uation	colour
1955	Birkenhead Brewery	India Pale Ale	21	1037.2	1007.2	3.90	80.65%	21
1955	Border Breweries	Border Bright Ale	19	1035.3	1007.7	3.58	78.19%	19
1964	Camerons	Bitter Ale	22	1037.4	1011.3	3.26	69.79%	35
1955	Catterall & Swarbrick	XL Pale Ale	22	1034.1	1005.1	3.77	85.04%	19
1959	Duttons	Pale Ale	24	1035.9	1009.4	3.31	73.82%	17
1964	Hammond	Prize Medal	24	1035.5	1012.8	2.84	63.94%	25
1955	Hey & Son	Gold Cup Ale	25	1037.6	1006.6	4.03	82.45%	19

Northern bottled Pale Ale 1034° to 1038° 1955 - 1964								
Year	**Brewer**	**Beer**	**Price per pint d**	**OG**	**FG**	**ABV**	**App. Atten-uation**	**colour**
1955	Hydes	Pale Ale	21	1034.9	1004	4.03	88.54%	23
1955	Lion Brewery, Birmingham	Bitter Beer	22	1034.7	1005.6	3.79	83.86%	17
1960	Marston	Burton Keg	21	1036	1006.8	3.65	81.11%	20
1959	Matthew Brown	Bitter Beer	22	1035.1	1004.4	3.84	87.46%	18
1955	Moors & Robson	Pale Ale	16	1034.1	1007.3	3.48	78.59%	14
1955	Newcastle Breweries	Amber Ale	20	1034.9	1007.5	3.56	78.51%	30
1959	Ramsdens	Stone Trough Ale	20	1035.7	1006.2	3.84	82.63%	24
1959	Samuel Smith	Taddy Bitter Ale	21	1035.7	1003.8	3.99	89.36%	17
1955	Tennant Bros.	Lion Pale Ale	22	1035.7	1008.5	3.53	76.19%	22
1955	Tetley	Bitter	25	1037.1	1004	4.32	89.22%	23
1959	Threllfall	Blue Label Pale Ale	23	1037.7	1005.6	4.01	85.15%	20
1959	Thwaites	Pale Ale	24	1037.2	1007.4	3.73	80.11%	22
1959	Webster	Dukes Ale	20	1035.3	1006.8	3.56	80.74%	19
1959	Whitakers	Light Shire Ale	10.5	1035.4	1011.8	3.05	66.67%	24
	Average		***21.2***	***1035.8***	***1007.1***	***3.67***	***80.10%***	***21.3***

Source:
Whitbread Gravity book held at the London Metropolitan Archives, document number LMA/4453/D/02/002.

We're now at beers of Best Bitter strength.

Bottled Pale Ale 1038° to 1045° 1946 - 1952								
Year	Brewer	Beer	Price per pint d	OG	FG	ABV	App. Atten-uation	colour
1948	Allsopp	John Bull Ale	26	1038.2	1008.2	3.90	78.53%	75
1952	Ansell	Spotlight	20	1038.3	1006.7	4.11	82.51%	19
1947	Dare	Bitter	28	1038.6	1006.7	4.15	82.64%	13
1949	Davenport	Pale Ale	19	1039.5	1006.6	4.28	83.29%	21
1950	Hammerton	Stock Ale	26	1040.7	1006.8	4.41	83.29%	28
1950	Ind Coope	John Bull Ale		1042.5	1012.2	3.93	71.29%	90
1946	Mann Crossman	Rustic Ale	16	1041.5	1010.6	4.01	74.46%	19.5
1947	Mann Crossman	Rustic Ale	16	1039.1	1008.1	4.03	79.28%	20.5
1947	Mann Crossman	Rustic Ale	17	1044.7	1009.3	4.60	79.19%	20
1948	Mann Crossman	Rustic Ale	22	1041.9	1009.8	4.17	76.61%	21.5
1949	Mann Crossman	Rustic Ale	22	1043.3	1007	4.73	83.83%	19.5
1950	Mann Crossman	Rustic Ale	21	1041.7	1009.8	4.14	76.50%	23
1952	McMullen	Macs No.1 Pale Ale	21	1038.2	1007.2	4.03	81.15%	30
1951	Peter Walker Ltd	Pale Ale	21	1038.5	1007.3	4.06	81.04%	24
1947	Robert Porter	Bulldog Sparkling Light Beer	25	1040.1	1004.05	4.71	89.90%	19.5
1950	Tennant Bros.	Pale Ale		1039.4	1012.2	3.52	69.04%	27
1946	Tollemache	Light Tolly	17	1038.4	1007.9	3.96	79.43%	14
1947	Tollemache	Light Bitter	16	1038.6	1006.3	4.20	83.68%	19.5
	Average		***20.8***	***1040.2***	***1008.2***	***4.16***	***79.76%***	***28.5***
Source: Whitbread Gravity book held at the London Metropolitan Archives, document number LMA/4453/D/02/002.								

I'm not so sure there's much to be learned from that small geographically diverse set. Not sure about Allsopp's John Bull Ale. It looks awfully dark for a Pale Ale.

For the next time period I've split them geographically again.

London bottled Pale Ale 1038° to 1045° 1953 - 1963								
Year	Brewer	Beer	Price per pint d	OG	FG	ABV	App. Atten-uation	colour
1954	Charrington	Pale Ale	19	1038.2	1008.5	3.86	77.75%	21
1963	Charrington	Toby Heavy Ale	23	1039.3	1009.3	3.89	76.34%	25
1955	Courage	Export	28	1039.4	1008.3	4.04	78.93%	24
1953	Fullers	London Pride	26	1044.5	1012.1	4.20	72.81%	22
1959	Fullers	London Pride	26	1042.3	1009.2	4.30	78.25%	26
1957	Mann Crossman	Rustic Ale	24	1043.2	1005.5	4.92	87.27%	23
1953	Meux	Treble Gold Ale	24	1042.4	1009.1	4.33	78.54%	32
1959	Meux	Treble Gold Ale	31	1042.3	1012.7	3.83	69.98%	24
	Average		***25.1***	***1041.5***	***1009.3***	***4.17***	***77.48%***	***24.6***
Source: Whitbread Gravity book held at the London Metropolitan Archives, document number LMA/4453/D/02/002.								

As you'll see when you look at the next set, the London beers have a lower degree of attenuation.

Northern bottled Pale Ale 1038° to 1045° 1953 - 1964								
Year	Brewer	Beer	Price per pint d	OG	FG	ABV	App. Atten-uation	colour
1956	Alnwick Brewery	Hotspur Export Ale	30	1042.1	1010.6	4.09	74.82%	26
1959	Bentleys	Special Pale Ale	22	1038.5	1006.2	4.04	83.90%	26
1957	Clubs Brewery Pontyclun	Triple Crown Ale	30	1044.6	1007.8	4.79	82.51%	24
1953	Duttons	DPA Pale Ale	24	1038.9	1005.2	4.39	86.63%	20
1955	Greenall Whitley	Pale Ale	26	1039.1	1008.1	4.03	79.28%	20
1959	Greenall Whitley	Champion Pale Ale	24	1039.5	1011.5	3.50	70.89%	22
1961	Greenall Whitley	Champion Pale Ale	26	1039.7	1008.2	3.94	79.35%	18
1964	Hey	Gold Cup Ale	28	1038.2	1007.2	3.88	81.15%	19
1959	Hydes	Anvil Gold Ale	28	1042.7	1006	4.59	85.95%	20
1959	John Smith	Magnet Pale Ale	26	1044.5	1010.2	4.29	77.08%	24
1964	John Smith	Magnet Pale Ale	29	1043.5	1007.2	4.54	83.45%	16
1955	Moors & Robson	Red Cap Bitter Beer	20	1038.1	1008.1	3.90	78.74%	15
1959	Ramsdens	Riding Ale	23	1042.8	1008.5	4.46	80.14%	19
1955	Shipstone	Pale Ale		1040.9	1009.3	4.10	77.26%	20
1961	Stone, Wm.	Treble B	30	1040.3	1007.5	4.10	81.39%	18
1959	Tetley	Bitter Ale	21	1039	1006.1	4.11	84.36%	23
1964	Tetley	Bitter Ale	25	1040	1005.6	4.30	86.00%	25
1959	Timothy Taylor	Landlord	28	1042.1	1010.9	3.90	74.11%	13
1953	Westoe	Export	30	1042.2	1008.3	4.41	80.33%	23
	Average		***26.1***	***1040.9***	***1008.0***	***4.18***	***80.39%***	***20.6***
Source: Whitbread Gravity book held at the London Metropolitan Archives, document number LMA/4453/D/02/002.								

The Northern examples were on average a little pale and more highly attenuated than the London ones. But also, surprisingly, slightly more expensive.

Midlands bottled Pale Ale 1038° to 1045° 1953 - 1964								
Year	Brewer	Beer	Price per pint d	OG	FG	ABV	App. Atten-uation	colour
1955	Hewitt Bros.	Pale Ale	23	1040.8	1008.4	4.21	79.41%	28
1964	Mansfield	Pale Ale	28	1040.8	1009.8	3.88	75.98%	21
1954	Marston	PA	19	1044.3	1005.1	5.12	88.49%	20
1953	Mitchell & Butler	Allbright Ale	19.5	1040.9	1009.5	4.08	76.77%	21
1957	Worthington	PA	21	1043.5	1004.6	5.08	89.43%	20
1961	Worthington	E	24	1040.7	1003.5	4.86	91.40%	20
1961	Worthington	Cannister	26	1043.7	1005.3	5.01	87.87%	19
1960	Thornley	TK Pale Ale	32	1043.8	1009.5	4.29	78.31%	22
	Average		***24.1***	***1042.3***	***1007.0***	***4.57***	***83.46%***	***21.4***
Source: Whitbread Gravity book held at the London Metropolitan Archives, document number LMA/4453/D/02/002.								

The Midlands beers are, on average, the cheapest, edging out the London ones by 1d per pint.

Southern bottled Pale Ale 1038° to 1045° 1953 - 1964								
Year	**Brewer**	**Beer**	**Price per pint d**	**OG**	**FG**	**ABV**	**App. Atten-uation**	**colour**
1959	Brickwoods	Pale Ale	28	1044.3	1011.4	4.27	74.27%	24
1956	Bullard	Pale Ale	24	1038.6	1007.4	4.06	80.83%	20
1960	Cheltenham & Hereford Brewery	West Country Ale	30	1044.1	1011.7	4.05	73.47%	28
1959	Flowers	Brewmaster	34	1041.1	1009.2	4.14	77.62%	15
1960	Georges	Export Port Ale	30	1043.4	1012.8	3.83	70.51%	18
1958	Hall & Woodhouse	"Forum" Best Pale Ale	32	1040.4	1009.3	3.89	76.98%	27.5
1960	Ind Coope	Double Diamond	30	1038.4	1012.4	3.36	67.71%	18
1964	Ind Coope	Long Life	38	1044.9	1008	4.81	82.18%	17.5
1953	McMullen	Lady Mac	23	1043.5	1008.3	4.58	80.92%	24
1954	Shepherd Neame	Abbey Ale	28	1044	1010.4	4.36	76.36%	22
1961	Shepherd Neame	Abbey Ale	30	1042.9	1014.1	3.60	67.13%	16
1953	Simonds	Tavern Pale Ale	30	1044.9	1012.3	4.23	72.61%	21
1955	Strong	Pale Ale	24	1044.3	1011.5	4.26	74.04%	19
1960	Strong	Special Pale Ale		1041.3	1009.7	3.95	76.51%	23
1953	Young & Son Portsmouth	Imperial Pale Ale		1042.1	1010.9	4.05	74.11%	26
	Average		29.3	***1042.5***	***1010.6***	***4.10***	***75.02%***	***21.3***
Source: Whitbread Gravity book held at the London Metropolitan Archives, document number LMA/4453/D/02/002.								

The Southern beers are the most expensive of the lot, averaging almost 30d a pint, almost 5d per pint more than the London average and 6d more than the Midlands ones. That's quite a difference.

London bottled Pale Ale 1045° to 1055° 1948 - 1951								
Year	**Brewer**	**Beer**	**Price per pint d**	**OG**	**FG**	**ABV**	**App. Atten-uation**	**colour**
1951	Barclay Perkins	Golden Hop Ale	25	1046	1018.8	3.51	59.13%	23
1949	Charrington	Toby Ale	26	1047	1011.6	4.60	75.32%	27
1950	Charrington	Toby Ale	27	1047.4	1011.4	4.68	75.95%	27
1951	Charrington	Toby Ale	26	1048.2	1012.4	4.65	74.27%	34
1948	Courage	Alton Pale Ale	31	1051.3	1003.5	6.27	93.18%	23
1950	Courage	Alton Pale Ale	31	1052.4	1003.3	6.44	93.70%	22
1948	Ind Coope	Double Diamond	26	1045.2	1009.4	4.48	79.20%	18
1950	Ind Coope	Double Diamond	29	1048.3	1010.9	4.86	77.43%	21
1950	Mann Crossman	Rustic Ale	24	1045.1	1011.5	4.36	74.50%	24
1949	Taylor Walker	Reserve Pale Ale	29	1051.2	1009.9	5.38	80.66%	25
1951	Taylor Walker	Reserve Pale Ale	29	1050.8	1010.4	5.26	79.53%	20.5
1950	Truman	Ben Truman Pale Ale	29	1052.1	1007	5.90	86.56%	24
1950	Watney	Red Barrel	28	1050.9	1014.2	4.76	72.10%	19
	Average		***27.7***	***1048.9***	***1010.3***	***5.01***	***78.58%***	***23.7***
Source: Whitbread Gravity book held at the London Metropolitan Archives, document number LMA/4453/D/02/002.								

It's striking that there were quite a few Pale Ales were knocking around that were over 1045° in the immediate post-war years. Remember average OG was around 1032° at that point.

There are some famous beers in this set: Toby Ale, Alton Pale Ale, Double Diamond, Ben Truman and, of course, Red Barrel. All were classy, top of the range Pale Ales. Some later became keg beers, still pretending to be classy.

Other bottled Pale Ale 1045° to 1055° 1946 - 1951								
Year	Brewer	Beer	Price per pint d	OG	FG	ABV	App. Atten-uation	colour
1948	Allsopp	Burton Pale Ale Export (bottled in Brussels)		1052.6	1007.1	5.95	86.50%	18
1948	Allsopp	Burton Pale Ale (bottled in Brussels)		1052.8	1008.9	5.73	83.14%	
1946	Bass	Red Triangle		1054.8	1010.1	5.83	81.57%	20
1948	Bass	PA	18.5	1054.2	1009.1	5.89	83.21%	17.5
1949	Bass	Export Pale Ale		1051	1010.6	5.26	79.22%	19.5
1949	Bass	PA	27	1054.1	1008.6	5.94	84.10%	
1948	Duncan Gilmour	Export Quality Golden PA		1053.1	1011.8	5.38	77.78%	21
1950	Imperial Brewing	Long Keeping Pale Ale		1047.7	1009	5.04	81.13%	
1951	John Smith	Magnet Ale	26	1047.1	1011.5	4.62	75.58%	24
1951	Mitchell & Butler	Export Pale Ale	21	1047.5	1010.3	4.84	78.32%	19
	Average		***23.1***	***1051.5***	***1009.7***	***5.45***	***81.06%***	***19.9***
Source: Whitbread Gravity book held at the London Metropolitan Archives, document number LMA/4453/D/02/002.								

There are a lot of Burton beers in this set, which isn't a shock. It was the home of Pale Ale, after all. The Allsopp beer was obviously intended for the Belgian market.

London bottled Pale Ale 1045° to 1055° 1953 - 1963								
Year	Brewer	Beer	Price per pint d	OG	FG	ABV	App. Atten-uation	colour
1953	Barclay Perkins	Golden Hop Ale	25	1048.7	1007.9	5.32	83.78%	27
1957	Charrington	Toby Ale	36	1047.8	1011.6	4.70	75.73%	20
1960	Charrington	Toby Ale	29	1046.5	1014.8	4.10	68.17%	23
1960	Courage	John Courage	30	1050.3	1011.85	5.00	76.44%	
1953	Ind Coope	Double Diamond	33	1048.7	1009.7	5.08	80.08%	23.5
1954	Ind Coope	John Bull Ale	30	1048.1	1014.8	4.31	69.23%	115
1955	Ind Coope	Double Diamond	32	1048.5	1012.7	4.65	73.81%	19
1959	Ind Coope	Double Diamond	32	1047.5	1011.9	4.62	74.95%	20
1961	Ind Coope	Long Life	32.5	1045.1	1009.1	4.68	79.82%	15
1962	Ind Coope	Double Diamond	30	1047.3	1011.7	4.62	75.26%	16
1953	Meux	Treble Gold Pale Ale	33	1046.9	1007.9	5.08	83.16%	29
1953	Taylor Walker	Reserve Pale Ale	36	1046.5	1011.1	4.60	76.13%	22
1957	Taylor Walker	Pale Ale (bottled in Belgium)		1048.7	1011.2	4.88	77.00%	27

London bottled Pale Ale 1045° to 1055° 1953 - 1963								
Year	**Brewer**	**Beer**	**Price per pint d**	**OG**	**FG**	**ABV**	**App. Atten-uation**	**colour**
1959	Taylor Walker	Reserve Special Pale Ale	31	1053.5	1014	5.13	73.83%	23
1953	Truman	Ben Truman	29	1049.9	1006.9	5.62	86.17%	20
1959	Truman	Ben Truman	32	1049.9	1010	5.20	79.96%	17
1963	Truman	Ben Truman	33	1049.3	1013.4	4.66	72.82%	20
1955	Watney	Red Barrel	31	1049.2	1014.7	4.47	70.12%	22
1960	Watney	Red Barrel	30	1048.9	1015.2	4.37	68.92%	23
	Average		***31.1***	***1048.5***	***1011.6***	***4.80***	***76.07%***	***26.8***

Source:
Which Beer Report, 1960, pages 171 - 173.
Whitbread Gravity book held at the London Metropolitan Archives, document number LMA/4453/D/02/002.

More of the top-class London Pale Ales, though at least one was an export beer. That excepted, most of these beers seem to be competing for the same slot in, predominantly, the London market. A strong, bottled beer, at a premium price.

Midlands bottled Pale Ale 1045° to 1055° 1955 - 1961								
Year	**Brewer**	**Beer**	**Price per pint d**	**OG**	**FG**	**ABV**	**App. Atten-uation**	**colour**
1955	Ansell	Special Pale Ale	27	1046.3	1009	4.86	80.56%	18
1959	Ansell	Pale Ale	27	1046.1	1009.6	4.56	79.18%	18
1956	Bass	Blue Triangle	34	1051.9	1012.4	5.14	76.11%	21
1956	Bass	Red Triangle	34	1053.5	1004.1	6.48	92.34%	20
1961	Bass	Red Triangle	36	1054.3	1002.7	6.78	95.03%	18
1964	Bass	Blue Triangle	34	1051.2	1010.1	5.36	80.27%	21
1964	Bass	Red Triangle	34	1053.9	1008.6	5.92	84.04%	21
1955	Home Brewery	Home Ale	25	1046.1	1013.8	4.19	70.07%	20
1955	Mitchell & Butler	Export Pale Ale	26	1045.7	1011.8	4.40	74.18%	20
1959	Mitchell & Butler	Export Pale Ale	26	1046.6	1012.4	4.27	73.39%	19
1959	Worthington	India Pale Ale	32	1051.6	1011.5	5.22	77.71%	18
1961	Worthington	Green Shield	37	1052.1	1008.8	5.65	83.11%	20
1961	Worthington	White Shield	37	1053.8	1008.7	5.89	83.83%	20
	Average		**29.6**	**1050.2**	**1009.5**	**5.29**	**80.75%**	**19.5**

Source:
Whitbread Gravity book held at the London Metropolitan Archives, document number LMA/4453/D/02/002.

A mix here of classic Burton Pale Ales, from Bass and Worthington, and a couple of random other Midlands breweries. Ansell and Mitchell & Butler were based in Birmingham, Home Ales in Nottingham.

The Burton brewed beers are mostly quite pale and highly-attenuated.

Northern bottled Pale Ale 1045° to 1055° 1953 - 1961								
Year	**Brewer**	**Beer**	**Price per pint d**	**OG**	**FG**	**ABV**	**App. Atten-uation**	**colour**
1953	Duttons	Special	28	1045	1007.2	4.93	84.00%	28
1959	Hammond	Export Unity	29	1046	1012.2	4.22	73.48%	21
1955	John Smith	Magnet Pale Ale	24	1045.3	1012.6	4.24	72.19%	25
1959	Ramsdens	Golden Ale	27	1047.3	1012.3	4.54	74.00%	22
1959	Samuel Smith	Taddy Pale Ale	28	1046.5	1006.3	5.03	86.45%	15
1961	Tennant Bros.	Don Jan Ale	28	1046.6	1012.2	4.30	73.82%	14
1961	United Caledonian	Piper Extra Export	28	1048.3	1012.4	4.49	74.33%	23
1953	Vaux	Special Export	30	1046.9	1010.4	4.75	77.83%	30
	Average		***27.8***	***1046.5***	***1010.7***	***4.56***	***77.01%***	***22.3***
Source: Whitbread Gravity book held at the London Metropolitan Archives, document number LMA/4453/D/02/002.								

This time the pricing is how you would expect, with the Northern beers averaging a good bit less than the London ones, over 3d per pint.

Southern bottled Pale Ale 1045° to 1055° 1953 - 1961								
Year	**Brewer**	**Beer**	**Price per pint d**	**OG**	**FG**	**ABV**	**App. Atten-uation**	**colour**
1953	Cobbold	Cardinal Ale	27	1045.7	1010.3	4.60	77.46%	22
1960	Cobbold	Cardinal Ale	30	1048.6	1015.8	4.10	67.49%	24
1956	Flowers	Brewmaster Ale	30	1045.8	1009.7	4.70	78.82%	18
1958	Flowers	Brewmaster Export Beer	36	1045.4	1008	4.68	82.38%	16
1962	Flowers	Brewmaster Export PA	36	1046.6	1015.6	3.87	66.52%	18
1959	Fremlin	Country Ale	36	1050.2	1005.3	5.88	89.44%	26
1965	Fremlin	Gold Top English Stock Bitter Ale	33	1046.3	1003.3	5.63	92.87%	24
1960	Greene King	Abbot Ale	30	1048.6	1006.7	5.24	86.21%	19
1959	Hunt Edmunds	Supreme Pale Ale	28	1047.1	1010.7	4.73	77.28%	15
1953	McMullen	Macs No. 3	30	1048.7	1011	4.90	77.41%	32
1959	McMullen	Mac's No 3	32	1047.7	1007.1	5.30	85.12%	21
1960	Morland	Viking Ale	28	1045.1	1012	4.14	73.39%	30
1959	Simonds	Tavern Export Ale	34	1045.8	1013	4.25	71.62%	18
	Average		***30.2***	***1047.0***	***1009.1***	***4.88***	***78.92%***	***22.7***
Source: Whitbread Gravity book held at the London Metropolitan Archives, document number LMA/4453/D/02/002.								

The Southern beers average out much like the London ones. More expensive than the Northern ones, but also a little higher in ABV.

Strong bottled Pale Ales, not that much different in strength from pre-WW I beers, were still available. Mostly brewed in Burton. The classic Bass Pale Ale still weighed in over 6% ABV in the 1950s. As did Worthington White Shield.

London bottled Pale Ale over 1055° 1950 - 1965								
Year	Brewer	Beer	Price per pint d	OG	FG	ABV	App. Atten-uation	colour
1965	Courage	Bulldog Pale Ale	61.5	1066.9	1020.1	6.08	69.96%	19
1965	Ind Coope	Double Diamond (sold in Belgium)		1056.1	1011.2	5.86	80.04%	20
1950	Truman	Ben Truman Pale Ale		1060.9	1010.1	6.65	83.42%	13
1955	Truman	Pale Ale		1061	1011.1	6.52	81.80%	31
1949	Watney	Pale Ale (purchased in Brussels)		1059.8	1015.5	5.76	74.08%	18
1950	Watney	Pale Ale		1059.9	1017.2	5.55	71.29%	18.5
1953	Watney	Export Pale Ale	48	1059.8	1019.5	5.22	67.39%	23
1955	Watney	Pale Ale		1061	1017.5	5.65	71.31%	23
	Average			***1060.7***	***1015.3***	***5.91***	***74.91%***	***20.7***
Source: Whitbread Gravity book held at the London Metropolitan Archives, document number LMA/4453/D/02/002.								

I've just noticed a slight error in my grouping here. Double Diamond probably and Ben Truman certainly, were brewed in Burton. Interesting that the Burton-brewed beers have distinctly higher degree of attenuation than the others.

When looking at this next set, I twigged something else. The strongest type of Pale Ale, especially when brewed in Burton, was also the palest.

Burton bottled Pale Ale over 1055° 1950 - 1965								
Year	Brewer	Beer	Price per pint d	OG	FG	ABV	App. Atten-uation	colour
1950	Bass	PA	37	1056.1	1004.6	6.76	91.80%	19
1950	Bass	PA	31	1057.1	1007.6	6.48	86.69%	19
1950	Bass	PA		1058	1008.3	6.51	85.69%	21
1953	Bass	Blue Triangle	36	1058.7	1013.8	5.85	76.49%	18.5
1953	Bass	Blue Triangle		1060.8	1010.5	6.58	82.73%	21
1955	Bass	Red Triangle		1063.2	1009.6	7.02	84.81%	19
1955	Bass	Blue Triangle		1063.5	1003.1	7.96	95.12%	19
1960	Bass	Blue Triangle		1061.1	1012.7	6.32	79.21%	17
1965	Bass	Blue Label sold in Belgium		1068.8	1014	7.17	79.65%	18
1951	Worthington	India Pale Ale	29	1056.7	1007.2	6.48	87.30%	18
1953	Worthington	India Pale Ale		1061.1	1013.5	6.21	77.91%	27
1955	Worthington	Green Shield		1063.3	1009.4	7.06	85.15%	18
1955	Worthington	White Shield		1063.7	1002.9	8.02	95.45%	18
	Average			***1060.9***	***1009.0***	***6.80***	***85.23%***	***19.4***
Source: Whitbread Gravity book held at the London Metropolitan Archives, document number LMA/4453/D/02/002.								

All but two of this set have a colour under 20 (Lovibond 1" cell) that is, below 5 SRM. If you look back at the previous tables, you'll see that this is a recurring theme for Pale Ales brewed in Burton. They're all very pale, especially considering their strength.

Some of these beers are much like 19th-century Burton IPA. The Bass Blue Triangle from 1955 in particular. Red Triangle and Blue triangle the same beer, just bottled differently. Red Triangle was bottle-conditioned, Blue Triangle brewery-conditioned. It was similar with Worthington, where White Shield was bottle-conditioned, Green Shield wasn't.

Other bottled Pale Ale over 1055° 1950 - 1965

Year	Brewer	Beer	Price per pint d	OG	FG	ABV	App. Atten-uation	colour
1963	Fremlin	Tower Pale Ale (sold in Belgium)		1065.9	1008.2	7.58	87.56%	19
1951	Hancocks	55 Export Ale	29	1055.7	1020.9	4.50	62.48%	22
1950	John Smith	Pale Ale		1058.6	1012.5	6.01	78.67%	20.5
1951	John Smith	Pale Ale		1059.4	1016.9	5.52	71.55%	22
1955	John Smith	Pale Ale		1060.2	1013.4	6.10	77.74%	24
1960	John Smith	Pale Ale (sold in Belgium)		1055.5	1013.7	5.22	75.32%	17
1965	John Smith	Pale Ale (sold in Belgium)		1056.1	1011.8	5.54	78.97%	13
1949	Simonds	Bulldog Pale Ale (bought in Brussels)		1069.8	1011.9	7.59	82.95%	25
1953	Simonds	Bulldog Pale Ale	43.5	1066.4	1019.6	6.08	70.48%	25
1955	Simonds	Bulldog Pale Ale		1067	1018	6.38	73.13%	20
1965	Simonds	Martins PA (sold in Belgium)		1068	1019.7	6.04	71.03%	17
1958	Ushers	Gold Best Bright Ale	34	1068.4	1012.3	7.01	82.02%	23
	Average			***1062.6***	***1014.9***	***6.13***	***75.99%***	***20.6***

Source:
Whitbread Gravity book held at the London Metropolitan Archives, document number LMA/4453/D/02/002.

Bulldog has an almost legendary status as a classic UK beer you couldn't usually find on sale in the UK.

Most of these beers were brewed for the Belgian market. Which explains their strength. Though it wasn't explicitly stated in ever Whitbread Gravity Book entry, I'm sure all those John Smith's beers were destined for Belgium. The lack of a price is one pointer. Which often indicates that a beer wasn't purchased in the UK.

Quite a few breweries were involved in the export trade to Belgium, and not just obvious ones. Fremlin wasn't particularly big, but I suppose being located in Kent, Belgium wasn't so far away. Simonds had long been in the export trade, having supplied the British military. John Smith? No idea how they got into the Belgian market.

But it must have been worth money to them, because they were prepared to fly beer over if necessary:

> **"YORKS BREWERY FLIES THE BEER TO BELGIUM**
> THE AIRLIFT to Europe has begun again from Yorkshire. But this time the load is not coal or flour—but beer!

Belgium's dock strike threatened to cut off imports of Tadcaster-brewed beer, so the brewery decided to fly direct to Antwerp from Sherburn airfield.

By to-morrow the equivalent 100,000 bottles special brew will have been flown by Halifax transport aircraft. After delivering, the plane brings back empties to Sherburn.

Week-end trips
The Halifax made three trips to Antwerp during the week-end, and took off again from Sherburn to-day with load of 36-gallon casks. It was due back to make a second run to-day.

With yesterday's load to Antwerp went the brewery's bottling manager, Mr. A. J. Edwards, of Tadcaster. He will superintend unshipping at Antwerp airport until the "beer-lift" finishes.

A brewery director said to-day: We were forced to take this step retain our hold on a valuable export market. We shall continue flying beer to Belgium as long as it is necessary."

A Customs and Excise officer is now at Sherburn for Customs formalities so that the aircraft can make a direct 90-minute run to Belgium."
Yorkshire Evening Post - Monday 28 August 1950, page 1.

Pale Ale Grists

I'm splitting the grists into Northern, Southern and London again. In the hope of perhaps spotting some regional trends.

Moving from the top to bottom of England, starting with the North.

Not a huge number of different malts being employed. As you'd expect, all use a base of pale malt. You might be surprised at how few of the beers contain crystal malt, but I'm not. Crystal malt in Pale Ale is a shockingly recent development.

Northern Pale Ale grists 1947 - 1964: malts							
Year	**Brewer**	**Beer**	**OG**	**pale malt**	**crystal malt**	**high dried malt**	**enzymic malt**
1947	Boddington	IP	1037.0	80.20%			2.97%
1951	Boddington	IP	1040.0	86.44%			2.54%
1966	Boddington	IP	1038.5	80.37%			2.77%
1961	Clarke	1/5 BB	1036.1	81.53%			1.27%
1956	Tennant	BB	1032.9	72.74%	4.34%		2.65%
1956	Tennant	Best B	1039.9	71.74%			2.45%
1956	Tennant	Queens Ale	1043.9	66.00%			3.00%
1946	Tetley	B	1042.1	66.27%			
1953	Truman (Burton)	P1 B	1050.7	75.84%	0.84%	12.64%	2.53%
1953	Truman (Burton)	P1	1044.6	80.77%		14.42%	2.88%
1964	Truman (Burton)	P1	1042.7	84.17%	2.16%		2.16%
1964	Truman (Burton)	P1 B	1049.6	86.09%	0.00%		2.61%

Sources:
Boddington brewing record held at Manchester Central Library, document number M693/405/130.
Boddington brewing record held at Manchester Central Library, document number M693/405/133.
Clarke brewing record held at Manchester Central Library, document number M693/405/137.
Tennant brewing record held at Sheffield City Archive, document number MD7518/38/34.
Tetley brewing record held at the West Yorkshire Archives, document number WYL756/ACC3349/565
Truman brewing record held at the London Metropolitan Archives, document number B/THB/C/355.
Truman brewing record held at the London Metropolitan Archives, document number B/THB/C/374.

Enzymic malt, on the other hand, is present in all but the Tetley's Bitter. It really is weird how popular that malt was after WW II.

Adjuncts were pretty common in Bitters, as you'll see below.

Northern Pale Ale grists 1947 - 1964: adjuncts					
Year	**Brewer**	**Beer**	**flaked maize**	**flaked barley**	**wheat**
1947	Boddington	IP		5.9%	
1951	Boddington	IP			
1966	Boddington	IP	2.1%		2.8%
1961	Clarke	1/5 BB	6.8%		
1956	Tennant	BB	6.6%		
1956	Tennant	Best B	10.6%		
1956	Tennant	Queens Ale	15.0%		
1946	Tetley	B		14.1%	
1953	Truman (Burton)	P1 B	5.9%		
1953	Truman (Burton)	P1			
1964	Truman (Burton)	P1	4.3%		
1964	Truman (Burton)	P1 B	7.8%		

All but two of the beers contained some sort of adjunct. Mostly in the form of flaked maize. This was an incredibly common ingredient, and had been pretty much from the first moment it became legal with the Free Mash Tun Act of 1880.

Northern Pale Ale grists 1947 - 1964: sugars

Year	Brewer	Beer	no. 1 sugar	no. 2 sugar	no. 3 sugar	cara-mel	glu-cose	lac-tose	malt extract	other sugar
1947	Boddington	IP							3.96%	6.93%
1951	Boddington	IP							4.24%	6.78%
1966	Boddington	IP							4.62%	7.39%
1961	Clarke	1/5 BB				0.21%	3.40%		3.40%	3.40%
1956	Tennant	BB		5.29%				1.32%	1.76%	5.29%
1956	Tennant	Best B		5.43%				1.09%	1.63%	7.07%
1956	Tennant	Queens Ale	6.00%					2.00%		8.00%
1946	Tetley	B								19.68%
1953	Truman	P1 B	2.25%							
1953	Truman	P1			1.92%					
1964	Truman	P1	5.76%							1.44%
1964	Truman	P1 B	3.48%							

You can see that sugar made up between 10% and 20% of the grists, with the one exception of Truman. All of their beers had well under 10%. That No. 1 and No. 2 invert are in so many beers is to be expected. They're the classic Pale Ale sugars. Every single beer contains sugar of some sort.

There's quite a lot of malt extract, too. Another favourite, along with enzymic malt, of the post-war era.

Weirdest is the lactose in all of Tennant's Pale Ales. I've not come across another brewery that did that.

Next it's the turn of Southern Pale Ales.

Southern Pale Ale grists 1947 - 1965: malts							
Year	Brewer	Beer	OG	pale malt	crystal malt	mild malt	enzymic malt
1947	Adnams	PA	1034.1	86.54%			
1955	Adnams	PA	1036.0	88.24%			
1965	Adnams	BB	1037.0	85.48%			2.82%
1964	Eldridge Pope	IPA	1043.2	76.49%	5.97%		
1949	Elgood	PA	1037.7	79.41%		8.82%	
1953	Elgood	BPA	1031.0	90.91%			
1955	Flowers	PX	1030.3	81.25%			
1955	Flowers	IPA	1034.2	93.00%			
1947	Shepherd Neame	BA	1034.3	86.90%			
1947	Shepherd Neame	BB	1031.3	74.42%			
1956	Shepherd Neame	PA	1035.5	99.28%			
1952	Strong	SAK	1030.5	28.93%		54.96%	
1952	Strong	PA	1036.6	82.02%			
1952	Strong	SPA	1045.4	74.96%			
1952	Strong	GA	1033.5	81.69%			
1959	Ushers	IPA	1043.8	92.11%			
Sources: Adnams brewing records held at the brewery Elgood brewing record held at the brewery Ref Shakespeare Birthplace Trust DR227/215 Brewing Record Book No2 Shepherd Neame 1947 brewing book held at the brewery Shepherd Neame 1954 brewing book H/500 held at the brewery 79A01-A3-3-27 1075-275-6 Wiltshire archives at Chippenham							

There are even fewer malts in these Southern grists than the Northern ones. Crystal malt makes a single solitary appearance. As does enzymic malt. The majority contain just a single malt: pale. But it's not the only base malt, there's also some mild malt.

Southern Pale Ale grists 1947 - 1965: adjuncts					
Year	Brewer	Beer	OG	flaked barley	wheat malt
1947	Adnams	PA	1034.1	5.77%	
1955	Adnams	PA	1036.0		
1965	Adnams	BB	1037.0		
1964	Eldridge Pope	IPA	1043.2		4.88%
1949	Elgood	PA	1037.7		
1953	Elgood	BPA	1031.0		
1955	Flowers	PX	1030.3		3.75%
1955	Flowers	IPA	1034.2		
1947	Shepherd Neame	BA	1034.3	12.41%	
1947	Shepherd Neame	BB	1031.3	9.30%	
1956	Shepherd Neame	PA	1035.5		
1952	Strong	SAK	1030.5		
1952	Strong	PA	1036.6		
1952	Strong	SPA	1045.4		
1952	Strong	GA	1033.5		
1959	Ushers	IPA	1043.8		

There are even fewer than in the Northern grists. Just a little flaked barley in 1947 – when it was probably still compulsory – and a little wheat. Though I guess that, as it's malted, it doesn't really count as an adjunct.

Southern Pale Ale grists 1947 - 1965: sugars

Year	Brewer	Beer	no. 1 sugar	no. 3 sugar	invert	cara-mel	glu-cose	malt extract	other sugar
1947	Adnams	PA	7.69%						
1955	Adnams	PA	11.76%						
1965	Adnams	BB	11.40%						0.31%
1964	Eldridge Pope	IPA			9.40%			3.25%	
1949	Elgood	PA	5.88%					5.88%	
1953	Elgood	BPA			6.06%			3.03%	
1955	Flowers	PX			3.33%			1.67%	10.00%
1955	Flowers	IPA			4.00%			2.00%	1.00%
1947	Shepherd Neame	BA						0.69%	
1947	Shepherd Neame	BB		15.50%				0.78%	
1956	Shepherd Neame	PA						0.72%	
1952	Strong	SAK		1.93%		0.69%		1.93%	11.57%
1952	Strong	PA				0.29%	4.82%	4.82%	8.04%
1952	Strong	SPA	10.52%			0.06%	7.89%	3.95%	2.63%
1952	Strong	GA	7.26%			0.16%	5.45%	3.63%	1.82%
1959	Ushers	IPA			6.70%	0.08%	0.00%	1.12%	

Apart from two Shepherd Neame beers, every one contains some type of invert. And apart from Adnams, they all contained malt extract.

It's odd that a couple contain the dark No. 3 invert, especially the quantity in BB. The tiny quantities of caramel in some beers are for colour correction.

But what was going on in the capital? Let's take a look.

London Pale Ale grists 1947 - 1965: malts								
Year	**Brewer**	**Beer**	**OG**	**pale malt**	**crystal malt**	**mild malt**	**SA malt**	**enzymic malt**
1946	Barclay Perkins	XLK	1031.5	55.34%	8.74%		26.21%	
1947	Barclay Perkins	PA (bottling)	1032.5	86.54%				
1947	Barclay Perkins	PA export	1055.5	92.31%				
1965	Beasley	IPA	1034.0	32.88%	8.22%	32.88%		2.05%
1948	Fuller	PA	1029.6	79.48%				
1955	Fuller	PA	1033.2	80.47%				
1960	Fuller	PA	1032.2	92.80%				
1963	Watney	Red Barrel	1039.2	88.00%	4.00%			
1947	Whitbread	IPA	1032.4	82.69%	9.62%			
1947	Whitbread	PA	1034.2	74.50%	10.93%			
1955	Whitbread	IPA	1034.7	82.69%	5.77%			
1955	Whitbread	PA	1039.5	75.47%	5.66%			
1960	Whitbread	WPA	1035.0	82.69%	5.77%			
1960	Whitbread	PA	1038.6	75.50%	5.96%			
1965	Whitbread	W	1036.4	76.36%	6.36%			
1965	Whitbread	PA	1039.5	82.22%	6.12%			

Sources:
Barclay Perkins brewing record held at the London Metropolitan Archives, document number ACC/2305/01/627.
Beasley brewing record held at the London Metropolitan Archives, document number ACC/2305/26/115.
Fullers brewing records held at the brewery.
Watney Quality Manual.
Whitbread brewing records held at the London Metropolitan Archives, document numbers LMA/4453/D/01/115, LMA/4453/D/01/122, LMA/4453/D/01/127, LMA/4453/D/01/132.

Lots more crystal malt in this set. But bugger all else. A couple of examples of other base malts in mild and SA. Plus one enzymic malt. I've noticed something: London breweries – and the large ones in general – weren't into enzymic malt. But there is quite a lot of crystal malt.

Ooh, look at the adjuncts:

London Pale Ale grists 1947 - 1965: adjuncts						
Year	**Brewer**	**Beer**	**OG**	**wheat malt**	**flaked maize**	**flaked barley**
1946	Barclay Perkins	XLK	1031.5			
1947	Barclay Perkins	PA (bottling)	1032.5			5.77%
1947	Barclay Perkins	PA export	1055.5			
1965	Beasley	IPA	1034.0	2.05%		8.22%
1948	Fuller	PA	1029.6			16.14%
1955	Fuller	PA	1033.2		13.81%	
1960	Fuller	PA	1032.2			
1963	Watney	Red Barrel	1039.2			
1947	Whitbread	IPA	1032.4			
1947	Whitbread	PA	1034.2			
1955	Whitbread	IPA	1034.7			
1955	Whitbread	PA	1039.5			
1960	Whitbread	WPA	1035.0			
1960	Whitbread	PA	1038.6			
1965	Whitbread	W	1036.4			17.27%
1965	Whitbread	PA	1039.5			

Isn't that fascinating? Not many at all. If you remove the non-voluntary flaked barley from the 1940s.

London Pale Ale grists 1947 - 1965: sugars									
Year	**Brewer**	**Beer**	**OG**	**no. 1 sugar**	**no. 2 sugar**	**no. 3 sugar**	**glucose**	**malt extract**	**other sugar**
1946	Barclay Perkins	XLK	1031.5			9.71%			
1947	Barclay Perkins	PA (bottling)	1032.5	7.69%					
1947	Barclay Perkins	PA export	1055.5	7.69%					
1965	Beasley	IPA	1034.0		5.48%			5.48%	2.74%
1948	Fuller	PA	1029.6	0.83%	0.83%				2.72%
1955	Fuller	PA	1033.2		2.00%		1.20%		2.51%
1960	Fuller	PA	1032.2		2.56%		1.53%		3.10%
1963	Watney	Red Barrel	1039.2			5.00%		3.00%	
1947	Whitbread	IPA	1032.4	7.69%					
1947	Whitbread	PA	1034.2	14.57%					
1955	Whitbread	IPA	1034.7	11.54%					
1955	Whitbread	PA	1039.5	18.87%					
1960	Whitbread	WPA	1035.0	11.54%					
1960	Whitbread	PA	1038.6	18.54%					
1965	Whitbread	W	1036.4						
1965	Whitbread	PA	1039.5	11.66%					

Invert sugar was very popular. There's one type of invert or another in all but one of these beers. Mostly No. 1 and No. 2, as you would expect. Not as much malt extract as in the provincial beers, though.

Scottish Pale Ale

In Scotland Pale Ale was supreme, at least for the time being. The vast majority of beer brewed was one of the three Pale Ales: 60/- (Light), 70/- (Heavy) and 80/- (Export). These were generally brewed to gravities of 1030°, 1037° and 1044°.

The types of Pale Ale were much more standardised than in England. Every Scottish brewer stuck to brewing beers of these three types. Which makes life much simpler for me.

The main differences with English Pale Ales were a lower hopping rate and a poorer degree of attenuation. Combined, these traits made Scottish Pale Ales appear more malty and sweeter than their English equivalents.

Scottish brewers used a very limited range of malts. Those that had given up brewing Stout generally used nothing other than pale malt. This was augmented by maize, usually in flaked form, and various sugars.

60/- or Light

As genuine Mild had all but disappeared in Scotland, 60/- often took its place in Scotland. Being quite often coloured dark brown with caramel at racking time, it looked the part. It also shared a low gravity and low rate of hopping with English Mild.

In 1945, 60/- was by far the most popular style in Scotland, but in the 1950's a decline set in. By 1965 it had been replaced by 70/- as the favourite Scots beer. Light's decline continued in the 1970s and by 1980 was on its last legs.

Draught Scottish 60/- Pale Ale 1949 - 1959

Year	Brewer	Beer	Price per pint (d)	OG	FG	ABV	App. Atten-uation	colour
1949	Aitken	60/-	15	1030.5	1007	3.05	77.05%	
1958	Bernard	No. 3		1031	1010	2.72	67.74%	
1949	Campbell, Hope & King	90/-		1031.5	1006	3.31	80.95%	
1948	Fowler	54/- Ale		1028	1007	2.72	75.00%	
1949	Mackay	90/-		1031	1004	3.51	87.10%	
1951	Maclay	PA 6d		1031	1012	2.51	61.29%	
1953	Steel Coulson	P. 60/-	14	1030				
1947	Usher	PA 60/-		1029.5	1010.5	2.45	64.41%	
1959	Wm. Younger	XXP Bitter	22	1030.4	1005.7	3.21	81.25%	21
	Average			***1030.3***	***1007.8***	***2.94***	***74.35%***	

Sources:
Thomas Usher Gravity Book held at the Scottish Brewing Archive, document number TU/6/11.
Whitbread Gravity book held at the London Metropolitan Archives, document number LMA/4453/D/02/002.
T & J Bernard's brewing records held at the Scottish Brewing Archive.
Maclay brewing record held at the Scottish Brewing Archive, document number M/6/1/1/28
document from the Steel Coulson archive held at the Scottish Brewing Archives

All 60/- was brewed to a very similar OG, but, as the rate of attenuation was all over the shop, the ABVs vary considerably.

Bottled Scottish 60/- Pale Ale 1949 - 1959								
Year	**Brewer**	**Beer**	**Price per pint d**	**OG**	**FG**	**ABV**	**App. Atten-uation**	**colour**
1949	Aitchison	PA 90/-		1029	1007	2.85	75.86%	
1956	Aitchison & Co	Aitchie Blue Seal Pale Ale	32	1030	1010.2	2.56	66.00%	26
1949	Aitken	90/- Ale		1030	1006.5	3.05	78.33%	
1964	Aitken	Sparkling Ale	24	1032.6	1007.8	3.10	76.07%	40
1947	Bernard	60/- Ale		1031	1003.5	3.58	88.71%	
1949	Calder Alloa	Beer		1029	1006.5	2.92	77.59%	
1947	Campbell, Hope & King	60/- Ale		1033.5	1010	3.04	70.15%	
1949	Deuchar, R	PA 60/-		1030	1008	2.85	73.33%	
1955	Deucher, James	Lochside Pale Ale	24	1032.2	1006	3.40	81.37%	26
1946	Dryborough	60/- Ale		1029.5	1007.5	2.85	74.58%	
1964	Drybrough	Starbright Ale	24	1030.3	1010.4	2.49	65.68%	20
1946	Fowler	60/- Ale		1029	1009	2.59	68.97%	
1949	Fowler	XP (extra Pale)	18.5	1029.5	1009	2.65	69.49%	
1946	Gordon & Blair	60/- Ale		1028	1006	2.85	78.57%	
1949	Jeffrey & Co	PA 60/-		1029.5	1006.5	2.98	77.97%	
1947	Mackay	"90" Pale Ale		1027.5	1006.5	2.72	76.36%	
1946	Maclay	60/- Ale		1028	1008.5	2.52	69.64%	
1947	McEwan	Blue Label Ale		1029	1009.5	2.52	67.24%	
1955	McEwan	Blue Label Ale	20	1031.2	1008.7	2.91	72.12%	45
1964	McEwan	Blue Label Ale	24	1030.9	1011.3	2.45	63.43%	30
1947	McLennan & Urquhart	Ale		1030.5	1012.5	2.32	59.02%	
1946	Morrison	60/- Ale		1028.5	1008	2.65	71.93%	
1946	Murray	60/- Ale		1028.5	1007	2.79	75.44%	
1959	Murray	"Wee Murray" Pale Ale	20	1032.7	1011.2	2.69	65.75%	30
1946	Steel Coulson	60/- Ale		1028.5	1006.5	2.85	77.19%	
1953	Steel Coulson	Elephant PA	19.5	1033.4	1007.5	3.36	77.54%	34
1960	Tennent	Pale Ale	20	1029.9	1011.8	2.26	60.54%	26
1964	United Caledonian	Pale Ale (Red Cap)	24	1032	1008.6	2.93	73.12%	40
1946	Usher	60/- Ale		1029.5	1008.5	2.72	71.19%	
1955	Usher	Pale Ale	24	1030.8	1008.8	2.85	71.43%	33
1964	Ushers	Pale Ale	24	1032	1012.2	2.47	61.87%	30
1949	Young	90/- Ale		1030.5	1009	2.78	70.49%	
1946	Younger, Geo	60/- Ale		1029.5	1007.5	2.85	74.58%	
1955	Younger, Geo.	Treble Top Ale	26.25	1031.2	1006.6	3.19	78.85%	37.5
1959	Younger, Geo.	Sparkling Ale	24	1031.8	1024.5	0.93	22.96%	45
1946	Younger, Robert	60/- Ale		1027.5	1010.5	2.19	61.82%	
1946	Younger, Wm.	60/- Ale		1029	1008	2.72	72.41%	
1955	Younger, Wm.	90/- Holyrood Ale	24	1031.6	1006.7	3.23	78.80%	35
1959	Younger, Wm.	Pale Ale	24	1029.9	1008	2.74	73.24%	24

Sources:
Thomas Usher Gravity Book held at the Scottish Brewing Archive, document number TU/6/11.
Whitbread Gravity book held at the London Metropolitan Archives, document number LMA/4453/D/02/002.

Before WW II, 90/- usually meant a low-gravity bottled Pale Ale. Confusingly, it continued to be used for what was effectively bottled 60/-.

70/- or Heavy

While 60/- was the most popular style in Scotland in 1945, by 1965 70/- had overtaken it in drinkers' affections.

Draught Scottish 70/- Pale Ale 1947 - 1965								
Year	Brewer	Beer	Price per pint (d)	OG	FG	ABV	App. Atten-uation	colour
1958	Bernard	No. 2		1036	1011	3.24	69.44%	
1951	Maclay	SPA		1038	1015	3.04	60.53%	
1964	McEwans	Best Scotch	17	1038.1	1007.1	3.87	81.36%	30
1953	Steel Coulson	PXA P. 70/-	19	1034				
1960	Tennant	Best Bitter	16	1038.3	1006.1	4.20	84.20%	
1947	Usher	PA 70/-		1037.5	1008.5	3.77	77.33%	
1964	Vaux	Best Scotch	17	1036.3	1006.6	3.71	81.82%	30
1965	Vaux Lorimer	Best Scotch	18	1036.4	1006.3	3.76	82.69%	26
1950	Wm. Younger	Pale Ale	16	1039.8				27
1951	Wm. Younger	Pale Ale	16	1036.9				27
1964	Wm. Younger	XXPS	17	1038.8	1009.2	3.70	76.29%	24
	Average		***17.0***	***1037.3***	***1008.7***	***3.66***	***76.71%***	***27.3***

Sources:
Thomas Usher Gravity Book held at the Scottish Brewing Archive, document number TU/6/11.
Truman Gravity Book held at the London Metropolitan Archives, document number B/THB/C/252
Whitbread Gravity book held at the London Metropolitan Archives, document number LMA/4453/D/02/002.
T & J Bernard's brewing records held at the Scottish Brewing Archive.
Maclay brewing record held at the Scottish Brewing Archive, document number M/6/1/1/28
document from the Steel Coulson archive held at the Scottish Brewing Archives
Which Beer Report, 1960, pages 171 - 173.

The OGs of 70/- vary a little more than 60/-, but they still all fall in a fairly narrow band. Bottled version of 70/- look very much like draught versions:

Bottled Scottish 70/- 1947 - 1950						
Year	Brewer	Beer	OG	FG	ABV	App. Atten-uation
1947	Murray	70/- Ale	1032.5	1006.5	3.38	80.00%
1947	Usher	70/- Ale	1036.5	1008.5	3.63	76.71%
1948	Aitken	Heavy Ale	1040.5	1006.5	4.43	83.95%
1949	Aitken	Heavy Beer	1034.5	1011.5	2.97	66.67%
1948	Usher	PA 70/-	1037.5	1011.5	3.37	69.33%
1949	Usher	PA 70/-	1036	1013.5	2.91	62.50%
1950	Usher	PA 70/-	1039.5	1011	3.69	72.15%
	Average		***1036.7***	***1009.9***	***3.48***	***73.04%***

Source:
Thomas Usher Gravity Book held at the Scottish Brewing Archive, document number TU/6/11.

80/- or Export

In the immediate post-war years, Export wasn't hugely popular, presumably on account of its relatively high price. Though its popularity increased a little as the 1950s and 1960s progressed, it was still very much a minority taste.

Draught Scottish 80/- Pale Ale 1947 - 1960								
Year	Brewer	Beer	Price per pint (d)	OG	FG	ABV	App. Atten-uation	colour
1951	Maclay	Exp		1043	1014	3.84	67.44%	
1964	McEwans	Special	20	1043.6	1007.6	4.50	82.57%	20
1959	Wm. Younger	Keg Bitter	19	1043.7	1007.8	4.68	82.15%	55
1960	Wm. Younger	Younger's Bitter	18	1043.9	1010.8	4.30	75.40%	
1947	Gordon & Blair	Pale Ale	20	1045.5	1004.5	5.36	90.11%	
1958	Bernard	Special No. 1		1046	1013	4.28	71.74%	
	Average		***19.3***	***1044.3***	***1009.6***	***4.49***	***78.23%***	

Sources:
Thomas Usher Gravity Book held at the Scottish Brewing Archive, document number TU/6/11.
Whitbread Gravity book held at the London Metropolitan Archives, document number LMA/4453/D/02/002.
T & J Bernard's brewing records held at the Scottish Brewing Archive.
Maclay brewing record held at the Scottish Brewing Archive, document number M/6/1/1/28
Which Beer Report, 1960, pages 171 - 173.

It's too small a sample to learn much about the colour. Though Scottish brewers' habit of colouring the same beer to multiple shades would have made even a large sample quite random. It would all just depend where the sample was purchased.

Export was pretty common as a bottled beer, in a form much the same as the draught version.

Bottled Scottish 80/- 1947 - 1949							
Year	Brewer	Beer	Price	OG	FG	ABV	App. Atten-uation
1949	Aitchison	"Best Cellar"		1042	1010.5	4.09	75.00%
1947	Aitchison	80/- Ale	16	1042	1008	4.42	80.95%
1947	Bernard	80/- Ale	16	1034	1006	3.64	82.35%
1947	Dryborough	80/- Ale	16	1034	1008	3.37	76.47%
1947	Gordon & Blair	80/- Ale	16	1045	1006	5.09	86.67%
1947	Maclachlan	80/- Ale	16	1042	1008.5	4.36	79.76%
1947	McEwan	80/- Ale	16	1043.5	1010	4.35	77.01%
1947	Morrison	80/- Ale	16	1037.5	1004	4.37	89.33%
1947	Steel Coulson	80/- Ale	16	1034.5	1007	3.57	79.71%
1947	Younger, Geo	80/- Ale	16	1039.5	1009	3.96	77.22%
1947	Younger, Robert	80/- Ale		1038.5	1009.5	3.76	75.32%

Bottled Scottish 80/- 1947 - 1949							
Year	**Brewer**	**Beer**	**Price**	**OG**	**FG**	**ABV**	**App. Atten-uation**
1947	Younger, Wm.	80/- Ale	16	1042	1012	3.89	71.43%
1948	Usher	80/- Ale		1044.5	1010.5	4.42	76.40%
1949	Belhaven	Export		1040.5	1009.5	4.03	76.54%
1949	Mackay	Export	10.25	1036.5	1008.5	3.63	76.71%
1948	Calder Alloa	Export Ale		1045.5	1015	3.95	67.03%
1949	Young	Export Ale		1037.5	1010.5	3.50	72.00%
1948	Younger, Geo	Heavy Export Ale		1048.5	1016	4.21	67.01%
1949	Younger, Wm	Monk Pale Ale Export		1046	1011	4.55	76.09%
1947	Usher	PA 80/-		1044.5	1013	4.08	70.79%
1947	Steel Coulson	Real Export		1039	1005.5	4.37	85.90%
1948	McEwan	Red Label Sparkling Beer		1040.3	1007.4	4.28	81.64%
1949	Bernard	Special Export Ale		1041	1007	4.43	82.93%
1948	Usher	XP		1044.5	1015	3.82	66.29%
	Average		***15.5***	***1041.0***	***1009.5***	***4.09***	***77.11%***
Sources: Thomas Usher Gravity Book held at the Scottish Brewing Archive, document number TU/6/11. Whitbread Gravity book held at the London Metropolitan Archives, document number LMA/4453/D/02/002.							

The rate of attenuation is all over the shop, from 66% to almost 90%. A couple of the beers aren't even strong enough to be 70/-, let alone 80/- as claimed. You'd expect an authentic interpretation of the style to be at least 1040°.

Strong Pale Ale

A handful of strong bottled Pale Ales, with gravities over 1050°, were brewed in Scotland. There doesn't appear to have been any generic name for this class of beer.

Bottled Scottish Strong Pale Ale 1947 - 1950						
Year	**Brewer**	**Beer**	**OG**	**FG**	**ABV**	**App. Atten-uation**
1947	Gordon & Blair	Unique	1050	1015.6	4.46	68.80%
1950	Calder Alloa	Pale Ale	1054.7	1014.2	5.26	74.04%
1947	Steel Coulson	Five X Edinburgh Ale	1054	1015	5.06	72.22%
Sources: Thomas Usher Gravity Book held at the Scottish Brewing Archive, document number TU/6/11. Whitbread Gravity book held at the London Metropolitan Archives, document number LMA/4453/D/02/002.						

Other Shilling Pale Ales

60/-, 70/- and 80/- were pretty well defined in terms of gravity. But there were other Shilling Pale Ales that were more random. 90/-, for example, isn't stronger than 80/-, as you would expect, but around the same strength as 60/-. 105/- could be same strength as a 60/-, 70/- or 80/-. There's no logic to it whatsoever.

The only one of this type of beer to show any consistency is 120/-, which was a round the same gravity as Export.

Random Scottish Shilling Pale Ales 1947 - 1949						
Year	Brewer	Beer	OG	FG	ABV	App. Atten-uation
1949	Aitken	90/- Ale	1030	1006.5	3.05	78.33%
1949	Young	90/- Ale	1030.5	1009	2.78	70.49%
1947	Younger, Wm.	90/- Sparkling Ale	1032	1009	2.98	71.88%
1949	Aitchison	PA 90/-	1029	1007	2.85	75.86%
1947	Aitchison	105/- Ale	1036	1008	3.64	77.78%
1947	Maclachlan	105/- Ale	1044	1010.5	4.35	76.14%
1947	Murray	105/- Ale	1032	1004.5	3.58	85.94%
1947	Younger, Wm.	105/- Ale	1036.5	1005.5	4.04	84.93%
1947	Youngs	105/- Ale	1037	1008	3.77	78.38%
1948	Usher	105/- Ale	1037.5	1007.5	3.90	80.00%
1948	Usher	120/-	1045.5	1009	4.75	80.22%
1948	Usher	120/-	1044	1011.5	4.22	73.86%
1947	Campbell, Hope & King	120/- Ale	1044	1008	4.69	81.82%
1947	Fowler	120/- Ale	1039.5	1011	3.69	72.15%
Source:						
Thomas Usher Gravity Book held at the Scottish Brewing Archive, document number TU/6/11.						

Scottish Pale Ale Grists

Scottish brewers were, for the most part pretty dull when it came to recipes. Most only had the one.

I've only bothered with one of a brewery's Pale Ale range, as all were parti-gyled together. Except at the ever contrary William Younger. Not only weren't their Pale Ales parti-gyled together, they all had slightly different recipes. The crazy bastards.

Scottish Pale Ale grists 1948 - 1965: malts and adjuncts								
Year	Brewer	Beer	OG	pale malt	black malt	enzymic malt	flaked maize	flaked barley
1958	Bernard	Pale 1/1	1031	75.20%	0.82%		13.08%	
1948	Drybrough	P 60/-	1030	79.11%	0.78%	1.65%		10.55%
1954	Drybrough	60/-	1032	74.52%	2.40%	0.64%	6.01%	6.01%
1960	Drybrough	60/-	1031	74.95%	0.44%		12.49%	
1965	Drybrough	60/-	1031	74.45%	0.06%		12.07%	
1951	Maclay	PA 6d	1030	86.33%				
1956	Maclay	PA 6d	1030	74.82%			11.51%	
1965	Maclay	PA 6d	1030	74.82%			11.51%	
1962	Thomas Usher	P 1/4	1036	69.23%			6.29%	
1957	Younger, Robert	60/-	1030	77.03%			13.75%	
1960	Younger, Robert	60/-	1030	71.39%			19.99%	
1949	Younger, Wm.	XXP Btg	1031	92.86%				7.14%
1949	Younger, Wm.	XXP	1031.5	88.24%				11.76%

Scottish Pale Ale grists 1948 - 1965: malts and adjuncts								
Year	**Brewer**	**Beer**	**OG**	**pale malt**	**black malt**	**enzymic malt**	**flaked maize**	**flaked barley**
1949	Younger, Wm.	Ext	1047	87.50%				12.50%
1958	Younger, Wm.	XXPQ	1033	60.00%			26.67%	
1958	Younger, Wm.	XXPSL	1038	58.62%			27.59%	
1958	Younger, Wm.	EXT	1046	60.94%			29.69%	
1958	Younger, Wm.	XXPS Btg	1038	62.16%			32.43%	

Sources:
T & J Bernard brewing record held at the Scottish Brewing Archive, document number TJB6/1/1/1.
Drybrough brewing record held at the Scottish Brewing Archive, document number D/6/1/1/6.
Drybrough brewing record held at the Scottish Brewing Archive, document number D/6/1/1/7.
Drybrough brewing record held at the Scottish Brewing Archive, document number D/6/1/1/8.
Maclay brewing record held at the Scottish Brewing Archive, document number M/6/1/1/28.
Maclay brewing record held at the Scottish Brewing Archive, document number M/6/1/1/35.
Maclay brewing record held at the Scottish Brewing Archive, document number M/6/1/1/44.
Thomas Usher brewing record held at the Scottish Brewing Archive, document number TU/6/9/1.
Robert Younger brewing record held at the Scottish Brewing Archive, document number RY/6/1/2.
Robert Younger brewing record held at the Scottish Brewing Archive, document number RY/6/1/3.
William Younger brewing record held at the Scottish Brewing Archive, document number WY/6/1/2/88.
William Younger brewing record held at the Scottish Brewing Archive, document number WY/6/1/3/112.

I've lumped the malts and adjuncts together because there aren't many of either. Mostly it's just pale malt and flaked maize or barley. A couple of examples have a small amount of black malt for colour. But there's no crystal malt in sight.

William Younger loved to stuff their beers with adjuncts. Before WW II most of their beers were 40% grits. The beers above aren't quite that bad, but those from the 1950s all still have over 25% flaked maize.

Two sugar tables for this set.

Scottish Pale Ale grists 1948 - 1965: sugars							
Year	Brewer	Beer	OG	no. 1 sugar	invert	Avona	Hydrol
1958	Bernard	Pale 1/1	1031		6.54%	4.36%	
1948	Drybrough	P 60/-	1030			2.64%	
1954	Drybrough	60/-	1032			3.21%	3.21%
1960	Drybrough	60/-	1031		6.81%	1.51%	
1965	Drybrough	60/-	1031		7.38%	0.67%	
1951	Maclay	PA 6d	1030	9.59%			
1956	Maclay	PA 6d	1030	7.67%			
1965	Maclay	PA 6d	1030	7.67%			
1962	Thomas Usher	P 1/4	1036		17.48%		
1957	Younger, Robert	60/-	1030		4.58%		3.67%
1960	Younger, Robert	60/-	1030		3.81%		3.81%
1949	Younger, Wm.	XXP Btg	1031				
1949	Younger, Wm.	XXP	1031.5				
1949	Younger, Wm.	Ext	1047				
1958	Younger, Wm.	XXPQ	1033				
1958	Younger, Wm.	XXPSL	1038		2.30%		
1958	Younger, Wm.	EXT	1046		3.13%		
1958	Younger, Wm.	XXPS Btg	1038				

Invert sugar is as popular as ever. No. 1 being what you'd expect in Pale Ales. The unspecific "invert" is most likely either No. 1 or No. 2 invert. Avona and Hydrol are enigmatic proprietary sugars.

Scottish Pale Ale grists 1948 - 1965: sugars again								
Year	Brewer	Beer	OG	cane	candy	caramel	malt extract	other sugar
1958	Bernard	Pale 1/1	1031					
1948	Drybrough	P 60/-	1030				0.88%	4.39%
1954	Drybrough	60/-	1032				0.80%	3.21%
1960	Drybrough	60/-	1031			1.51%	0.76%	1.51%
1965	Drybrough	60/-	1031				2.68%	2.68%
1951	Maclay	PA 6d	1030			0.24%		3.84%
1956	Maclay	PA 6d	1030			0.24%	1.92%	3.84%
1965	Maclay	PA 6d	1030			0.24%	1.92%	3.84%
1962	Thomas Usher	P 1/4	1036			0.00%	2.10%	4.90%
1957	Younger, Robert	60/-	1030			0.05%	0.92%	
1960	Younger, Robert	60/-	1030			0.05%	0.95%	
1949	Younger, Wm.	XXP Btg	1031					
1949	Younger, Wm.	XXP	1031.5					
1949	Younger, Wm.	Ext	1047					
1958	Younger, Wm.	XXPQ	1033	8.89%	4.44%			
1958	Younger, Wm.	XXPSL	1038	6.90%	4.60%			
1958	Younger, Wm.	EXT	1046	6.25%				
1958	Younger, Wm.	XXPS Btg	1038	5.41%				

A more normal lot of sugars. Though exactly what is meant by cane and candy isn't 100% clear. I assume that cane refers to some partially refined cane sugar. There's lots of malt extract again, always in tiny quantities. The largest amount used is under 3% of the total grist.

Pale malt, flaked adjunct and sugar. That's all there is to Scottish Pale Ale grists.

Stout

Guinness had by no means a monopoly on Stout brewing. Pretty much every brewery in the UK had at least one Stout in their portfolio. Mostly in bottled form. Some London brewers were still producing cask Stout well into the 1950s, but, other than in Northern Ireland, it had died out in the rest of the UK. Until the 1960s, that is, when keg Draught Guinness began to spread outside Ireland.

Many Stout types were brewed in the UK. Sweet Stout and Guinness weren't the only options. Sure, there were loads of Stouts of varying degrees of ridiculous sweetness. Especially in Scotland. In contrast, there were also powerful Imperial Stouts and dry, more Guinness-like Stouts brewed in England.

These may have often been remnants of an earlier beer culture, but there was still a huge variety in the character of Stouts.

There are so many examples of bottled Stouts of different character, that I've split them up into three groups: weak, standard and strong.

Draught Stout

Although it had disappeared from most of England between the wars, draught Stout was still available in some parts of the UK. Northern Ireland, obviously, where cask and later keg Guinness was available. In London, too, local brewers still sold cask Stout in some of their tied houses. By 1965, the only available draught Stout was Keg Guinness.

Sweet Stout

Sweet Stouts were very much on the rise, though these came in different forms. Most obvious are the lactose-laced Milk Stouts in the Mackeson mould.

But other brewers achieved sweetness in different ways. For example through the addition of glucose at the end of primary fermentation. Tennant's of Sheffield brewed a Stout of this type that you'll find in the recipe section. Some kept the FG artificially high by stopping fermentation prematurely.

Many of the sweetest beers occur in the weak Stout category.

Weak Stout

I'm defining as weak Stout as anything under 1040°. Which, let's face it, is pretty damn weak for a beer whose name literally means "strong".

While watery Stouts are often associated with a huge amount of sweetness, there were quite dry low gravity Stouts. They were many and they were varied.

London Weak Stout >70% attenuation								
Date	Year	Beer	Price per pint d	OG	FG	ABV	App. Atten-uation	colour
1951	Barclay Perkins	Stout	18	1035.1	1010.4	3.20	70.37%	275
1951	Charrington	Anchor Stout	18	1037.4	1010.5	3.49	71.93%	300
1950	Courage	London Stout	17	1033	1008	3.24	75.76%	275
1950	Courage	Brown Stout	17	1030.2	1008.1	2.86	73.18%	300
1957	Fullers	Nourishing Stout	22	1033	1009	3.11	72.73%	240
1951	Mann Crossman	Oatmeal Stout	18	1036.1	1010.7	3.29	70.36%	310
1950	Meux	Special Stout	24	1038.7	1011.5	3.52	70.28%	250
1952	Whitbread	WS		1038.3	1008.5	3.94	77.81%	175
	Average		***19.1***	***1035.2***	***1009.6***	***3.33***	***72.80%***	***265.6***
Source: Whitbread Gravity book held at the London Metropolitan Archives, document number LMA/4453/D/02/002.								

This set, in terms of attenuation, looks like traditional London Stout. The big difference is a much lower gravity that those beers had, not just before WW I, but also between the wars.

Midlands Weak Stout >70% attenuation								
Date	Year	Beer	Price per pint d	OG	FG	ABV	App. Atten-uation	colour
1954	Bents Brewery	Imperial Stone Stout	22	1039.8	1006.5	4.34	83.67%	200
1958	Everards	VB Brown Ale	26	1038.8	1008.8	3.75	77.32%	110
1959	Home	Home Stout	26	1038.5	1011.1	3.55	71.17%	400
1953	Mitchell & Butler	Nourishing Stout	20	1039.2	1006.5	4.26	83.42%	175
1951	Groves & Whitnall	Red Rose Stout	26	1036.8	1008.1	3.73	77.99%	
	Average		***24***	***1038.6***	***1008.2***	***3.92***	***78.71%***	***221.3***
Source: Whitbread Gravity book held at the London Metropolitan Archives, document number LMA/4453/D/02/002.								

It's almost as if they had a contest to see who could get away with the most watery Imperial. I suppose the Bents version did just about scramble over 4% ABV. In its early days, it must have been a much stronger beer. How I wish I knew its history.

Northern Weak Stout >70% attenuation								
Date	**Year**	**Beer**	**Price per pint d**	**OG**	**FG**	**ABV**	**App. Atten-uation**	**colour**
1954	Hey	White Rose Stout	24	1038.1	1010.8	3.54	71.65%	210
1951	Higson	Stout	22	1038.9	1008.9	3.90	77.12%	
1951	Peter Walker	Stout	22	1038.1	1009.1	3.76	76.12%	175
1953	Threlfalls	Extra Stout	39	1038.1	1008	3.91	79.00%	125
1952	Thwaites	Cream Stout	24	1039.6	1008.7	4.01	78.03%	
1952	Masseys	Prize Stout	27	1038.3	1006.7	4.11	82.51%	330
	Average		***26.3***	***1038.5***	***1008.7***	***3.87***	***77.40%***	***210.0***
Source: Whitbread Gravity book held at the London Metropolitan Archives, document number LMA/4453/D/02/002.								

Not a huge number of examples. Not very dark ones, either. Yet the average price is much the same as the beers in the same gravity band you'll see below.

Southern Weak Stout >70% attenuation								
Date	**Year**	**Beer**	**Price per pint d**	**OG**	**FG**	**ABV**	**App. Atten-uation**	**colour**
1952	Arnold & Hancock	Stout	24	1028.3	1003.9	3.17	86.22%	125
1956	Bullard	Double Stout (no lactose)	24	1038.7	1008.1	3.98	79.07%	275
1958	Cheltenham & Hereford Brewery	Gloster Stout	24	1037.2	1009.8	3.43	73.66%	275
1953	Greene King	Stout	19	1034.4	1008.6	3.35	75.00%	330
1954	JW Green	Oatmeal Stout	22	1039.1	1007.4	4.12	81.07%	228
1953	Star Brewery	Stout	19	1031.7	1009.5	2.87	70.03%	350
1952	Strong	Black Bess Stout	19	1036	1007.3	3.73	79.72%	125
1958	Stroud Brewery	Nourishing Stout	20	1033.1	1008.9	3.02	73.11%	250
1950	Wadworth	Barley Malt		1039.7	1009.8	3.88	75.31%	225
1957	Young & Co.	Stout	24	1037.3	1009.6	3.59	74.26%	500
1956	Young, Crawshay & Young	Double Stout	22	1037.8	1011.2	3.44	70.37%	400
	Average		***21.7***	***1035.8***	***1008.6***	***3.51***	***76.17%***	***280.3***
Source: Whitbread Gravity book held at the London Metropolitan Archives, document number LMA/4453/D/02/002.								

The beer from Arnold & Hancock is one of the weakest Stouts I've ever seen. Weaker even than the weakest wartime Stouts. It really is taking the piss.

Celtic fringe Weak Stout >70% attenuation								
Date	**Year**	**Beer**	**Price per pint d**	**OG**	**FG**	**ABV**	**App. Atten-uation**	**colour**
1956	Ely Brewery	Cardiff Stout	24	1034.9	1005.4	3.84	84.53%	300
1951	Hancocks	Extra Stout	18	1037.1	1006.3	4.01	83.02%	
1951	Hancocks	Oatmeal Stout	15.5	1037	1010.1	3.49	72.70%	
1955	Beamish & Crawford	Irish Stout (no lactose)		1039.5	1009.6	3.88	75.70%	212
1951	Castletown	Manx Oyster Stout	30	1039.6	1011.2	3.68	71.72%	
	Average		***21.9***	***1037.6***	***1008.5***	***3.78***	***77.53%***	***256.0***
Source: Whitbread Gravity book held at the London Metropolitan Archives, document number LMA/4453/D/02/002.								

It's worth noting that the Irish example – Beamish & Crawford – is one of the least attenuated beers in this set. I'm sure that the two Hancocks examples are the same beer, just with different labels. The London brewers usually had oats in all their Stouts so they could legally sell some as Oatmeal Stout.

London Weak Stout 60-70% attenuation								
Year	**Brewer**	**Beer**	**Price per pint d**	**OG**	**FG**	**ABV**	**App. Atten-uation**	**colour**
1950	Barclay Perkins	Stout	18	1032.7	1010.9	2.82	66.67%	330
1950	Barclay Perkins	Victory Stout	24	1039.2	1013.2	3.36	66.33%	275
1951	Courage	London Stout	20	1032.7	1010.7	2.85	67.28%	225
1951	Hammerton	Oatmeal Stout	21	1039.7	1012.7	3.49	68.01%	275
1950	Ind Coope	Allsopp Special Stout	18	1034.4	1010.4	3.11	69.77%	800
1959	Ind Coope	"Dry Club" Stout	26	1038.7	1013.2	3.30	65.89%	240
1950	Mann Crossman	London Stout	17	1036.8	1013.9	2.96	62.23%	300
1950	Mann Crossman	Oatmeal Stout	16	1032.4	1011.5	2.70	64.51%	275
1951	Taylor Walker	Nourishing Stout	17	1032.8	1012.7	2.59	61.28%	300
1957	Taylor Walker	Nourishing Stout	22	1033.3	1012.9	2.63	61.26%	300
1951	Truman	Eagle Stout	18	1034.5	1013.1	2.76	62.03%	200
1953	Truman	Eagle Stout	19	1034	1012.3	2.80	63.82%	250
1954	Truman	Oatmeal Stout	18	1034.4	1012.8	2.79	62.79%	300
1950	Watney	Reids Family Stout	21	1037	1012.2	3.21	67.03%	225
1951	Watney	Family Stout	20	1036.4	1012	3.16	67.03%	200
1952	Watney	Extra Stout	29	1039.4	1012.2	3.52	69.04%	200
1954	Watney	Dairymaid Stout	21	1033.8	1012.6	2.74	62.72%	325
1959	Whitbread	Oatmeal Stout	24	1038.6	1012.4	3.39	67.88%	225
	Average		***20.5***	***1035.6***	***1012.3***	***3.01***	***65.31%***	***291.4***
Source: Whitbread Gravity book held at the London Metropolitan Archives, document number LMA/4453/D/02/002.								

Watney had a confusing array of Stouts, some still branded as Reid, a brewery that closed in 1898. How many actual different Stouts they brewed is another matter. They might all be the same beer with different labels. Al lot of that went on.

Midlands Weak Stout 60-70% attenuation								
Year	**Brewer**	**Beer**	**Price per pint d**	**OG**	**FG**	**ABV**	**App. Atten-uation**	**colour**
1957	Dare, Birmingham	Sugar Sweet Stout	32	1038.1	1014.4	3.06	62.20%	250
1956	Worthington	XX Stout	28	1036.7	1013.8	2.96	62.40%	300
	Average		***30.0***	***1037.4***	***1014.1***	***3.01***	***62.30%***	***275.0***
Source: Whitbread Gravity book held at the London Metropolitan Archives, document number LMA/4453/D/02/002.								

The word "sweet" often appears in the names of Stouts. Even ones like the Dare's example above, which doesn't look like it was that sweet. Clearly Sweet Stout sold.

Northern Weak Stout 60-70% attenuation								
Year	**Brewer**	**Beer**	**Price per pint d**	**OG**	**FG**	**ABV**	**App. Atten-uation**	**colour**
1955	Brains	Extra Stout	22	1039.1	1014.6	3.16	62.66%	215
1959	Darley	Barley Cream Stout	25	1039.4	1012.2	3.52	69.04%	250
1952	Duncan Gilmour	Milk Round Stout	22	1038.1	1012.4	3.32	67.45%	175
1955	Hancocks	Extra Stout	22	1034.1	1012.2	2.83	64.22%	200
1959	John J. Hunt	Regal Stout	30	1039.4	1013.3	3.37	66.24%	275
1957	Mitchells, Lancaster	Oatmeal Stout (lactose absent)	26	1036.4	1011.2	3.26	69.23%	200
1959	Peter Walker	Summit Stout	24	1037.4	1013.5	3.09	63.90%	250
1959	Russell	Imperial Stout	28	1039.4	1014.2	3.26	63.96%	200
1953	United Breweries	Double Stout	20	1038.2	1014.6	3.05	61.78%	225
1953	Vale of Neath Brewery	Mellow Stout	26	1035.7	1014.2	2.77	60.22%	600
1959	Ward	Malt Stout	25	1039.7	1013	3.45	67.25%	300
1954	Whitaker	Standard Stout	24	1037.2	1014.3	2.96	61.56%	250
1957	Yates & Jackson	Oatmeal Stout (lactose absent)	31	1035.3	1011.1	3.13	68.56%	425
	Average		***25.0***	***1037.6***	***1013.1***	***3.17***	***65.08%***	***274.2***
Source: Whitbread Gravity book held at the London Metropolitan Archives, document number LMA/4453/D/02/002.								

The words breweries used to describe their Stouts are fascinating: cream, mellow, regal, malt. You don't see such variety in the names of other styles. Oh, and imperial. Here's another not very imperial Imperial Stout.

Southern Weak Stout 60-70% attenuation								
Year	**Brewer**	**Beer**	**Price per pint d**	**OG**	**FG**	**ABV**	**App. Atten-uation**	**colour**
1951	Benskin	Brown Stout	20	1039.2	1013.6	3.31	65.31%	330
1953	Brickwoods	Oatmeal Stout	21	1039	1014	3.23	64.10%	300
1951	Charrington	Anchor Stout	17	1035	1012	2.97	65.71%	315
1959	Cheltenham & Hereford	Gloster Stout	22	1035.5	1012.6	2.96	64.51%	375
1953	Cobbold	Double Stout	19	1036.6	1011.9	3.19	67.49%	315
1956	East Anglian Breweries	Ely Oatmeal Stout	22	1038	1011.7	3.40	69.21%	350
1953	Fremlin	Nourishing Stout	19	1031.7	1010.1	2.79	68.14%	225
1954	Greene King	Stout	19	1034.3	1012.7	2.79	62.97%	450
1959	Groves, Weymouth	Nourishing Stout	22	1036.1	1012.5	3.05	65.37%	240
1951	Lovibond	Special Stout	18	1036.6	1014.2	2.89	61.20%	315
1952	McMullen	Macs Stout	21	1039	1012.1	3.48	68.97%	260
1954	McMullen	Mac Stout	23	1039.4	1012.6	3.47	68.02%	275
1953	Octagon Brewery	Special Stout	24	1036.9	1012.2	3.19	66.94%	250
1950	Samuel Smith	Taddy Stout	22	1039.3	1012.9	3.41	67.18%	400
1951	Simonds	Luncheon Stout	18	1034.1	1013.1	2.71	61.58%	250
1959	Strong	Black Bess Stout	22	1034.1	1012.2	2.83	64.22%	300
1953	Tamplin	Double Oatmeal Stout	18	1032.1	1010.3	2.82	67.91%	400
1954	Tollemache	Oatmeal Stout	19	1030.9	1012.1	2.43	60.84%	275
1953	Ushers Trowbridge	Oatmeal Stout	15	1033.8	1012.7	2.72	62.43%	250
1959	Young & Co	Query Stout	32	1039.2	1013.6	3.31	65.31%	375
	Average		***20.7***	***1035.8***	***1012.6***	***3.01***	***64.84%***	***310.8***
Source: Whitbread Gravity book held at the London Metropolitan Archives, document number LMA/4453/D/02/002.								

"Nourishing" is a word that occurs often in Stout names. Usually pretty weedy ones. It's a hangover from the Victorian idea of Stout as an invigorating drink. In the 19th century Invalid Stout was common. Nourishing Stout is the 20th-century equivalent.

Scottish Weak Stout 60-70% attenuation								
Year	**Brewer**	**Beer**	**Price per pint d**	**OG**	**FG**	**ABV**	**App. Atten-uation**	**colour**
1955	Blair	Sweet Stout	30	1033.1	1010.9	2.87	67.07%	300
1959	Machlachan	Stout	28	1035.4	1013.1	2.88	62.99%	175
1955	Morison	Sweet Stout	27	1035.7	1012.3	3.02	65.55%	325
1959	Younger, Wm.	Sweet Stout	28	1033.3	1013.1	2.61	60.66%	300
	Average		***28.3***	***1034.4***	***1012.4***	***2.85***	***64.07%***	***275.0***
Source: Whitbread Gravity book held at the London Metropolitan Archives, document number LMA/4453/D/02/002.								

Sweet Stout was a big thing in Scotland. As the fact that three of the four examples above are specifically called that. Though these beers aren't ***that*** sweet. We'll be seeing the really sweet ones later.

London Weak Stout 50-60% attenuation								
Year	Brewer	Beer	Price per pint d	OG	FG	ABV	App. Atten-uation	colour
1951	Barclay Perkins	Stout	18	1035	1015.6	2.50	55.43%	275
1957	Barclay Perkins	Stout	22	1033.8	1014.4	2.50	57.40%	210
1957	Courage & Barclay	London Stout	22	1034.9	1016.3	2.39	53.30%	340
1957	Friary	Malt Stout	24	1036.1	1017.5	2.39	51.52%	300
1953	Friary	Double Stout	20	1034.7	1014.6	2.59	57.93%	330
1951	Ind Coope	Special Stout	29	1037.1	1015.3	2.81	58.76%	300
1956	Ind Coope	Sweet Stout (lactose present)	28	1038.5	1016.5	2.83	57.14%	250
1959	Ind Coope	Allsopp's Sweet Stout	28	1037.8	1015.4	2.89	59.26%	275
1951	Taylor Walker	Nourishing Stout	17	1033.9	1014.1	2.55	58.41%	330
1950	Truman	Eagle Stout	9d	1034.1	1014.8	2.49	56.60%	225
1950	Truman	Best Stout	16	1038.6	1019	2.52	50.78%	250
1954	Truman	Oatmeal Stout	24	1035.5	1015.9	2.52	55.21%	350
1950	Watney	Glasgow Special Stout	26	1032.1	1013.7	2.37	57.32%	300
1951	Watney	Dairymaid Sweet Stout	18	1032.7	1015.1	2.27	53.82%	
	Average		***22.5***	***1035.3***	***1015.6***	***2.55***	***55.96%***	***287.3***
Source: Whitbread Gravity book held at the London Metropolitan Archives, document number LMA/4453/D/02/002.								

I'd be interested to know what Friary Single Stout was like if Double Stout is just 1035°. Not sure why Watney had a Glasgow Stout. They never bought a Glasgow brewery, as far as I'm aware.

Midlands Weak Stout 50-60% attenuation								
Year	Brewer	Beer	Price per pint d	OG	FG	ABV	App. Atten-uation	colour
1959	Hole	Sweet Castle Stout	28	1038.7	1018.7	2.57	51.68%	350
1952	Northampton Brewery	Jumbo Stout	18	1037.8	1016.8	2.70	55.56%	100
1953	Offilers	Nourishing Stout	30	1037.7	1017.3	2.63	54.11%	250
1959	Offilers	Nourishing Stout	28	1035.9	1015	2.69	58.22%	275
1959	Phipps	Jumbo Stout	23	1036	1015.2	2.68	57.78%	275
1959	Phipps	Ratcliffe Stout	23	1037	1017.9	2.46	51.62%	425
1959	Warwick & Richardson	Milk Maid Stout	30	1039.6	1018.6	2.70	53.03%	250
	Average		***25.7***	***1037.5***	***1017.1***	***2.63***	***54.57%***	***275.0***
Source: Whitbread Gravity book held at the London Metropolitan Archives, document number LMA/4453/D/02/002.								

I'd put money on the two Phipps beers being identical. Inevitably, with the low degree of attenuation, all the beers are well under 3% ABV. I'm delighted to see two Newark beer.

Milk Maid Stout was what my mum drank.

Northern Weak Stout 50-60% attenuation								
Year	Brewer	Beer	Price per pint d	OG	FG	ABV	App. Atten-uation	colour
1953	Daniell & Sons	Double Stout	20	1037.1	1016.3	2.68	56.06%	350
1957	Ely Brewery	Gold & Silver Stout	24	1039.9	1017.3	2.91	56.64%	275
1959	Hope & Anchor	Jubilee Stout	30	1039.2	1015.7	3.03	59.95%	200
1957	Hull Brewery	Black Beauty Sweet Stout	24	1037.5	1018.5	2.44	50.67%	250
1953	Tennant Bros.	Malt Stout	24	1036.6	1015.1	2.77	58.74%	330
1959	Tennant Bros.	Glucose Stout	25	1039.8	1018.8	2.70	52.76%	225
1957	Thwaites	Cream Stout (lactose absent)	24	1033.1	1014.7	2.37	55.59%	225
	Average		***24.4***	***1037.6***	***1016.6***	***2.70***	***55.77%***	***265.0***
Source: Whitbread Gravity book held at the London Metropolitan Archives, document number LMA/4453/D/02/002.								

Glucose Stouts were produced by more breweries. From looking at the Tennant's recipe, where there's no mention of glucose, it must have been added after primary fermentation. Malt Stout looks like the same beer, just without the glucose.

Southern Weak Stout 50-60% attenuation								
Year	Brewer	Beer	Price per pint d	OG	FG	ABV	App. Atten-uation	colour
1956	Adams	Double Stout	22	1036.6	1015.2	2.76	58.47%	275
1953	Benskin	Brown Stout	21	1037.6	1018.3	2.48	51.33%	275
1953	Fremlin	Kents Best Special Stout	26	1039.2	1018	2.73	54.08%	375
1954	JW Paddey	Paddey's Stout	24	1037.2	1015.9	2.74	57.26%	275
1956	Lacons	Extra Stout	22	1034.5	1015.5	2.45	55.07%	300
1956	Morgans	Viking Stout	22	1035.4	1016	2.50	54.80%	150
1957	Simonds	Luncheon Stout	22	1033.6	1014.9	2.41	55.65%	275
1959	Ushers	Sweet Stout	28	1034.6	1015.5	2.46	55.20%	425
1959	Ushers	Oatmeal Stout	20	1033.6	1016.4	2.21	51.19%	225
1959	Wadworth	Special Double Stout	24	1037.6	1016	2.78	57.45%	350
1953	Young & Son Portsmouth	Victory Stout	17	1033.1	1013.3	2.55	59.82%	175
	Average		***22.5***	***1035.7***	***1015.9***	***2.55***	***55.48%***	***281.8***
Source: Whitbread Gravity book held at the London Metropolitan Archives, document number LMA/4453/D/02/002.								

Luncheon Stout is a blast from the past. It was a common name in Victorian times for a lowish gravity, bottled Stout. It's intriguing how long the term Brown Stout – the original name for Stout – hung around. When Stout had long since stopped being brown.

Scottish Weak Stout 50-60% attenuation								
Year	Brewer	Beer	Price per pint d	OG	FG	ABV	App. Atten-uation	colour
1955	Fowler	Stout	30	1038	1018.6	2.49	51.05%	400
1955	Maclachlan	Extra Sweet Stout	30	1035.8	1014.8	2.71	58.66%	225
1955	McEwan	Sweet Stout	30	1038.4	1018.6	2.55	51.56%	375
1959	Murray, Wm	Extra Sweet Stout	28	1039.6	1018.3	2.74	53.79%	175
1954	Steel Coulson	Elephant Stout	29	1038.9	1017.5	2.76	55.01%	315
1954	Younger, Geo.	Extra Stout	28	1037.5	1018	2.51	52.00%	625
1955	Younger, Geo.	Extra Stout	30	1038.5	1015.8	2.93	58.96%	575
1953	Younger, Robert	Sweet Stout	29	1035.7	1017.2	2.38	51.82%	200
	Average		***29.3***	***1037.8***	***1017.4***	***2.63***	***54.11%***	***361.3***

Source:
Whitbread Gravity book held at the London Metropolitan Archives, document number LMA/4453/D/02/002.

As we get lower down the attenuation scale, the number of Scottish examples is increasing. Sweet is certainly a good description of these Stouts.

Scottish Weak Stout < 50% attenuation								
Year	Brewer	Beer	Price per pint d	OG	FG	ABV	App. Atten-uation	colour
1959	Aitchison	Dalkeith Sweet Stout	30	1037.3	1021.3	2.05	42.90%	600
1959	Aitken	Stout	28	1039.4	1022.3	2.19	43.40%	250
1954	Jeffrey	Nourishing Stout	28	1036.1	1019.3	2.16	46.54%	250
1954	McEwan	Sweet Stout	28	1036.1	1019.3	2.16	46.54%	350
1954	McLennan & Urquhart	Dalkeith Stout		1037.1	1019.7	2.23	46.90%	450
1955	Tennent	Stout	30	1034.7	1019.3	1.98	44.38%	325
1955	Younger, Geo	Sweetheart Stout	32.5	1036.4	1024.5	1.52	32.69%	225
1956	Younger, Geo	Sweetheart Stout	30	1037.6	1024.6	1.66	34.57%	225
1959	Younger, Geo	Sweetheart Stout	28	1036.4	1024.4	1.53	32.97%	275
1959	Younger, R	Sweet Stout	28	1035.5	1018.3	2.21	48.45%	250
1951	Younger, Wm.	Sweet Stout	28	1035.7	1019.5	2.08	45.38%	150
1955	Younger, Wm.	Sweet Stout	30	1034.9	1017.5	2.24	49.86%	200
	Average		***29.1***	***1036.4***	***1020.8***	***2.00***	***42.88%***	***295.8***

Source:
Whitbread Gravity book held at the London Metropolitan Archives, document number LMA/4453/D/02/002.

Now we're at the really sweet ones. And also non-alcoholic ones. Sweetheart Stout is barely as strong as shandy. Yet it costs more than Stouts three times as strong. It's incredibly poor value for money. It's also one of a handful of Stouts from the 1950s that's still in production.

Other Weak Stout < 50% attenuation								
Year	Brewer	Beer	Price per pint d	OG	FG	ABV	App. Atten-uation	colour
1955	Benskin	Double Stout	22	1036.1	1018.3	2.29	49.31%	275
1957	Isleworth	Stout	22	1021.8	1011.8	1.29	45.87%	300
1954	Tollemache	Double Stout	23	1037.6	1021.8	2.02	42.02%	350
1950	Wenlock	Oatmeal Stout	30	1030.5	1015.3	1.96	49.84%	200
	Average		***24.3***	***1031.5***	***1016.8***	***1.89***	***46.76%***	***281.3***

Source:
Whitbread Gravity book held at the London Metropolitan Archives, document number LMA/4453/D/02/002.

That Isleworth Stout really is a joke. Weaker than shandy. In fact, there's no chance of getting pissed with any of these beers.

Standard Stout

My definition of standard Stout is one of a gravity in the range 1040° - 1050°. The majority of Stout after WW II falls in this group. And all the big sellers, beers like Guinness Extra Stout and Mackeson.

Guinness Standard Stout >70% attenuation								
Year	Brewer	Beer	Price per pint d	OG	FG	ABV	App. Atten-uation	colour
1950	Guinness	Extra Stout	23	1048.6	1008.6	5.21	82.30%	100
1951	Guinness	Extra Stout	30	1049.1	1007.5	5.43	84.73%	100
1951	Guinness	Extra Stout	31	1047.7	1008.1	5.16	83.02%	112
1952	Guinness	Extra Stout	28	1047.4	1007.5	5.20	84.18%	100
1953	Guinness	Extra Stout	36	1046.3	1002.8	5.70	93.95%	100
1953	Guinness	Extra Stout	31	1047.4	1008.7	5.04	81.65%	175
1954	Guinness	Extra Stout	31	1047.5	1006.6	5.34	86.11%	200
1954	Guinness	Extra Stout	28	1047.4	1007.1	5.26	85.02%	225
1957	Guinness	Extra Stout	34	1047.3	1008.6	5.04	81.82%	150
1958	Guinness	Extra Stout	33	1046.3	1009.2	4.83	80.13%	200
	Average		***30.5***	***1047.5***	***1007.47***	***5.22***	***84.29%***	***146.2***

Source:
Whitbread Gravity book held at the London Metropolitan Archives, document number LMA/4453/D/02/002.

I've no idea where these samples of Guinness were brewed. My guess would be that most are from Park Royal, as Whitbread was based in London. But the Dublin-brewed version was available in the UK, especially in the North and Scotland.

The rate of attenuation amongst the Guinness examples has a fair spread, from 80.13% to 93.95% apparent. There are plenty of examples from other breweries with a higher degree of attenuation of the least attenuated version of Guinness. What I'm trying to say is that

Guinness wasn't unique in its dryness.

Judging by its price, Guinness was a premium product. It averages 30.5d per, almost 5d per pint more than the Northern Stouts below. But that makes sense, if you think about it. Two breweries – Guinness and the bottling/reselling brewery – both needed to make a profit from it.

Northern Standard Stout >70% attenuation

Year	Brewer	Beer	Price per pint d	OG	FG	ABV	App. Atten-uation	colour
1951	Hancocks	77 Export Stout	28	1045.9	1010.3	4.63	77.56%	200
1954	JW Lees	Archer Stout	24	1040.7	1008.5	4.19	79.12%	225
1951	JW Lees	Archer Stout	26	1041.7	1009.6	4.17	76.98%	
1951	JW Lees	Archer Stout	26	1040	1009.5	3.96	76.25%	
1959	Cornbrook Brewery	Barley Stout	25	1046.3	1013.8	4.21	70.19%	250
1959	Holt, Joseph	Brown Stout	27	1045.2	1007.5	4.91	83.41%	325
1959	Ardwick Brewery	Chesters Special Sweet Stout	30	1045.5	1012.5	4.28	72.53%	200
1954	Thwaites	Cream Stout	26	1044.3	1013.2	4.03	70.20%	200
1954	Chester Brewery	Extra Stout	24	1042.7	1006.5	4.72	84.78%	250
1954	Magee Marshall	Extra Stout	22	1043.5	1006.4	4.84	85.29%	200
1959	Threlfalls	Extra Stout	26	1044.4	1010.5	4.40	76.35%	175
1954	Threlfalls	Extra Stout	26	1046.9	1011.5	4.60	75.48%	225
1959	Matthew Brown	Lion Oatmeal Stout	26	1040.4	1005.2	4.59	87.13%	150
1957	Matthew Brown	Lion Oatmeal Stout	24	1041.4	1006.7	4.52	83.82%	250
1959	Lion Brewery	Lion Prize Stout	28	1046.3	1011.3	4.38	75.59%	175
1952	Nimmo	Nimmo's Stout	24	1045	1011.4	4.36	74.67%	80
1952	Matthew Brown	Oatmeal Stout	23	1041.1	1007.8	4.33	81.02%	175
1959	Massey	Prize Stout	25	1040.8	1004.2	4.78	89.71%	475
1950	Stone, Wm.	Samson Stout	24	1043.1	1012.11	4.02	71.90%	330
1953	Camerons	Sovereign Stout	26	1044.3	1009.6	4.51	78.33%	315
1954	Hydes	Special Stout (Lactose present)	24	1043.2	1010.9	4.19	74.77%	225
1959	Chesters	Special Sweet Stout	28	1044.6	1013.2	4.07	70.40%	200
1959	Robinson	Unicorn Black Stout	29	1041.8	1008.1	4.38	80.62%	240
1959	Hey's	White Rose Stout	28	1046.6	1008.7	4.94	81.33%	325
1952	Greenall Whitley	Wilderspool Extra Stout	26	1040.4	1011	3.81	72.77%	125
	Average		***25.8***	***1043.4***	***1009.6***	***4.39***	***78.01%***	***231.1***

Source:
Whitbread Gravity book held at the London Metropolitan Archives, document number LMA/4453/D/02/002.

There are several beers that look quite similar to Guinness: Massey, Matthew Brown, Magee Marshall, Chesters and Holts. Though some do have a lower OG. All are from the Northwest of England. Is that a coincidence, or were drier Stouts more popular in that part of the country?

I was surprised to see a beer described as a Sweet Stout (Chesters) in this set and one containing lactose (Hydes). Especially as the latter had a 75% rate of attenuation. There can't have been that much lactose added or the FG would be higher.

Midlands Standard Stout >70% attenuation								
Year	Brewer	Beer	Price per pint d	OG	FG	ABV	App. Atten-uation	colour
1953	Mitchell & Butler	Extra Stout	24	1049	1008.2	5.32	83.27%	175
1952	Bent's Brewery	Imperial Stone Stout	23	1041.3	1007.1	4.45	82.81%	100
1951	Mitchell & Butler	Nourishing Stout	17	1042.8	1007.4	4.61	82.71%	150
1951	Mitchell & Butler	Nourishing Stout	18	1042.1	1007.3	4.53	82.66%	200
1951	Mitchell & Butler	Extra Stout	21	1048	1009	5.08	81.25%	125
1959	Hewitt Bros.	Oatmeal Stout	20	1042.3	1008.8	4.36	79.20%	300
1953	Mitchell & Butler	Extra Stout	24	1046.2	1009.8	4.74	78.79%	
1954	Mitchell & Butler	Extra Stout	24	1049	1011.2	4.92	77.14%	250
1952	Leicester Brewing & Malting	Milk Stout	29	1044.2	1010.2	4.42	76.92%	285
1952	Marston	Mylki Extra Stout	30	1043.9	1011.2	4.24	74.49%	
1952	Marston	Extra Stout	30	1042.1	1011.4	3.98	72.92%	235
1954	Marston	Mylki Stout	28	1043.1	1012	4.03	72.16%	250
1953	Worthington	XX Stout	24	1040	1012	3.63	70.00%	300
	Average		***24***	***1044.2***	***1009.7***	***4.49***	***78.02%***	***215.5***
Source: Whitbread Gravity book held at the London Metropolitan Archives, document number LMA/4453/D/02/002.								

Micthell & Butler's Stout is pretty highly-attenuated, though it varies quite a lot between the different samples. And quite a bit of variation in colour, too.

The name Mylki Stout implies something containing lactose, making an attenuation rate of over 70% something of a surprise.

Southern Standard Stout >70% attenuation								
Year	Brewer	Beer	Price per pint d	OG	FG	ABV	App. Atten-uation	colour
1953	Stroud Brewery	Cottswold Stout	24	1043.3	1010.4	4.27	75.98%	250
1952	Shrewesbury & Wem	Extra Stout	28	1041	1011.8	3.78	71.22%	330
1959	Hunt Edmunds	Country Stout	24	1043.3	1011.7	4.10	72.98%	225
1953	Starkey, Knight & Ford	Super Stout	28	1045.9	1013.4	4.21	70.81%	275
1954	Flowers	Table Stout		1046.4	1013.6	4.25	70.69%	350
	Average		***26***	***1044.0***	***1012.2***	***4.12***	***72.34%***	***286.0***
Source: Whitbread Gravity book held at the London Metropolitan Archives, document number LMA/4453/D/02/002.								

The attenuation amongst the Southern breweries is on the low side. And there aren't a huge number of them, either. Not sure what that tells us, but I find it interesting.

London Standard Stout >70% attenuation								
Year	**Brewer**	**Beer**	**Price per pint d**	**OG**	**FG**	**ABV**	**App. Atten-uation**	**colour**
1954	Watney	Reids Special Stout	25	1043.3	1008.5	4.53	80.37%	275
1951	Courage	Sturdy Extra Stout	24	1043.6	1008.6	4.55	80.28%	
1951	Watney	Special Stout	24	1045.3	1009.1	4.71	79.91%	200
1950	Watney	Reids Special Stout	24	1045.9	1009.6	4.72	79.08%	175
1950	Watney	Reids Stout	17	1042.9	1009.1	4.39	78.79%	150
1957	Watney	Special Stout	26	1042.3	1009.4	4.28	77.78%	200
1957	Watney	Reids Special Stout	36	1045.2	1011.8	4.33	73.89%	225
1950	Truman	Black Ben Stout	29	1048.8	1014.2	4.49	70.90%	125
1950	Truman	Black Ben Stout	29	1049	1014.3	4.50	70.82%	150
	Average		***26***	***1045.1***	***1010.5***	***4.50***	***76.87%***	***187.5***
Source: Whitbread Gravity book held at the London Metropolitan Archives, document number LMA/4453/D/02/002.								

In London, they were still brewing the type of Stout they always had, with a fairly standard degree of attenuation of around 75%. The only difference was that the gravity was considerably lower. Before WW I, an ordinary Stout would have had an OG of 1070° - 1080°. Between the wars, around 1055°.

The average price of this class of Stout is most regions is much the same: around 26d per pint. I'm surprised at how pale many examples are. I'd expect Stout to start at around 250 on this scale.

Northern Standard Stouts 65-70% attenuation								
Year	**Brewer**	**Beer**	**Price per pint d**	**OG**	**FG**	**ABV**	**App. Atten-uation**	**colour**
1954	Cornbrook Brewery	Barley Stout (Lactose present)	26	1047.2	1016.5	3.97	65.04%	300
1952	Duttons	Mercers Stout	26	1045.3	1014.1	4.04	68.87%	400
1959	Greenall Whitley	Sterling Stout	28	1046.8	1015.1	4.10	67.74%	225
1951	Groves & Whitnall	Red Rose Stout	28	1047.5	1014.6	4.26	69.26%	
1954	Groves & Whitnall	Red Rose Stout (Lactose present)	26	1048.8	1016.9	4.13	65.37%	300
1950	Hancocks	Export Stout	28	1044.4	1013.4	4.02	69.82%	340
1954	Hancocks	M Stout (Lactose present)	24	1043	1014.5	3.69	66.28%	350
1952	Hope & Anchor	Jubilee Stout	28	1041.7	1014	3.58	66.43%	175
1950	Hydes	Special Stout	40	1045.5	1014.2	4.05	68.79%	125
1959	Hydes	Special Anvil Stout	25	1041.4	1013.7	3.58	66.91%	200
1953	Mercers	Stout	26	1045.7	1013.8	4.13	69.80%	425
1959	Sam Smith	Taddy Stout	28	1047.1	1015.1	4.14	67.94%	225
1957	Samuel Smith	Sams Extra Stout (lactose absent)	28	1049.8	1016.6	4.30	66.67%	225
1953	Stones	Samson Stout	25	1046.6	1015	4.09	67.81%	375
1959	Stones	Samson Stout	26	1045.7	1014.2	4.08	68.93%	450

Northern Standard Stouts 65-70% attenuation								
Year	Brewer	Beer	Price per pint d	OG	FG	ABV	App. Atten-uation	colour
1959	Thwaites	Cream Stout	26	1044.3	1014.3	3.88	67.72%	225
1954	Vaux & Co	Sweet Strong Stout	28	1047.6	1016.4	4.03	65.55%	375
1952	Wilsons	Wembley Stout	23	1044.3	1014.5	3.86	67.27%	250
1959	Workington	John Peel Stout	26	1040.9	1013.7	3.52	66.50%	300
	Average		***27.1***	***1045.5***	***1014.8***	***3.97***	***67.51%***	***292.5***
Source: Whitbread Gravity book held at the London Metropolitan Archives, document number LMA/4453/D/02/002.								

I just spotted something odd: a lot of the FG's are very similar. Most are between 1014° and 1015.9°. Looks like customers expected a certain amount of body in their Stout.

It's surprising that in these reasonably-attenuated set that there should be at least three Stouts containing lactose. Though there could have been more as the Whitbread Gravity Book didn't always record its presence.

Southern Standard Stouts 65-70% attenuation								
Year	Brewer	Beer	Price per pint d	OG	FG	ABV	App. Atten-uation	colour
1953	Brickwoods	Black Bricky	33	1045.7	1015.1	3.96	66.96%	200
1956	East Anglian Breweries	Ely Silk Stout	28	1046.2	1015.4	3.98	66.67%	275
1952	Flowers	Stout	22	1044.1	1014.2	3.87	67.80%	300
1959	Flowers	Sable Stout	30	1044.3	1015	3.79	66.14%	250
1954	Hall & woodhouse	Glucose Stout	24	1042.7	1014.7	3.62	65.57%	375
1953	Plymouth Breweries	Oatmeal Stout	25	1047.9	1015.4	4.21	67.85%	275
1954	Tollemache	Beano Stout	19	1041	1012.6	3.68	69.27%	350
	Average		***25.9***	***1044.6***	***1014.6***	***3.87***	***67.18%***	***289.3***
Source: Whitbread Gravity book held at the London Metropolitan Archives, document number LMA/4453/D/02/002.								

The Southern examples also all have very similar FGs. I doubt that it's coincidental.

Midlands Standard Stouts 65-70% attenuation								
Year	**Brewer**	**Beer**	**Price per pint d**	**OG**	**FG**	**ABV**	**App. Atten-uation**	**colour**
1954	Ansell	New Best Stout	28	1049.7	1015.7	4.40	68.41%	125
1959	Ansell	Newcrest Stout	28	1046	1014	4.15	69.57%	190
1952	Atkinsons	Semi Sweet Stout	24	1046	1016.1	3.87	65.00%	300
1959	Bents	Red Label Stout	24	1048.3	1014.5	4.38	69.98%	250
1954	Chesham & Brackley	Raven Stout	30	1047.5	1015.8	4.10	66.74%	475
1959	Hanson, Julia	Special Stout	30	1044.9	1015.1	3.85	66.37%	225
1959	Marston	Mello Sweet Stout	30	1040.3	1013.6	3.45	66.25%	325
	Average		***27.7***	***1046.1***	***1015.0***	***4.03***	***67.47%***	***270.0***
Source: Whitbread Gravity book held at the London Metropolitan Archives, document number LMA/4453/D/02/002.								

Despite not really being in tooth-rotting country yet, many of the beers in this category have the words "sweet" of "glucose" in their name. Looks to me like sweetness was becoming a selling point for Stout. Quite a change from its 18th-century classification as a beer and hence heavily hopped.

London Standard Stouts 65-70% attenuation								
Year	**Brewer**	**Beer**	**Price per pint d**	**OG**	**FG**	**ABV**	**App. Atten-uation**	**colour**
1950	Hammerton	Oatmeal Stout	21	1040.7	1013.7	3.49	66.34%	315
1951	Hammerton	Oatmeal Stout	23	1047.1	1014.3	4.25	69.64%	375
1954	Meux	Special Stout (no lactose)	31.5	1040.2	1012.7	3.56	68.41%	300
1951	Truman	Black Ben Stout	29	1047.6	1014.9	4.23	68.70%	125
1953	Truman	Best Stout (Lactose present)	24	1044.4	1015.2	3.78	65.77%	100
1957	Whitbread	Mackeson Stout	32	1046.3	1015.9	3.93	65.66%	250
	Average		***26.8***	***1044.4***	***1014.5***	***3.87***	***67.42%***	***244.2***
Source: Whitbread Gravity book held at the London Metropolitan Archives, document number LMA/4453/D/02/002.								

The two Truman's Stouts are shockingly pale. Which drags the average for London Stouts right down.

Scottish Standard Stouts 65-70% attenuation								
Year	**Brewer**	**Beer**	**Price per pint d**	**OG**	**FG**	**ABV**	**App. Atten-uation**	**colour**
1950	Bernard	Export Stout	26	1045.5	1014.1	4.07	69.01%	150
1959	Bernard	Export Stout	26	1046.2	1015.8	3.93	65.80%	275
1950	McEwan	Imperial Stout	27	1043	1014.4	3.70	66.51%	
1954	Steel Coulson	Elephant Sweet Stout	29	1041.7	1014.1	3.57	66.19%	350
	Average		***27.0***	***1044.1***	***1014.6***	***3.82***	***66.88%***	***258.3***

Source:
Whitbread Gravity book held at the London Metropolitan Archives, document number LMA/4453/D/02/002.

How exactly is Mc Ewan's Stout Imperial at just 3.7% ABV? That's a Table Beer by 19th-century standards.

Of the beers in this category, Mackeson and Sam Smiths Extra Stout are the only two that still exist. Not such a shock as only Hydes, Sam Smiths and Thwaites are still around.

London Standard Stouts 60-65% attenuation								
Year	**Brewer**	**Beer**	**Price per pint d**	**OG**	**FG**	**ABV**	**App. Atten-uation**	**colour**
1954	Charrington	Punch Stout	30	1047.5	1017.3	3.90	63.58%	330
1952	Hammerton	Oatmeal Stout	29	1047.2	1017	3.90	63.98%	340
1959	Taylor Walker	Cannon Stout	29	1045.8	1018.1	3.57	60.48%	425
1951	Truman	Best Stout	22	1040.9	1015.3	3.31	62.59%	300
1959	Whitbread	Mackeson Stout	32	1046	1017.8	3.64	61.30%	400
	Average		***28.4***	***1045.5***	***1017.1***	***3.66***	***62.39%***	***359.0***

Source:
Whitbread Gravity book held at the London Metropolitan Archives, document number LMA/4453/D/02/002.

As we gradually move our way down the attenuation scale, you'll see the FGs rise and ABVs fall. Which is only logical. Though we've still got a way to go down that particular road.

Northern Standard Stouts 60-65% attenuation								
Year	**Brewer**	**Beer**	**Price per pint d**	**OG**	**FG**	**ABV**	**App. Atten-uation**	**colour**
1951	Birkenhead	BB Stout	26	1046.6	1017.1	3.81	63.30%	
1957	Boddingtons	Extra Stout (lactose absent)	28	1043.9	1015.6	3.66	64.46%	250
1953	Camerons	Sovereign Stout	28	1047.3	1018.6	3.70	60.68%	275
1950	Castletown	Manx Oyster Stout	26	1043.7	1015.4	3.66	64.76%	315
1951	Greenalls	Oatmeal Stout	21	1042.7	1016.1	3.43	62.30%	
1952	Groves & Whitnall	Red Rose Stout	26	1047.9	1017.9	3.87	62.63%	200
1959	Groves & Whitnall	Red Roses Stout	25	1047.5	1018.7	3.72	60.63%	250
1952	Hope & Anchor	Jubilee Stout	28	1040.5	1014.9	3.31	63.21%	215
1959	Nimmo	Nimmo's Stout	28	1048.2	1017.4	3.98	63.90%	300
1953	Samuel Smith	Sams Stout	22	1043.9	1015.7	3.64	64.24%	175
1959	Vaux	Red Label Stout	28	1043.9	1015.5	3.67	64.69%	300
1954	Whitworth Son & Nephew	Sweet Stout	28	1044.7	1017.6	3.50	60.63%	375
1954	Wilsons	Wembly Extra Stout	26	1044.3	1017.4	3.47	60.72%	325
	Average		***26.2***	***1045.0***	***1016.8***	***3.65***	***62.78%***	***270.9***
Source: Whitbread Gravity book held at the London Metropolitan Archives, document number LMA/4453/D/02/002.								

There's a considerable variation in price, not always that directly related to strength. The cheapest, Greenall's Oatmeal Stout was just 21d – 8.75p in modern money – while the dearest, Mackeson cost 32d (13.33p). That's almost 50% more, despite there being little difference in ABV. As national, heavily-advertised brand, it shouldn't be a surprise that Mackeson demanded a premium price. The same seems to be true to a lesser extent of Charrington's Punch Stout.

Southern Standard Stouts 60-65% attenuation								
Year	**Brewer**	**Beer**	**Price per pint d**	**OG**	**FG**	**ABV**	**App. Atten-uation**	**colour**
1955	Devenish	Double Weymouth Sweet Stout	28	1042.8	1015.6	3.51	63.55%	400
1959	Flowers	Table Stout	30	1043.3	1016	3.53	63.05%	250
1953	Georges	Glucose Stout	28	1045.5	1017.6	3.60	61.32%	175
1953	Hunt Edmunds	Country Stout	26	1043.8	1015.4	3.67	64.84%	275
1954	Plymouth Breweries	Brown Imperial Stout	25	1048.6	1018.5	3.89	61.93%	375
1954	Plymouth Breweries	Oatmeal Stout	25	1048.7	1019.2	3.81	60.57%	400
1953	Young & Son	Victory Oyster Stout	26	1046.5	1016.4	3.89	64.73%	315
	Average		***26.9***	***1045.6***	***1017.0***	***3.70***	***62.86%***	***312.9***
Source: Whitbread Gravity book held at the London Metropolitan Archives, document number LMA/4453/D/02/002.								

There's a very good spread of beer from every corner of the UK. In this particular set there are ones from the West Country (Devenish, Plymouth, Georges, Young), Oxfordshire (Hunt Edmunds) and Luton (Flowers).

Midlands Standard Stouts 60-65% attenuation

Year	Brewer	Beer	Price per pint d	OG	FG	ABV	App. Atten-uation	colour
1952	Atkinsons	Punch Stout	24	1045.3	1017.3	3.61	61.81%	175
1954	Bent's	Red Label Stout	26	1049.2	1017.8	4.06	63.82%	300
1959	Butler, Wm	Black Satin Sweet Stout	29	1042.2	1016.6	3.30	60.66%	300
1953	Davenport	Celebration Stout	22	1041.9	1014.7	3.52	64.92%	315
1953	Hole	Castle Stout	24	1041	1015	3.36	63.41%	315
1953	Joule	Royal Stout	28	1046.3	1018.2	3.63	60.69%	300
1959	Joule	Royal Stout	28	1047.1	1018	3.76	61.78%	250
1959	Wrekin	MS Stout	28	1042.3	1016.2	3.37	61.70%	250
	Average		***26.1***	***1044.4***	***1016.7***	***3.58***	***62.35%***	***275.6***

Source:
Whitbread Gravity book held at the London Metropolitan Archives, document number LMA/4453/D/02/002.

The average prices of each set are remarkably close to each other, around 26d. Except for London, which the average was 28d.

Scottish Standard Stouts 60-65% attenuation

Year	Brewer	Beer	Price per pint d	OG	FG	ABV	App. Atten-uation	colour
1954	Calder	Scotch Stout	28	1040.9	1015.9	3.23	61.12%	250
1956	Deuchar R	Edinburgh Sweet Stout	30	1042.9	1016.8	3.37	60.84%	300
	Average		***29.0***	***1041.9***	***1016.4***	***3.30***	***60.98%***	***275.0***

Source:
Whitbread Gravity book held at the London Metropolitan Archives, document number LMA/4453/D/02/002.

Only two Scottish examples both have attenuation close to the bottom end of this category.

There are an awful lot of analyses of Stout in the Whitbread Gravity Book. Especially Sweet and Milk Stout. These were rivals to their own Mackeson brand, a beer which was incredibly important for the company in the 1950's.

Of the beers in this category, just 5 examples have the word "sweet" or "glucose" in their name. Almost as many, 4, are Oatmeal Stouts. More surprisingly, there are two Oyster Stouts. How modern.

London Standard Stouts 50-60% attenuation								
Year	**Brewer**	**Beer**	**Price per pint d**	**OG**	**FG**	**ABV**	**App. Atten-uation**	**colour**
1957	Barclay Perkins	Stout	30	1042.5	1020	2.89	52.94%	300
1953	Beasley	Arsenal Extra Stout	28	1049.2	1022	3.50	55.28%	400
1954	Courage	Hodgsons Stout	28	1044	1019.1	3.21	56.59%	350
1957	Hammerton	Oatmeal Stout	30	1047.1	1021.6	3.28	54.14%	350
1957	Harman's	Ship Stout	24	1049.8	1022.8	3.47	54.22%	375
1950	Mann Crossman	Cream Label Stout	26	1043.7	1021.8	2.81	50.11%	330
1952	Taylor Walker	Cannon Stout	30	1046.7	1019.4	3.52	58.46%	375
1957	Taylor Walker	Cannon Stout	32	1043.5	1018.8	3.18	56.78%	350
1950	Truman	Best Stout	22	1041.3	1017.2	3.11	58.35%	200
1956	Truman	Malt Stout (Lactose present)	29	1045	1021.2	3.06	52.89%	225
1954	Wenlock	Special Stout	28	1047.2	1022.8	3.14	51.69%	300
1959	Whitbread	Mackeson Stout	32	1046.2	1020.8	3.27	54.98%	250
	Average		***28.6***	***1044.6***	***1020.2***	***3.15***	***54.94%***	***265.0***
Source: Whitbread Gravity book held at the London Metropolitan Archives, document number LMA/4453/D/02/002.								

You'll notice that some of the same London Stouts have occurred in earlier tables. That's because the FG and hence rate of attenuation was all over the shop in some beers, for example Mackeson. Talking of Mackeson, I've lumped it with London beers, but it was brewed in multiple locations, pretty much in every brewery Whitbread owned. Though this particular beer I do know was brewed at Chiswell Street.

Midlands Standard Stouts 50-60% attenuation								
Year	**Brewer**	**Beer**	**Price per pint d**	**OG**	**FG**	**ABV**	**App. Atten-uation**	**colour**
1952	Hardys	Blackamoor Sweet Stout	26	1045.6	1021.7	3.07	52.41%	475
1959	Hardys	Blackamoor Sweet Stout	32	1044	1021.2	2.93	51.82%	450
1955	Phipps	Velvet Stout	32	1045	1018.2	3.46	59.56%	475
1959	Phipps	Velvet Stout	32	1049.2	1023.1	3.36	53.05%	475
1959	Shipstone	Ship Sweet Stout	30	1044.8	1018.6	3.38	58.48%	275
1955	Thornley	Special Glucose Stout	28	1040.6	1018.7	2.82	53.94%	375
	Average		***30.0***	***1044.9***	***1020.3***	***3.17***	***54.88%***	***420.8***
Source: Whitbread Gravity book held at the London Metropolitan Archives, document number LMA/4453/D/02/002.								

The Hardy and Shipstone Stout look very similar. Which should be a shock as they were both brewed for the same market: Nottingham. Given their modest level of alcohol, these beers are poor value for money. A Brown Ale of a similar ABV would have cost about 10d less.

Northern Standard Stouts 50-60% attenuation								
Year	**Brewer**	**Beer**	**Price per pint d**	**OG**	**FG**	**ABV**	**App. Atten-uation**	**colour**
1959	Birkenhead	B.B. Stout	25	1047	1022.3	3.18	52.55%	400
1959	Carlisle State	Sweet Stout	22	1046.6	1022.5	3.10	51.72%	425
1957	Greenall Whitley	Wilderspool Stout	30	1049.7	1021.3	3.55	57.14%	275
1956	Hey	White Rose Stout (no lactose)	31	1047.2	1019.9	3.52	57.84%	425
1952	Hope & Anchor	Jubilee Stout	28	1040.7	1017.1	3.04	57.99%	125
1957	Hope & Anchor	Jubilee Stout (lactose present)	30	1040.4	1016.3	3.11	59.65%	225
1959	John Smith	Magnet Stout	24	1047.9	1021.2	3.44	55.74%	250
1959	Northern Club Federation	F.B. Sweet Stout	26	1048.1	1021.9	3.37	54.47%	500
1957	Robinsons	Black Unicorn Stout (lactose present)	28	1043.2	1017.7	3.29	59.03%	250
1954	Russells	Imperial Stout	24	1041.6	1016.8	3.20	59.62%	175
1956	Webster	Velvet Stout	28	1045.1	1022.3	2.93	50.55%	425
1959	Webster	Velvet Stout	26	1040.1	1019.8	2.61	50.62%	300
1959	Whitakers	Special Standard Stout	24	1043.1	1019.7	3.01	54.29%	400
1959	Wilsons	Extra Stout	26	1045.4	1020.4	3.22	55.07%	250
	Average		***26.6***	***1044.7***	***1019.9***	***3.18***	***55.45%***	***316.1***
Source: Whitbread Gravity book held at the London Metropolitan Archives, document number LMA/4453/D/02/002.								

There are rather fewer examples in this set. Implying that they liked their Stouts more attenuated in the North.

Southern Standard Stouts 50-60% attenuation								
Year	**Brewer**	**Beer**	**Price per pint d**	**OG**	**FG**	**ABV**	**App. Atten-uation**	**colour**
1954	Adnams	Black Velvet Sweet Stout (no lactose)	28	1043.7	1020.9	2.93	52.17%	675
1959	Eldridge Pope	Sweet Double Stout	28	1044.2	1020.2	3.09	54.30%	250
1959	Georges	Glucose Stout	28	1045	1018.7	3.39	58.44%	225
1954	Greene King	Sweet Stout	26	1046.6	1020.3	3.39	56.44%	450
1954	Lamb Brewery	Double Stout	28	1047.2	1022.8	3.14	51.69%	300
1955	Rayments	Town Stout (no lactose)	22	1040.2	1019.9	2.61	50.50%	225
1953	Simonds	Velvet Stout	26	1046.2	1022.5	3.05	51.30%	225
1959	Simonds	Velvet Stout	32	1047.9	1022	3.33	54.07%	275
1953	Star Brewery	Double Stout	23	1045.3	1019.8	3.28	56.29%	400
1959	Starkey, Knight & Ford	Super Stout	28	1043	1018.2	3.20	57.67%	350
1952	Tollemache	Double Stout	23	1043	1019.3	3.05	55.12%	315
1953	Wadworth	Special Double Stout	26	1043.6	1020	3.04	54.13%	315
	Average		***26.5***	***1044.7***	***1020.4***	***3.12***	***54.34%***	***333.8***
Source: Whitbread Gravity book held at the London Metropolitan Archives, document number LMA/4453/D/02/002.								

There seem to be quite a few beers called Velvet Stout. I'm surprised no-one trademarked the name. As, unlike Milk Stout, it doesn't really refer to any specific characteristic of the beer.

Scottish Standard Stouts 50-60% attenuation								
Year	**Brewer**	**Beer**	**Price per pint d**	**OG**	**FG**	**ABV**	**App. Atten-uation**	**colour**
1955	Aitken	Stout	30	1040.3	1019.5	2.67	51.61%	325
1959	Deuchar, R	Edinburgh Sweet Stout	28	1043.5	1019.7	3.06	54.71%	275
1954	Younger, Wm.	Capital Stout (Lactose present)	32	1046.5	1019.7	3.45	57.63%	250
1959	Younger, Wm.	Capital Stout	30	1043.7	1021.6	2.84	50.57%	376
	Average		***30.0***	***1043.5***	***1020.1***	***3.01***	***53.63%***	***306.5***
Source: Whitbread Gravity book held at the London Metropolitan Archives, document number LMA/4453/D/02/002.								

As we get to the lower end of the attenuation scale we'll be seeing more and more Scottish examples. They really liked their Stout sweet North of the border.

Standard Stouts < 50% attenuation								
Year	**Brewer**	**Beer**	**Price per pint d**	**OG**	**FG**	**ABV**	**App. Atten-uation**	**colour**
1954	Simonds	Velvet Stout	29	1047.5	1023.8	3.04	49.89%	350
1956	Thornley	Gluco Stout	28	1042.3	1021.2	2.71	49.88%	400
1959	Calders	Scotch Stout	28	1042.2	1021.5	2.66	49.05%	300
1954	Aitken	A Stout	28	1041.4	1021.2	2.59	48.79%	375
1957	Courage	Hodgsons Stout	30	1043.3	1022.2	2.71	48.73%	325
1956	Tennant Bros.	Glucose Stout	26	1040.4	1021	2.49	48.02%	225
1951	Mann Crossman	Cream Label Stout	24	1045.2	1023.5	2.78	48.01%	310
1955	Rayment	????? Stout	22	1040	1020.8	2.47	48.00%	275
1959	Hall & Woodhouse	Glucose Stout	28	1041	1021.5	2.50	47.56%	190
1952	Warwick & Richardson	Milk Maid Stout	28	1040.7	1021.7	2.44	46.68%	200
1953	Warwick & Richardson	Milk Maid Stout	28	1040.5	1022.2	2.35	45.19%	225
1959	Everards	Meadows Sweet Extra Stout	28	1041	1022.8	2.33	44.39%	325
1955	Brutton, Mitchell, Toms Ltd.	Ruby Stout (lactose present)	26	1040.9	1023.6	2.22	42.30%	475
1959	JW Lees	Archer Stout	28	1041.5	1024.1	2.23	41.93%	325
	Average		***27.2***	***1042.0***	***1022.2***	***2.54***	***47.03%***	***307.1***
Source: Whitbread Gravity book held at the London Metropolitan Archives, document number LMA/4453/D/02/002.								

The final set in this category is barley fermented at all. And pretty weak. Only one is above 3% ABV.

Glucose Stout was another popular name. Though it did at least refer to something specific: an addition of glucose. This must have been done at the end of fermentation and the beer pasteurised. There would be no other way of preventing the glucose from simply being consumed by the yeast.

Strong Stout

I'm calling anything over 1050° strong Stout. Before the war ordinary Stout – stuff like draught London Stout and Guinness Extra Stout – would have fallen into this category. After the war, only special Stouts were as strong as this. It's sobering to think that Guinness Extra Stout was the same strength as Foreign Extra Stout until 1916.

Barclay Perkins continued to brew the most old-fashioned sort of strong Stout. Their Russian Stout, though brewed in weaker form during the 1940s, returned to full strength in the 1950s, also retaining its Brettanomyces secondary fermentation. It wasn't the only really strong Stout, but they were becoming quite rare.

Strong Stouts >65% attenuation

Year	Brewer	Beer	Price per pint d	OG	FG	ABV	App. Atten-uation	colour
1953	Barclay Perkins	Russian Stout	45	1101	1018	10.97	82.18%	500
1950	Barclay Perkins	Russian Stout	45	1100.1	1021.1	10.41	78.92%	350
1955	Bass	Imperial Stout		1078.8	1018.4	7.90	76.65%	375
1955	Worthington	Imperial Stout		1078.2	1017.3	7.97	77.88%	325
1953	Bass	Imperial Stout	45	1078.2	1025.1	6.90	67.90%	375
1953	Samuel Smith	Sam's Extra Stout	28	1077.8	1020	7.54	74.29%	225
1958	Guinness	Foreign Extra Stout		1074.4	1015.9	7.65	78.63%	250
1950	Watney	Reids Stout		1072.9	1021	6.75	71.19%	265
1955	Watney	Reids Stout		1072.1	1018	7.06	75.03%	325
1955	Guinness	Export Stout		1071.4	1013.3	7.61	81.37%	175
1950	Unknown	Imperial Stout		1066.8	1017	6.49	74.55%	350
1955	Murray	Export Stout	45	1064.6	1015.8	6.36	75.54%	350
1953	Castletown	Manx Maid Stout	45	1064.1	1022.3	5.41	65.21%	320
1950	Tennent	Milk Stout (Export)		1063.2	1020	5.60	68.35%	340
1955	Castletown	Manx Oyster Stout		1063	1013	6.53	79.37%	250
1955	Hope & Anchor	Royal Jubilee Stout		1059.5	1019.9	5.13	66.55%	325
1953	Brickwoods	Black Bricky	36	1054.8	1015.5	5.10	71.72%	175
1953	Young & Co	No. 1 Stout	33	1052.1	1016.3	4.64	68.71%	1400
1956	Hammonds	Senior Sovereign Sweet Stout	31	1050.4	1016.2	4.43	67.86%	300
	Average		***39.2***	***1070.7***	***1018.1***	***6.87***	***73.79%***	***367.1***

Source:
Whitbread Gravity book held at the London Metropolitan Archives, document number LMA/4453/D/02/002.

The biggest surprise is how many strong Stouts were still knocking around after WW II. There are six different brands with gravities over 1070. Kicking off with the granddaddy of them all, Barclay's Russian Stout. Which had returned to its classic 1100 OG. In the early 1950's it's the only beer I can think of which still retained its 19th-century strength. Hang on.

That 1958 Guinness FES is another.

The Bass and Worthington examples are obviously the same beer: P2. Just as Bass Red Triangle and Worthington White Shield were the same beer. I'm not sure why they insisted on keeping both brands long after the beers had become the same. Something similar was going on at Watney, where they were still branding Stouts as Reid half a century after the brewery closed.

Royal Jubilee Stout played a key role in the merger mania of the 1950's. Hope & Anchor of Sheffield wanted to sell it in Canada and struck a deal whereby they brewed Canadian Black Label Lager under licence in return. This drew the UK market to the attention of Eddie Taylor, owner of the Black Label brand. He'd been successful in merging brewing operations in Canada and saw an opportunity to do the same in Britain. The structure of the industry was transformed in a decade.

Most of the stronger examples in the table have pretty decent attenuation. In the case of Russian Stout, you could say by cheating. With a secondary Brettanomyces fermentation measured in years, it was always going to be a dry beer. The same is probably true of Guinness FES, which I still believe was at least partially aged in vats in the 1950s.

I'm struck by how good value Russian Stout was. It's the same price – 45d per pint – as the Bass, Murray and Castletown Stouts all of which are much weaker. Given that Russian Stout took more than two years from mash tun to glass, that's impressive.

It's surprise to find a Milk Stout and a Sweet Stout in a set with more than 65% attenuation. The names allocated to Stouts in the 1950's do show a trend towards sweetness. Things like Glucose Stout or – a real favourite this one – Nourishing Stout.

One last point. None of these even vaguely resembles the very sweet, low ABV beers British Stouts were supposed to have become around 1900, if you'd believe some beer historians.

Strong Stouts <65% attenuation

Year	Brewer	Beer	Price per pint d	OG	FG	ABV	App. Atten-uation	colour
1953	Simonds	Archangel Stout	49.5	1084.6	1041.2	5.57	51.30%	150
1956	Bass	Imperial Stout	54	1077.5	1027.9	6.43	64.00%	350
1950	Calder Alloa	Milk Stout		1069.3	1029.7	5.10	57.14%	250
1958	Hope Brewery	Export Vitamin Stout	45	1066.2	1024.2	5.25	63.44%	300
1956	Steward & Patteson	Stout	45	1064.6	1027.4	4.79	57.59%	350
1953	Steward & Patteson	Double Stout	42	1063.8	1031.4	4.16	50.78%	650
1955	Truman	Stout		1062	1022	5.18	64.52%	225
1957	Tennent	Stout		1059.4	1020.8	4.99	64.98%	300
1953	Bellhaven	Heavy Stout	45	1059	1029.6	3.77	49.83%	300
1956	Whitbread	EMS		1056.7	1020.3	4.71	64.20%	325
1956	Atkinsons	Double Punch Stout	46.5	1051.8	1018.9	4.25	63.51%	500
	Average		***46.7***	***1065.0***	***1026.7***	***4.93***	***59.21%***	***336.4***

Source:
Whitbread Gravity book held at the London Metropolitan Archives, document number LMA/4453/D/02/002.

More than half of the examples are only just below my arbitrary ceiling for this group. One, Bass Imperial Stout, also appears in the other table. Of the five examples with attenuation below 60%, it's significant that two are Scottish. Scottish Stout genuinely seems to have gone mostly sweet quite early. From what I've seen in brewing records the trend started in the 19th century.

Archangel Stout must have been an interesting drink. With an FG of over 1040° - that's higher than the OG of many Stouts – it must have been quite treacly. Which is just how an Arctic Ale is supposed to be.

Would you be allowed to call a beer Export Vitamin Stout today? I doubt it. They probably wouldn't even let Nourishing or Invalid Stout pass, the miserable bastards.

Notice how few beers there are in this group. You could argue there are only really five. Which is all there would be left if I shifted the boundary from 65% to 63% attenuation.

Stout Grists

Stout was the one style where it was common to have multiple coloured malts. Though, as we'll see later, that wasn't always the case.

I'm grouping the breweries geographically, starting with the North.

Northern Stout grists 1951 - 1966: malts

Year	Brewer	Beer	OG	pale malt	brown malt	black malt	amber malt	choc. Malt	crystal malt
1951	Boddington	Stout	1040	42.23%		4.49%	30.16%		15.08%
1966	Boddington	Stout	1038.5	45.70%		4.53%	24.37%		12.19%
1952	Lees	Stout	1038	51.22%	3.66%	3.66%		7.32%	7.32%
1958	Lees	Archer	1036	36.92%	13.85%	9.23%			
1963	Lees	Archer	1036	39.34%	14.75%	9.84%			
1956	Tennant	Glucose Stout	1040	58.27%		3.94%	7.87%		4.72%

Sources:
Boddington brewing record held at Manchester Central Library, document number M693/405/130.
Boddington brewing record held at Manchester Central Library, document number M693/405/133.
Lees brewing records held at the brewery.
Tennant brewing record held at Sheffield City Archive, document number MD7518/38/34.

Every beer contains at least two coloured grains. Though the only one common to every example is black malt. No big surprise there. Enzymic malt is totally absent. Surely with so many dark grains extra enzymes would be more needed than for other beers.

Northern Stout grists 1951 - 1966: adjuncts					
Year	Brewer	Beer	OG	wheat	oats
1951	Boddington	Stout	1040		
1966	Boddington	Stout	1038.5	3.05%	
1952	Lees	Stout	1038		7.32%
1958	Lees	Archer	1036		4.62%
1963	Lees	Archer	1036		4.92%
1956	Tennant	Glucose Stout	1040		

There aren't a huge amount of adjuncts, just oats in the Lees Stouts and wheat in Boddingtons.

Northern Stout grists 1951 - 1966: sugars									
Year	Brewer	Beer	no. 2 sugar	black invert	cara-mel	glu-cose	lac-tose	malt extract	other sugar
1951	Boddington	Stout			4.02%				4.02%
1966	Boddington	Stout			4.06%			2.03%	4.06%
1952	Lees	Stout			9.76%				9.76%
1958	Lees	Archer		6.15%	4.62%		12.31%		12.31%
1963	Lees	Archer		6.56%	4.92%		13.11%		6.56%
1956	Tennant	Glucose Stout	3.15%		11.02%	11.02%			

Not much in the way of invert sugar in this set, but plenty of other sugars. Every example contains caramel of some kind. The glucose was added after primary fermentation to Tennant's Stout, making a massively sweet beer which must have been pasteurised.

Looking South, there are also plenty of different malts in the grists.

Southern Stout grists 1947 - 1965: malts									
Year	**Brewer**	**Beer**	**OG**	**pale malt**	**black malt**	**amber malt**	**choc. Malt**	**crystal malt**	**mild malt**
1948	Adnams	DS	1037			4.96%	4.96%	4.96%	69.40%
1955	Adnams	DS	1036				8.11%	16.22%	64.86%
1965	Adnams	DS	1038				8.11%	16.22%	64.86%
1964	Eldridge Pope	DS	1039.3	54.55%			13.64%	15.34%	
1964	Elgood	Stout	1029.9	47.62%	4.76%				28.57%
1955	Flowers	Stout	1039.8	66.67%	7.41%			3.70%	
1947	Shepherd Neame	SS	1027.1	60.94%	9.38%				
1952	Shepherd Neame	SS	1030.2	87.48%	2.55%				
1956	Shepherd Neame	SS	1026.3	74.07%	11.11%				
1952	Strong	Stout	1036.6	25.42%	7.63%			5.08%	38.14%
1959	Ushers Trowbridge	Watney Dairy Maid Sweet Stout	1034		9.68%				75.27%

Sources:
Adnams brewing record held at the brewery
Elgood brewing record held at the brewery
Ref Shakespeare Birthplace Trust DR227/215 Brewing Record Book No2
Shepherd Neame brewing record held at the brewery
79A01-A3-3-27
1075-275-6 Wiltshire archives at Chippenham

Other than Shepherd Neame and Usher, every brewery employed multiple coloured malts. Mild malt was quite often used as a base in Stout, presumably because you weren't going to notice the character of the pale malt with all those darker grains.

Southern Stout grists 1947 - 1965: adjuncts							
Year	**Brewer**	**Beer**	**OG**	**flaked maize**	**wheat malt**	**flaked barley**	**malted oats**
1948	Adnams	DS	1037			9.91%	
1955	Adnams	DS	1036				
1965	Adnams	DS	1038				
1964	Eldridge Pope	DS	1039.3				3.41%
1964	Elgood	Stout	1029.9				
1955	Flowers	Stout	1039.8		7.41%		
1947	Shepherd Neame	SS	1027.1				9.38%
1952	Shepherd Neame	SS	1030.2				4.60%
1956	Shepherd Neame	SS	1026.3				3.70%
1952	Strong	Stout	1036.6				
1959	Ushers Trowbridge	Watney Dairy Maid Sweet Stout	1034	3.23%			

There a few more adjuncts in this set, but, if you remove the oats for Oat Stouts, there's not much left. Just one example each of flaked barley and flaked maize, and another of wheat malt.

Southern Stout grists 1947 - 1965: sugars								
Year	**Brewer**	**Beer**	**OG**	**no. 3 sugar**	**caramel**	**lactose**	**malt extract**	**other sugar**
1948	Adnams	DS	1037	3.30%	2.51%			
1955	Adnams	DS	1036	5.41%				5.41%
1965	Adnams	DS	1038	5.41%				5.41%
1964	Eldridge Pope	DS	1039.3				3.41%	9.66%
1964	Elgood	Stout	1029.9					19.05%
1955	Flowers	Stout	1039.8			7.41%	2.47%	4.94%
1947	Shepherd Neame	SS	1027.1				3.13%	17.19%
1952	Shepherd Neame	SS	1030.2		1.53%		0.77%	3.07%
1956	Shepherd Neame	SS	1026.3		4.94%		1.23%	4.94%
1952	Strong	Stout	1036.6	5.08%				18.64%
1959	Ushers Trowbridge	Watney Dairy Maid Sweet Stout	1034		6.09%			5.73%

Malt extract is popular in this group. Other than that, it's all a bit scattergun. There's just one example of lactose, which is lightly surprising given the popularity of Milk Stout at the time.

Now it's the turn of the home of Stout, London.

London Stout grists 1947 - 1964: malts											
Year	**Brewer**	**Beer**	**OG**	**pale malt**	**brown malt**	**black malt**	**amber malt**	**choc. Malt**	**crystal malt**	**mild malt**	**SA malt**
1947	Barclay Perkins	IBS	1043.5		7.99%		7.99%		7.10%	12.43%	24.85
1947	Barclay Perkins	BS	1040.4		10.71%		6.25%		6.25%	8.93%	28.57
1947	Barclay Perkins	LS	1030.5		10.41%		6.62%		6.62%	17.98%	24.61
1946	Fullers	P	1029.3	58.01%		11.60%					
1958	Fullers	NS	1032.1	53.73%		13.43%			8.96%		
1947	Whitbread	WS	1035.3	9.49%	6.65%			7.59%		60.76%	
1952	Whitbread	WS	1038.3		6.67%			8.57%		78.10%	
1958	Whitbread	WOS	1039.3		7.48%			8.41%		69.16%	
1964	Whitbread	WOS	1037.8		8.72%			8.72%		70.93%	

Sources:
Barclay Perkins brewing record held at the London Metropolitan Archives, document number ACC/2305/01/627.
Fullers brewing records held at the brewery
Whitbread brewing record held at the London Metropolitan Archives, document number, LMA/4453/D/09/130.
Whitbread brewing record held at the London Metropolitan Archives, document number, LMA/4453/D/09/132/
Whitbread brewing record held at the London Metropolitan Archives, document number, LMA/4453/D/09/134.
Whitbread brewing record held at the London Metropolitan Archives, document number, LMA/4453/D/09/138.

It's no shock to find brown malt still in use in London. Brewers there were very loyal to it. Whitbread continued to use it in the Stouts brewed at their Chiswell Street brewery right up until it closed in 1974. On the other hand, there's no black malt in the Barclay Perkins or Whitbread Stout. IBS is Imperial Russian Stout, incidentally. The session strength version.

London Stout grists 1947 - 1964: adjuncts							
Year	Brewer	Beer	OG	malted oats	flaked maize	roast barley	flaked barley
1947	Barclay Perkins	IBS (Scot.)	1043.5			12.43%	
1947	Barclay Perkins	BS	1040.4			12.50%	
1947	Barclay Perkins	LS	1030.5			11.36%	
1946	Fullers	P	1029.3				5.80%
1958	Fullers	NS	1032.1		8.96%		
1947	Whitbread	WS	1035.3	0.95%			
1952	Whitbread	WS	1038.3				
1958	Whitbread	WOS	1039.3	4.67%			
1964	Whitbread	WOS	1037.8	6.10%			

You may have noticed that, despite the fairy tale that roast barley is the defining feature of Stout, Barclay Perkins is the only brewery in any of the sets to have used it.

London Stout grists 1947 - 1964: sugars							
Year	Brewer	Beer	OG	no. 3 sugar	caramel	malt extract	other sugar
1947	Barclay Perkins	IBS (Scot.)	1043.5	22.49%	4.73%		
1947	Barclay Perkins	BS	1040.4	22.62%	4.17%		
1947	Barclay Perkins	LS	1030.5	16.40%	4.73%	1.26%	
1946	Fullers	P	1029.3		5.25%		19.34%
1958	Fullers	NS	1032.1				14.93%
1947	Whitbread	WS	1035.3	10.13%			4.43%
1952	Whitbread	WS	1038.3	3.81%			2.86%
1958	Whitbread	WOS	1039.3	8.10%			2.18%
1964	Whitbread	WOS	1037.8	3.49%			2.03%

No. 3 invert is a popular choice again. Other than at Fullers. The majority of the sugar in their Stouts was something called Special Dark. It was probably something similar to No. 4 invert. Barclay Perkins LS is the only one to include malt extract.

Strong Ales

There was still a diverse range of Strong Ales brewed in the UK. Though some of the Southern Draught Old Ales would scarcely have counted as strong in Continental Europe. Genuinely strong beers – in fact some of the strongest made anywhere in the world – were produced in Britain. Beers like Bass No. 1 or Tennant's Gold Label.

Most really strong beers were only available in bottled form. Finishing off the session with a Barley Wine was a known phenomenon. Hardy Ale's sales suffered badly when Eldridge Pope's pubs were split from the brewery in the 1990s. Surprisingly, a large proportion of Hardy Ale had been consumed in their pubs.

There's no real way of splitting apart Barley Wine and Old Ale, other than going by what the brewer called the beer. There's considerable overlap. Though a beer of below 7% ABV was unlikely to be called a Barley Wine.

Old Ale

After WW II, the term Old Ale rarely referred to a beer that had been aged for any length of time. Mostly, it was just something stronger than usual. And how much stronger that was varied from region to region and brewery to brewery. There was one feature they all had in common: a dark colour.

In the Southeast, Old Ale was effectively a stronger version of Dark Mild. And was often parti-gyled with it.

In the North, it was often something stronger. Old Tom, for example. Or Old Something. Strong, dark beers often had an Old prefix. Often the difference between these stronger types and Barley Wine is blurred.

Bottled Old Ale 1950 - 1965								
Year	**Brewer**	**Beer**	**Price per pint d**	**OG**	**FG**	**ABV**	**App. Atten-uation**	**colour**
1950	Barclay Perkins	No. 1 Southwarke Ale	32	1052.4	1021.1	4.04	59.73%	80
1953	Bentley's Yorkshire Brewery	Old Timothy	45	1075.6	1014.7	7.98	80.56%	100
1953	Bullard	Old Ale	48	1080.5	1026.2	7.06	67.45%	68
1952	Courage	Double Courage	43.5	1068.4	1010.8	7.55	84.21%	150
1953	Duttons	O.B.J.	32	1060.9	1013.7	6.15	77.50%	83
1959	George Gale	Prize Old Ale		1089.3	1006.9	10.95	92.27%	60
1953	Greene King	Suffolk Ale	36	1062.8	1020.7	5.46	67.04%	56
1953	John Smith	Magnet Old Ale	42	1072.5	1022.9	6.44	68.41%	83
1953	JW Green	Dragon's Blood	45	1073.6	1028.1	5.88	61.82%	56
1953	McMullen	Old Time Ale	45	1062.1	1015.1	6.12	75.68%	105
1958	Mitchell & Butler	Amba Pale Old Ale	45	1056.3	1012.4	5.49	77.98%	18
1953	Steward & Patteson	Old Ale	48	1080.3	1011	9.13	86.30%	80
1959	Websters	Old Tom	26	1045.1	1012.5	4.23	72.28%	150
1965	Wrekin	Old Ale	31	1039.8	1012.7	3.39	68.09%	90
1953	Youngs, Crawshay & Youngs	Old John	54	1075.2	1025.3	6.47	66.36%	80
	Average		***40.9***	***1066.3***	***1016.9***	***6.4***	***73.71%***	***83.9***
Sources: Whitbread Gravity book held at the London Metropolitan Archives, document number LMA/4453/D/02/002.								

Old Ale Grists

For this set I've selected only beers which had Old Ale in their name, or that I know were sold as Old Ale. None of these is of the stronger Northern type.

Old Ale grists: malts							
Year	Brewer	Beer	OG	pale malt	mild malt	amber malt	crystal malt
1949	Adnams	XXXX	1051.0		78.94%	5.38%	5.38%
1953	Adnams	XXXX	1053.0		79.02%	6.08%	6.08%
1959	Adnams	XXXX	1046.0		74.82%		13.60%
1964	Eldridge Pope	Strong Old Ale	1051.2	76.49%			5.97%
1964	Eldridge Pope	XXXX	1053.2	71.68%			13.94%
1957	Younger, Robert	Old Edinburgh Ale	1044	77.53%			

Sources:
Adnams brewing records held at the brewery.
Robert Younger brewing record held at the Scottish Brewing Archive, document number RY/6/1/2.
Eldridge Pope brewing records.

Despite its dark colour, not a huge amount of coloured malt shows up in their grists. Which isn't uncommon for British dark beers. There's nothing darker than amber or crystal malt. It's not surprising that Adnams XXXX should have a base of mild malt as it was, effectively, a strong Mild Ale.

Old Ale grists: adjuncts and invert sugar							
Year	Brewer	Beer	OG	flaked maize	wheat flour	no. 3 sugar	invert
1949	Adnams	XXXX	1051.0			9.57%	
1953	Adnams	XXXX	1053.0			8.10%	
1959	Adnams	XXXX	1046.0			4.53%	
1964	Eldridge Pope	Strong Old Ale	1051.2		4.88%		9.40%
1964	Eldridge Pope	XXXX	1053.2		4.65%		
1957	Younger, Robert	Old Edinburgh Ale	1044	13.20%			4.40%

There isn't much in the way of adjuncts, other than flaked maize at Robert Younger and the wheat flour Eldridge Pope seemed to put in all their beers.

No. 3 invert sugar is what you would expect to see in this type of beer and to be one of the main sources of colour. It's quite possible that what was listed simply as invert in the Eldridge Pope and Robert Younger records was also No. 3.

Old Ale grists: sugars							
Year	Brewer	Beer	Hydrol	HX	malt extract	caramel	other sugar
1949	Adnams	XXXX				0.73%	
1953	Adnams	XXXX				0.72%	
1959	Adnams	XXXX	4.53%	1.26%			1.26%
1964	Eldridge Pope	Strong Old Ale			3.25%		
1964	Eldridge Pope	XXXX		2.65%	3.54%		3.54%
1957	Younger, Robert	Old Edinburgh Ale	3.30%		1.10%	0.47%	

Caramel was another source of colour in some of the beers. While malt extract also pops up in a few. Plus the inevitable other weird sugars like Hydrol and HX.

Burton Ale

In London Burton Ale remained a standard draught beer. Though after the mid-1950's it increasingly became a winter seasonal. There were also stronger versions that the standard KK. These were mostly sold in bottles, but sometimes appeared on draught.

Before WW I draught Burton Ale, or KK as it was often known, was a very powerful dark beer with an OG of 1070°-1075°. The war knocked the stuffing out of Burton and in the 1920s and 1930s it had a gravity of around 1055°. The next war lopped off another ten gravity points or so.

Draught Burton Ale 1948 - 1954

Year	Brewer	Beer	Price per pint d	OG	FG	ABV	App. Atten-uation	colour
1951	Barclay Perkins	Strong Ale	27	1079	1011	8.96	86.08%	120
1951	Barclay Perkins	Burton	21	1043	1010.5	4.22	75.58%	100
1954	Barclay Perkins	KK	21	1043	1011.1	4.14	74.19%	120
1953	Charrington	Strong Ale	19	1039.9				144
1954	Charrington	KK	19	1048.1	1010.7	4.86	77.75%	130
1951	Charrington	Burton	20	1046.3	1012.1	4.44	73.87%	180
1948	Courage	Burton	21	1044.5	1008.5	4.69	80.90%	140
1951	Courage	XXX	20	1048.1	1015.5	4.22	67.78%	
1954	Courage	XXX	20	1046.2	1013.8	4.20	70.13%	200
1951	Ind Coope	Double Burton	24	1054.3	1013.9	5.25	74.40%	110
1953	Ind Coope	Strong Ale	19	1043.0				112
1951	Mann Crossman	Burton	19	1041.5	1007.6	4.41	81.69%	145
1948	Meux	Burton	20	1041	1006.4	4.51	84.39%	245
1951	Meux	XXX	20	1046.2	1013.1	4.29	71.65%	
1953	Meux	Strong Ale	20	1045.8				152
1951	Taylor Walker	Burton	21	1050	1014.3	4.63	71.40%	120
1954	Taylor Walker	KKK	21	1049.1	1017	4.15	65.38%	110
1951	Truman	Strong Ale	22	1047.7	1010.7	4.81	77.57%	
1953	Truman	Strong Ale	22	1045.6				
1954	Truman	SA	22	1049.1	1009.3	5.19	81.06%	110
1948	Watney	KKKK	21	1046.1	1010.5	4.63	77.22%	115
1954	Watney	KKKK	24	1055.2	1013.5	5.42	75.54%	140
1953	Wenlock	Strong Ale	20	1043.4				176
1949	Whitbread	Strong Ale	20	1046.7				104
1951	Whitbread	KKKK	23	1053.5				
1953	Whitbread	Strong Ale	23	1052.1				104
1954	Whitbread	KKKK	23	1051.2	1011.9	5.11	76.76%	100
	Average		***21.8***	***1049.4***	***1011.9***	***5.11***	***75.96%***	***128***

Sources:
Whitbread Gravity book held at the London Metropolitan Archives, document number LMA/4453/D/02/002.
Truman Gravity Book held at the London Metropolitan Archives, document number B/THB/C/252.

The lack of any analyses in the Whitbread Gravity Book is an indication that Burton was going out of fashion. By the 1960s, only a few London breweries still made a draught version. When Fullers replaced their Burton with ESB and Youngs changed the name of theirs to Winter Warmer the style was, in terms of its name, dead.

I've much less information of bottled versions of Burton Ale.

Bottled Burton Ale 1950 - 1960								
Year	**Brewer**	**Beer**	**Price per pint d**	**OG**	**FG**	**ABV**	**App. Atten-uation**	**colour**
1951	McMullen	Burton	20	1043.9	1011.2	4.24	74.49%	
1950	Watney	Strong Ale	36	1061.1	1014.5	6.07	76.27%	105
1955	Watney	Burton Ale	34	1054.1	1018.5	4.61	65.80%	100
1960	Watney	Burton Ale	32	1053.6	1019.7	4.38	63.25%	125
1951	Wenlock	Burton Ale	20	1045.5	1013.2	4.19	70.99%	
1953	Wenlock	Strong Ale	46.5	1065.9	1017.9	6.24	72.84%	105

Sources:
Whitbread Gravity book held at the London Metropolitan Archives, document number LMA/4453/D/02/002.

I've not bothered with any averages as the beers vary so much in strength.

Burton Ale Grists

I haven't a great number of examples for Burton Ale. Whitbread didn't appear to brew one for many years. Unless it was so infrequently I missed it. The Fullers beeers were parti-gyled with Mild, while the others were brewed single-gyle.

Burton Ale grists 1946 - 1958: malts								
Year	**Brewer**	**Beer**	**OG**	**pale malt**	**SA malt**	**amber malt**	**choc. Malt**	**crystal malt**
1946	Barclay Perkins	KK (bottling)	1047.4	73.47%				5.44%
1946	Barclay Perkins	KK (trade)	1042.5	36.99%	34.68%	4.62%		6.94%
1958	Whitbread	KKKK	1050.5	82.23%			0.90%	
1960	Whitbread	KKKK	1051.8	82.85%			0.87%	
1949	Fullers	BO	1041.5	80.43%				
1958	Fullers	OBE	1049.4	81.06%				

Sources:
Barclay Perkins brewing record held at the London Metropolitan Archives, document number ACC/2305/01/627.
Whitbread brewing records held at the London Metropolitan Archives, document numbers LMA/4453/D/01/126 and LMA/4453/D/01/127.
Fullers brewing records held at the brewery.

Considering that these were dark beers, this not a great deal of coloured malt in the grists. Fuller, typically, only used base malt.

Burton Ale grists 1946 - 1958: adjuncts and sugars								
Year	**Brewer**	**Beer**	**OG**	**flaked maize**	**flaked barley**	**no. 1 sugar**	**no. 2 sugar**	**no. 3 sugar**
1946	Barclay Perkins	KK (bottling)	1047.4		5.44%	14.51%		
1946	Barclay Perkins	KK (trade)	1042.5		4.62%			10.79%
1958	Whitbread	KKKK	1050.5					14.46%
1960	Whitbread	KKKK	1051.8					13.95%
1949	Fullers	BO	1041.5		15.40%		0.57%	
1958	Fullers	OBE	1049.4	9.01%			4.80%	

The No. 1 invert in Barclay Perkins KK (bottling) is a bit strange. In the brewing record a "3" has been crossed out and a "1" written in red. Obviously, it was a last-minute substitution.

Burton Ale grists 1946 - 1958: sugars								
Year	**Brewer**	**Beer**	**OG**	**PEX**	**CDM**	**glucose**	**caramel**	**other sugar**
1946	Barclay Perkins	KK (bottling)	1047.4				1.13%	
1946	Barclay Perkins	KK (trade)	1042.5				1.35%	
1958	Whitbread	KKKK	1050.5					2.41%
1960	Whitbread	KKKK	1051.8					2.33%
1949	Fullers	BO	1041.5	1.14%		0.57%	1.88%	
1958	Fullers	OBE	1049.4	2.40%	2.73%			

CDM stands for caramelised dextro-maltose. It's often found in dark beers. I've no idea what PEX was. Other than that Fullers used a lot of it.

Barley Wine

The term was originally coined by Bass, by at least the 1870s, to describe the strongest of its Burton Ales, No. 1. They weren't the only brewery to make a beer to a similar specification or name.

Barley Wine 1953 to 1959								
Year	**Brewer**	**Beer**	**Price per pint (d)**	**OG**	**FG**	**ABV**	**App. Atten-uation**	**colour (EBC)**
1959	Tamplin	Cheer-i-o No. 1 Barley Wine		1062.6	1016.1	6.05	74.28%	120
1953	Tamplin	Cheerio Barley Wine	36	1063.3	1015.1	6.28	76.15%	105
1953	Scarborough & Whitby	Barley Wine	43.5	1064.3	1024.3	5.17	62.21%	110
1954	Tollemache	Tolly Royal	43	1065.9	1013.7	6.82	79.21%	110
1953	Morgans	Barley Wine	42	1072.3	1024	6.27	66.80%	85
1953	Tollemache	Tolly Royal	48	1073.3	1023.6	6.45	67.80%	110
1953	Cobbold	Barley Wine	37.5	1073.8	1029.5	5.72	60.03%	100

Barley Wine 1953 to 1959								
Year	Brewer	Beer	Price per pint (d)	OG	FG	ABV	App. Atten-uation	colour (EBC)
1953	Everards	Barley Wine	51	1077.1	1017.2	7.84	77.69%	90
1956	Ind Coope	Arctic Barley Wine	54	1077.1	1019.7	7.49	74.45%	105
1959	Hall & Woodhouse	Stingo Barley Wine		1077.3	1010.4	8.81	86.55%	45
1954	Georges	Barley Wine	40	1078.2	1026	6.78	66.75%	95
1953	Tetley	Imperial Barley Wine	54	1078.9	1022.1	7.40	71.99%	80
1953	Ind Coope	Arctic Ale	54	1079	1018	7.98	77.22%	115
1959	Harvey	Elixzabethan Ale		1085.4	1030.5	7.12	64.29%	100
1953	Watney	Yorkshire Stingo	51	1089.6	1031.7	7.52	64.62%	110
1953	Benskin	Colne Spring Ale	60	1090.7	1008.2	10.95	90.96%	100
1955	Benskin	Colne Spring Ale	60	1091.8	1011.1	10.69	87.91%	75
1959	Ind Coope	Colne Spring Ale	47	1092.8	1009.3	11.08	89.98%	80
1953	Truman	No. 1 Burton Barley Wine	60	1095.4	1023.6	9.42	75.26%	65
1955	Tennant	No. 1 Barley Wine	57	1097.5	1022.6	9.84	76.82%	175
1954	Tennant	Gold Label No.1 Sparkling Barley Wine	60	1101.5	1021.1	10.60	79.21%	90
1955	Tennant	Gold Label Barley Wine	57	1102.4	1020.8	10.77	79.69%	45
1958	Tennant	Gold Label No.1 Barley Wine	57	1102.5	1017.9	10.58	82.54%	35
1953	Bass	Barley Wine	60	1104.6	1036.3	8.90	65.30%	80
1958	Bass	No. 1 Barley Wine	63	1106.8	1039.8	8.71	62.73%	100
	Average		***51.0***	***1084.2***	***1021.3***	***8.21***	***74.42%***	***93***
Sources: Whitbread Gravity book held at the London Metropolitan Archives, document number LMA/4453/D/02/002.								

Numbered Ales were common amongst Burton brewers. Truman also had a set topped by a No. 1 Barley Wine. The tradition spread outside Burton. William Younger in Edinburgh brewed a set, 1 to 4. But other brewers, like Tennant in Sheffield, just brewed a No. 1 Barley Wine, without bothering with the lower numbers. The term No. 1 became associated with Barley Wine.

Truman continued to brew their No. 1 Barley Wine in a particularly old-fashioned sort of way right through into the 1970s. A Keeping was brewed at their Burton brewery, where it was aged for a year or more. It was then shipped down to their London brewery where it was blended a weaker Running version. The trick was getting the level of acidity right in the finished blend.

Tennant of Sheffield brewed two Barley Wines for a time. Their Original No. 1 Barley Wine, which, as all other examples of the style, was dark in colour. Then, in the mid-1950s, they introduced a revolutionary new beer, Gold Label No. 1, the first pale Barley Wine. A powerful beer that, initially at least, was aged for 12 months in oak casks.

After Tennants were bought by Whitbread, Gold Label became a national brand. Promoted by advertising, it sold in surprisingly large volumes for such a strong beer. Its success prompted imitations and many other brewers produced pale Barley Wines.

Barley Wine Grists

Most of the examples here were brewed single-gyled, with the exception of the Eldridge Pope beers, which were parti-gyled with Pale Ales.

Barley Wine grists: malts

Year	Brewer	Beer	OG	pale malt	mild malt	black malt	amber malt	choc. malt	crystal malt
1953	Adnams	Tally Ho	1080		83.02%		4.88%		4.88%
1967	Adnams	Tally Ho	1075		75.20%				8.06%
1956	Tennant	Gold Label	1103.5	67.56%					
1956	Tennant	No. 1	1100.6	75.36%		2.54%			2.17%
1968	Whitbread	FSA	1079.6	87.86%				3.47%	
1967	Eldridge Pope	BW	1085.3	54.27%					8.74%
1967	Eldridge Pope	Hardy Ale	1110.2	59.84%					6.30%
1964	Truman	S1	1105.3	92.47%					2.05%
1964	Truman	R1	1093.6	88.73%					4.23%

Sources:
Adnams brewing records held at the brewery.
Tennant brewing record held at Sheffield City Archive, document number MD7518/38/34.
Whitbread brewing record held at the London Metropolitan Archives, document number LMA/4453/D/01/137.
Eldridge Pope brewing records.
Truman brewing record held at the London Metropolitan Archives, document number B/THB/C/374.

Not a great amount of coloured malt, but lots of crystal. It's likely to be an odd mix of malts, as some of these beers are pale and some dark. Tennant No. 1 was dark, while Gold Label was pale, which explains the difference in their grists.

Barley Wine grists: odd malts and adjuncts

Year	Brewer	Beer	OG	enzymic malt	lager malt	wheat malt	flaked maize
1953	Adnams	Tally Ho	1080				
1967	Adnams	Tally Ho	1075	2.69%			
1956	Tennant	Gold Label	1103.5	1.15%			18.32%
1956	Tennant	No. 1	1100.6				7.18%
1968	Whitbread	FSA	1079.6				
1967	Eldridge Pope	BW	1085.3		21.11%	11.46%	
1967	Eldridge Pope	Hardy Ale	1110.2		22.05%	11.81%	
1964	Truman	S1	1105.3				
1964	Truman	R1	1093.6				4.23%

There's more enzymic malt, an ingredient that was weirdly popular after WW II. The lager and wheat malt in the Eldridge Pope beers look like they're intended to keep the colour pale. Not a huge amount of adjuncts, though.

Barley Wine grists: sugars								
Year	Brewer	Beer	no. 1 sugar	no. 2 sugar	no. 3 sugar	malt extract	caramel	other sugar
1953	Adnams	Tally Ho			6.51%		0.70%	
1967	Adnams	Tally Ho			8.95%			5.10%
1956	Tennant	Gold Label	12.98%					
1956	Tennant	No. 1		11.96%		0.80%		
1968	Whitbread	FSA	8.67%					
1967	Eldridge Pope	BW				4.42%		
1967	Eldridge Pope	Hardy Ale						
1964	Truman	S1			5.48%			
1964	Truman	R1	2.82%					

Not as many sugars as you might expect. And mostly just numbered invert sugars.

Strong Ale

In addition to Old Ale, Burton Ale and Barley Wine, there were other strong beers that were simply called Strong Ale. These came in a variety of strengths and colours, being as diverse as their name was vague.

Some Strong Ales were much like a London Burton or a Southern draught Old Ale: 1045°-1050° and dark brown. Others more like the stronger Northern type of Old Ale: 1060°-1080° and also dark brown. Odd ones were either weaker or much stronger than those two types. And some are quite pale.

London Strong Ales 1953 - 1965								
Date	Year	Beer	Price per pint d	OG	FG	ABV	App. Atten-uation	colour
1953	Fullers	Strong Ale	48	1066.8	1020.3	6.04	69.61%	115
1948	Ind Coope	No. 3 Strong Ale	57	1040.8	1010.8	3.89	73.53%	90
1954	Mann Crossman	Dragon Ale	24	1051.2	1019.1	4.15	62.70%	150
1950	Watney	Strong Ale	36	1061.1	1014.5	6.07	76.27%	105
1964	Watney	Export Gold	57	1078	1012.1	8.67	84.49%	23
1953	Wenlock	Strong Ale	46.5	1065.9	1017.9	6.24	72.84%	105
1965	Whitbread	Final Selection	57	1079.2	1013.5	8.63	82.95%	68
	Average		***46.5***	***1063.3***	***1015.5***	***6.2***	***74.63%***	***93.7***
Source: Whitbread Gravity book held at the London Metropolitan Archives, document number LMA/4453/D/02/002.								

Not really much in common amongst that group. The Ind Coope example isn't strong at all. Even though most of them are dark, Watney Export Gold is very pale.

Next versions from the Midlands.

Midlands Strong Ales 1953 - 1963								
Date	**Year**	**Beer**	**Price per pint d**	**OG**	**FG**	**ABV**	**App. Atten-uation**	**colour**
1963	Bass	Gold Triangle	72	1063.6	1013	6.61	79.56%	19
1953	Holes	Strong Ale	42	1080.7	1021.5	7.73	73.36%	75
1959	Mansfield	Golden Drop	54	1055.4	1014.9	5.06	73.10%	80
1965	Midland Clubs	Strong Extra Special	24	1036.4	1007.6	3.60	79.12%	100
1953	Mitchell & Butler	Strong Ale	56	1106	1026.5	10.45	75.00%	63
1961	Offilers	Derby Strong	34	1045.4	1013.6	3.98	70.04%	75
	Average		***42***	***1064.8***	***1016.8***	***6.16***	***75.03%***	***78.6***
Source: Whitbread Gravity book held at the London Metropolitan Archives, document number LMA/4453/D/02/002.								

Not how you can describe a beer of 3.6% ABV Strong Extra Special. But, in the days before there was any indication of a beer's strength on the label, brewers could get away with a lot. Contrast that with the Mitchell & Butler beer which really was full strength.

I've rather more examples from the North.

Northern Strong Ales 1953 - 1963								
Date	**Year**	**Beer**	**Price per pint d**	**OG**	**FG**	**ABV**	**App. Atten-uation**	**colour**
1953	Alnwick Brewery	Strong Ale	43.5	1057.1	1013.4	5.69	76.53%	63
1953	Carlisle State Brewery	Cream Ale		1067.5	1009.4	7.63	86.07%	85
1963	Carlisle State Brewery	Strong Ale	36	1051.7	1014.2	4.69	72.53%	21
1953	Chester Brewery	Strong Ale	43.5	1069	1014.9	7.07	78.41%	75
1957	Ely Brewery Co., Cardiff	Little Gem Ale	42	1078.1	1021.5	7.07	72.47%	75
1953	Felinfoel	Strong Ale	33	1043.3	1014.5	3.73	66.51%	25
1953	Hammonds United Breweries	Guards Ale	45	1073	1011.9	8.02	83.70%	100
1952	Hancocks	Strong Ale	16	1031	1004.7	3.42	84.84%	65
1953	Hay & Co	Red Seal Special Ale	42	1054.2	1011	5.63	79.70%	60
1953	Holt Bros.	Strong Ale	36	1059.9	1018.1	5.42	69.78%	71
1953	Hydes	Strong Ale	51	1066.9	1014.7	6.81	78.03%	77
1959	Peter Walker	Merrie England Strong Ale	51	1073.8	1023.2	6.32	68.56%	75
1959	Ramsdens	Strong Ale	49	1064.8	1018.1	6.07	72.07%	70
1953	Wards Ltd	No. 1 Strong Ale	36	1065.1	1015.3	6.49	76.50%	48
1953	Whitakers	Ram Tam	45	1070	1020.1	6.49	71.29%	71
1959	Whitakers	Ram Tam	54	1070.6	1024.8	5.93	64.87%	70
1959	Whitakers	Strong Shire Ale	24	1042.2	1017	3.25	59.72%	70
	Average		***40.4***	***1061.1***	***1015.7***	***5.87***	***74.21%***	***65.9***
Source: Whitbread Gravity book held at the London Metropolitan Archives, document number LMA/4453/D/02/002.								

Another very mixed bag. With Hancocks "Strong Ale" at just 1031° being a particular joke. There are quite a few similar beers in the 1060°-1070° range from both sides of the Pennines. Most have a Dark Mild type of colour, but there are a couple of pale outliers.

Almost all of the Strong Ales in these tables were packaged in nip (third of a pint) bottles. The drinker at the bar would have been handing over a third of the price per pint. Which would have made it less of a shock.

We finish with a broad set of Southern Strong Ales.

Southern Strong Ales 1953 - 1962								
Date	**Year**	**Beer**	**Price per pint d**	**OG**	**FG**	**ABV**	**App. Atten-uation**	**colour**
1959	Adnams	Fisherman Strong Ale	28.5	1044.3	1014.3	3.88	67.72%	115
1953	Brickwoods	Little Bricky	36	1070	1022.1	6.22	68.43%	110
1956	Bullard	Strong Ale	48	1081.4	1026	7.20	68.06%	85
1959	Eldridge Pope	Dorset Special Ale		1076.1	1019.9	7.33	73.85%	90
1953	Flowers	Shakespeare Ale	46.5	1079.6	1024.7	7.14	68.97%	61
1959	John Groves	Stingo		1062.4	1009.5	6.93	84.78%	125
1959	King & Barnes	Golding Ale		1070.4	1017.1	6.95	75.71%	50
1959	King & Barnes	Strong Ale		1044	1011.8	4.18	73.18%	130
1953	Norman & Pring	Imperial Strong Ale	54	1081.2	1051.8	3.74	36.21%	105
1949	Octagon	OB Armada Ale XXXX	24	1043.7	1009.8	4.41	77.57%	28.5
1953	Octagon	Two in one Ale	43.5	1064.1	1015.7	6.31	75.51%	55
1953	Plymouth Breweries	Strong English Ale	43.5	1069.4	1023.2	5.99	66.57%	71
1953	Simonds	Old Berkshire Strong Ale	43.5	1076.7	1033.2	5.61	56.71%	105
1960	St. Austell	Smugglers Ale	45	1068	1019.6	6.05	71.18%	100
1953	Star Brewery	Strong Ale	48	1067.4	1015.8	6.73	76.56%	95
1959	Strong	Strong 'un		1040.3	1010.2	3.91	74.69%	100
1962	Strong	Royal Old English Ale	40	1058.2	1013.9	5.54	76.12%	45
1959	Stroud Brewery	Charter Brew	37	1058.5	1006.3	6.85	89.23%	65
1956	Wells & Winch	Christmas Ale	45	1065.2	1026.7	4.97	59.05%	115
	Average		***41.6***	***1064.3***	***1019.6***	***5.78***	***70.53%***	***86.9***
Source: Whitbread Gravity book held at the London Metropolitan Archives, document number LMA/4453/D/02/002.								

There are quite a few weak ones. Adnams Fisherman Ale looks like a bottled version of their XXXX Old Ale. Ditto for the King & Barnes Strong Ale. Most of the rest are in a reasonable 1060°-1080° range. Again, with a couple of exceptions they're all dark.

Strong Ale Grists

These are the Strong Ales that aren't assigned any specific style, such as Old Ale of Barley Wine. Most are simply called Strong Ale.

Random Strong Ale grists: malts									
Year	**Brewer**	**Beer**	**OG**	**pale malt**	**mild malt**	**brown malt**	**black malt**	**choc. Malt**	**crystal malt**
1951	Boddington	CC	1054.5	77.42%					12.90%
1966	Boddington	SA	1065.5	73.38%					10.79%
1954	Elgood	SA	1047.1	90.00%					
1955	Flowers	SA	1075.4	77.92%					3.90%
1959	Fuller	SA	1072.4	79.30%					
1946	Lees	"C" Ale	1052.0	75.07%			1.38%		
1953	Lees	"C" Ale	1052.0	73.56%		1.44%	1.44%	1.44%	2.88%
1955	Lees	Strong Ale	1068.0	60.72%	10.12%				2.53%
1959	Lees	Strong Ale	1070.0	73.52%					2.30%
1963	Lees	Strong Ale	1076.0	67.81%					2.26%
1952	Strong	SSB	1045.4	17.24%	57.48%				2.87%

Sources:
Lees brewing record held at the brewery.
79A01-A3-3-27
Elgood brewing record held at the brewery.
Ref Shakespeare Birthplace Trust DR227/215 Brewing Record Book No2
Boddington brewing records held at Manchester Central Library, document numbers M693/405/130 and M693/405/133.
Fullers brewing record held at the brewery.

Lots of crystal again, but little in the way of roasted malts, other than in Lees "C" Ale, which contains three.

Random Strong Ale grists: weird malts and adjuncts							
Year	**Brewer**	**Beer**	**OG**	**enzymic malt**	**wheat malt**	**flaked maize**	**flaked barley**
1951	Boddington	CC	1054.5				
1966	Boddington	SA	1065.5		4.32%		
1954	Elgood	SA	1047.1				
1955	Flowers	SA	1075.4				
1959	Fuller	SA	1072.4			9.39%	
1946	Lees	"C" Ale	1052.0				13.25%
1953	Lees	"C" Ale	1052.0				
1955	Lees	Strong Ale	1068.0	2.53%		10.12%	
1959	Lees	Strong Ale	1070.0	2.30%		9.19%	
1963	Lees	Strong Ale	1076.0	2.26%		9.04%	
1952	Strong	SSB	1045.4				

Lees and Fuller are the only breweries using unmalted adjuncts. Which I do find surprising. I thought their use was almost universal.

Random Strong Ale grists: sugars 1								
Year	Brewer	Beer	OG	no. 2 sugar	no. 3 sugar	invert	CWA	CDM
1951	Boddington	CC	1054.5					
1966	Boddington	SA	1065.5			2.88%		
1954	Elgood	SA	1047.1			5.00%		
1955	Flowers	SA	1075.4		7.79%			
1959	Fuller	SA	1072.4	6.96%				2.26%
1946	Lees	"C" Ale	1052.0			7.36%		
1953	Lees	"C" Ale	1052.0			3.85%		
1955	Lees	Strong Ale	1068.0			3.37%	6.75%	0.48%
1959	Lees	Strong Ale	1070.0			3.06%	6.13%	0.44%
1963	Lees	Strong Ale	1076.0			3.01%		0.54%
1952	Strong	SSB	1045.4		3.83%		1.92%	

Random Strong Ale grists: sugars 2								
Year	Brewer	Beer	OG	HX	caramel	glucose	malt extract	other sugar
1951	Boddington	CC	1054.5		1.08%		2.87%	5.73%
1966	Boddington	SA	1065.5		0.72%		2.88%	5.04%
1954	Elgood	SA	1047.1				5.00%	
1955	Flowers	SA	1075.4				5.19%	5.19%
1959	Fuller	SA	1072.4					2.09%
1946	Lees	"C" Ale	1052.0			2.94%		
1953	Lees	"C" Ale	1052.0		3.85%	3.85%		7.69%
1955	Lees	Strong Ale	1068.0	3.37%				
1959	Lees	Strong Ale	1070.0	3.06%				
1963	Lees	Strong Ale	1076.0	3.01%				12.06%
1952	Strong	SSB	1045.4		1.33%		3.83%	11.50%

Every beer except the 1951 Boddington CC contains invert sugar in some form. Accompanied by a dizzying array of other sugars. Every example has at least 10% sugar.

Scotch Ale

I'm only going to consider strong Scotch Ales as being in this category. Scottish Shilling Ales – 60/-, 70/- and 80/- are just types of Pale Ale.

Scottish breweries were dead dull for most of the 20th century, William Younger excepted. Most had a single recipe, from which they'd parti-gyle three Pale Ales – 60/-, 70/- and 80/- - plus possibly a Strong Ale. Sometimes they even managed to parti-gyle Stout with Pale Ale.

I'm classing Scotch Ale as two types. Which rather than pissing around with some abstract description, I'll define in reference to two William Younger beers: No. 1 and No. 3. Though the latter type seems to have been peculiar to them. Strong Ales from other Scottish breweries were mostly along the lines of No. 1.

The No. 1 type of Scotch Ale was around 1070° - 1080°, dark and not particularly well attenuated. At most breweries it was parti-gyled with Pale Ales and so was effectively a double-strength Scottish Pale Ale.

Scotch Ale 1947 - 1950

Year	Brewer	Beer	OG	FG	ABV	App. Atten-uation	colour
1950	Aitchison	Scotch Ale	1080	1020.8	7.73	74.00%	55
1948	Aitken	Strong Ale	1067.5	1021	6.04	68.89%	
1948	Ballingall	"Angus" Strong Ale	1073.5	1023.5	6.49	68.03%	
1948	Calder	Scotch Strong Ale	1065.5	1019	6.04	70.99%	
1950	Campbell	Royal Scotch Ale	1080.1	1014.2	8.66	82.27%	77
1948	Dryborough	Strong Ale	1060	1019.5	5.25	67.50%	
1947	Fowler	Heavy Ale	1081.4	1025.5	7.27	68.67%	
1948	Fowler	Twelve Guinea Ale	1080	1021.5	7.63	73.13%	
1949	Fowler	Extra Strong	1078	1012	8.68	84.62%	
1949	Fowler	Twelve Guinea Ale	1077.7	1030.3	6.13	61.00%	100
1948	Jeffrey	Strong Ale No. 1	1067	1025	5.43	62.69%	
1948	Jeffrey	Strong Ale	1065	1019.5	5.91	70.00%	
1948	Maclachlan	Strong Ale	1070.5	1024.5	5.96	65.25%	
1948	McEwan	Strong Ale	1078	1022.5	7.23	71.15%	
1950	McEwan	Scotch Ale	1088	1022.6	8.56	74.32%	63
1947	Murray	Heavy Ale	1066.3	1017.25	6.38	73.96%	
1948	Steel Coulson	Strong Ale	1063	1026	4.77	58.73%	
1947	Usher	Old Scotch Ale	1073.5	1020.5	6.90	72.11%	
1948	Usher	Strong Ale	1090.5	1024.5	8.63	72.93%	
1947	Younger, Wm.	No. 1 Strong Ale	1074	1022	6.76	70.27%	
1950	Younger, Wm.	Scotch Ale	1087.6	1017.5	9.21	80.02%	60
	Average		***1074.6***	***1021.4***	***6.94***	***70.98%***	***71.0***

Sources:
Whitbread Gravity book held at the London Metropolitan Archives, document number LMA/4453/D/02/002.
Thomas Usher Gravity Book held at the Scottish Brewing Archive, document TU/6/11.

You may have noticed that some of the examples were called Scotch Ale, others Strong Ale. The same beer might be given both names, depending on the market it was intended for. Generally, when sold in Scotland it would be called Strong Ale, when sold anywhere else, Scotch Ale.

Scotch Ale wasn't cheap. There were two reasons for that. First, it was strong and there was a lot of tax on it. Second, it was mostly sold in nip (a third of a pint) bottles, which was an expensive format. It was more than treble the price per pint of Mild Ale.

Scotch Ale 1950 - 1960

Year	Brewer	Beer	Price per pint d	OG	FG	ABV	App. Atten-uation	colour
1953	Aitchison	Strong Ale	45	1072.6	1021.5	6.64	70.39%	75
1953	Aitken	Strong Ale	43.5	1065.6	1018.3	6.15	72.10%	100
1955	Aitken	Strong Ale	45	1067	1020.3	6.06	69.70%	105

Scotch Ale 1950 - 1960								
Year	**Brewer**	**Beer**	**Price per pint d**	**OG**	**FG**	**ABV**	**App. Atten- uation**	**colour**
1953	Ballingall	Angus Strong Ale	48	1059.8	1017.2	5.53	71.24%	90
1953	Barnard	Strong Ale	43.5	1065.2	1018.2	6.11	72.09%	115
1952	Campbell	Royal Edinburgh Scotch Ale		1080.3	1011.1	9.12	86.18%	50
1953	Fowler	Strong Ale	45	1070.3	1017.6	6.87	74.96%	85
1955	Fowler	Twelve Guinea Ale	45	1068.1	1016.9	6.67	75.18%	120
1953	James Deucher	Lochside Strong Ale	38	1066.9	1014.9	6.79	77.73%	24
1955	James Deucher	Lochside Strong Ale	45	1069.6	1019.6	6.50	71.84%	31
1953	Jeffrey	Strong Ale	43.5	1064.3	1019.7	5.79	69.36%	83
1957	Jeffrey	Dishers Extra Strong Ale	64	1088.6	1017.1	9.40	80.70%	27
1953	Maclachlan	Strong Ale	43.5	1063.2	1016.2	6.12	74.37%	105
1955	Maclachlan	Strong Ale	45	1068.6	1023.4	5.86	65.89%	75
1953	McEwan	Strong Ale	45	1070.7	1019.5	6.66	72.42%	79
1955	McEwan	Strong Ale	45	1071.5	1020.8	6.59	70.91%	85
1953	Murray	Heavy Ale	43.5	1065.9	1019.2	6.07	70.86%	90
1955	Murray	Heavy Ale	45	1071.7	1021	6.59	70.71%	105
1953	Steel Coulson	Strong Ale	43.5	1069.5	1014.1	7.24	79.71%	83
1953	Tennent	Strong Ale	43.5	1066.4	1021.2	5.86	68.07%	95
1958	Tennent	Strong Ale	31.25	1068.4	1022.7	5.71	66.81%	100
1953	Usher	Strong Ale	43.5	1068.5	1020.1	6.29	70.66%	60
1953	WB Reid	Strong Ale	39	1065.9	1020.3	5.92	69.20%	72
1953	Younger, Geo.	Strong Ale	43.5	1067.6	1021.9	5.93	67.60%	90
1955	Younger, Geo.	Strong Ale	45	1067.6	1022.3	5.87	67.01%	100
1953	Younger, Robert	Strong Ale	43.5	1066.3	1016.8	6.45	74.66%	103
1952	Younger, Wm.	No. 1 Strong Ale		1083.5	1021.7	8.07	74.01%	72
1953	Younger, Wm.	No. 1 Strong Ale	43.5	1071.2	1024.2	6.09	66.01%	75
1955	Younger, Wm.	No. 1 Strong Ale	45	1071.4	1024.3	6.11	65.97%	80
1960	Younger, Wm.	No. 1 Strong Ale	48	1065.9	1019	6.10	71.17%	
	Average		***44.3***	***1069.4***	***1019.4***	***6.51***	***71.92%***	***81.9***
Sources:								
Whitbread Gravity book held at the London Metropolitan Archives, document number LMA/4453/D/02/002.								
Which Beer Report, 1960, pages 171 - 173.								

Scotch Ale was very popular in Belgium. So much so that some breweries made a Scotch specifically for the Belgian market. Including some, like John Smith and Truman, which weren't even in Scotland.

Scotch Ale for the Belgian market 1950 - 1955							
Year	**Brewer**	**Beer**	**OG**	**FG**	**ABV**	**App. Atten-uation**	**colour**
1950	John Smith	Scotch Ale	1080.3	1025.6	7.11	68.12%	65
1950	John Smith	Scotch Ale	1080.6	1025.6	7.15	68.24%	61
1952	John Smith	Scotch Ale	1078.6	1024	7.10	69.47%	77
1954	John Smith	Scotch Ale	1072.6	1022.1	6.56	69.56%	95
1955	John Smith	Scotch Ale	1072.3	1022	6.54	69.57%	75
1955	McEwan	Scotch Ale	1088.2	1020.2	8.92	77.10%	65
1952	McEwan	Scotch Ale	1090.3	1023.1	8.80	74.42%	62
1955	Truman	Scotch Ale	1083.4	1025.6	7.52	69.30%	80
1950	Younger, Geo.	Gordon Highland Scotch Ale	1091.2	1031.1	7.81	65.90%	45
1950	Younger, Geo.	Gordon Xmas Ale	1090.7	1032.3	7.58	64.39%	48
1952	Younger, Geo.	Gordon Highland Scotch Ale	1081.8	1026.5	7.19	67.60%	50
1954	Younger, Geo.	Gordon Highland Scotch Ale	1090.9	1028	8.20	69.20%	60
1955	Younger, Geo.	Gordon Highland Scotch Ale	1090.3	1029.9	7.86	66.89%	55
	Average		***1083.9***	***1025.8***	***7.56***	***69.21%***	***64.5***

Sources:
Whitbread Gravity book held at the London Metropolitan Archives, document number LMA/4453/D/02/002.

The colour of these beers is paler than for those intended for the UK market. The Gordon branded beers in particular aren't very dark at all. Gordon's beers are still available in Belgium, despite George Younger having closed many decades ago.

The second type of Scotch Ale was much weaker, usually with an OG in the mid-1040ºs.

Weaker Scotch Ale 1948 - 1960								
Year	**Brewer**	**Beer**	**Price per pint d**	**OG**	**FG**	**ABV**	**App. Atten-uation**	**colour**
1948	Gordon & Blair	"Unique" Scotch Ale		1043.5	1017	3.49	62.07%	
1953	Gordon & Blair	Strong Ale	43.5	1046.7	1006	5.32	87.15%	75
1950	McEwan	Double Scotch Ale	36	1057.7	1018	5.09	68.11%	80
1948	Steel Coulson	Elephant Brand Scotch Ale		1044	1012	4.22	73.86%	
1948	Younger, Robert	Strong Ale		1048	1015	4.34	69.79%	
1949	Younger, Wm.	Double Century Ale		1058.5	1018	5.32	70.09%	
1949	Younger, Wm.	draught No. 3	36	1041.7	1011	3.98	73.62%	55
1950	Younger, Wm.	Double Century Ale	36	1058.4	1020	4.96	65.58%	75
1953	Younger, Wm.	Century Ale	36	1056.4	1021	4.52	62.06%	71
1957	Younger, Wm.	Double Century Ale	32.5	1051.5	1019	4.25	63.88%	80
1960	Younger, Wm.	No. 3 Scotch Ale	45	1046.2	1013	4.30	71.75%	
	Average		***37.9***	***1050.2***	***1015.3***	***4.5***	***69.82%***	***72.7***

Sources:
Whitbread Gravity book held at the London Metropolitan Archives, document number LMA/4453/D/02/002.
Which Beer Report, 1960, pages 171 - 173.
Thomas Usher Gravity Book held at the Scottish Brewing Archive, document TU/6/11.

No. 3 in particular was very simple in strength and character to a London Burton Ale. In William Younger's London pubs it filled that slot.

Scotch Ale Grists

As mentioned above, most Scotch Ales were parti-gyled with Pale Ale, meaning that their grists might look eerily familiar. The one exception is William Younger, who brewed everything single-gyle.

Scotch Ale grists: malts

Year	Brewer	Beer	OG	pale malt	black malt	crystal malt	mild malt	enzymic malt
1948	Drybrough	Burns	1070	79.20%	1.18%			1.56%
1956	Drybrough	Burns	1073	75.12%	1.19%			1.57%
1960	Drybrough	Burns	1073	75.79%	1.13%			
1951	Maclay	SA	1075	86.33%				
1957	Maclay	SA	1077	73.24%				
1962	Thomas Usher	GSA	1077	85.71%				
1960	Younger, Robert	SA	1070	72.65%				
1949	Younger, Wm.	No. 3 Pale	1044	86.96%				
1949	Younger, Wm.	No. 1	1074	79.25%		2.83%	2.83%	
1949	Younger, Wm.	Double Century	1057	76.83%		3.66%	3.66%	
1958	Younger, Wm.	No. 3L	1044	64.95%				
1958	Younger, Wm.	Double Century	1057	61.48%				
1958	Younger, Wm.	No. 3N	1045	60.00%				
1958	Younger, Wm.	No. 1	1089	60.00%				
1958	Younger, Wm.	200/- BW	1100	76.12%				

Sources:
William Younger brewing record held at the Scottish Brewing Archive, document number WY/6/1/2/88.
William Younger brewing record held at the Scottish Brewing Archive, document number WY/6/1/3/112.
Robert Younger brewing record held at the Scottish Brewing Archive, document number RY/6/1/3.
Maclay brewing record held at the Scottish Brewing Archive, document number M/6/1/1/28.
Maclay brewing record held at the Scottish Brewing Archive, document number M/6/1/1/35.
Drybrough brewing record held at the Scottish Brewing Archive, document number D/6/1/1/6.
Drybrough brewing record held at the Scottish Brewing Archive, document number D/6/1/1/7.
Thomas Usher brewing record held at the Scottish Brewing Archive, document number TU/6/9/1.

There aren't a huge number of malts involved. A little black malt and enzymic malt in Burns Ale, some crystal and mild malt in a couple of the William Younger beers. Maclay Usher and Robert Younger used just pale malt alone.

Scotch Ale grists: adjuncts					
Year	**Brewer**	**Beer**	**OG**	**flaked maize**	**flaked barley**
1948	Drybrough	Burns	1070		10.42%
1956	Drybrough	Burns	1073	6.26%	5.01%
1960	Drybrough	Burns	1073	11.76%	
1951	Maclay	SA	1075		
1957	Maclay	SA	1077	11.27%	
1962	Thomas Usher	GSA	1077	9.89%	
1960	Younger, Robert	SA	1070	18.49%	
1949	Younger, Wm.	No. 3 Pale	1044		13.04%
1949	Younger, Wm.	No. 1	1074		11.32%
1949	Younger, Wm.	Double Century	1057	10.98%	
1958	Younger, Wm.	No. 3L	1044	30.93%	
1958	Younger, Wm.	Double Century	1057	31.97%	
1958	Younger, Wm.	No. 3N	1045	28.57%	
1958	Younger, Wm.	No. 1	1089	32.00%	
1958	Younger, Wm.	200/- BW	1100	17.91%	

Not much to see there. All but one beer contained some sort of flakes. Though the quantities in the 1958 William Younger beers are very high. 10-15% is more normal.

All the variety comes in the sugars.

Scotch Ale grists: sugars								
Year	**Brewer**	**Beer**	**OG**	**no. 1 sugar**	**invert**	**cane**	**Hydrol**	**Avona**
1948	Drybrough	Burns	1070					2.78%
1956	Drybrough	Burns	1073		2.50%		1.67%	1.67%
1960	Drybrough	Burns	1073		4.36%			1.74%
1951	Maclay	SA	1075	9.59%				
1957	Maclay	SA	1077	9.39%				
1962	Thomas Usher	GSA	1077					
1960	Younger, Robert	SA	1070		3.52%		4.40%	
1949	Younger, Wm.	No. 3 Pale	1044					
1949	Younger, Wm.	No. 1	1074					
1949	Younger, Wm.	Double Century	1057					
1958	Younger, Wm.	No. 3L	1044			4.12%		
1958	Younger, Wm.	Double Century	1057			1.64%		
1958	Younger, Wm.	No. 3N	1045		1.90%	1.90%		
1958	Younger, Wm.	No. 1	1089		8.00%			
1958	Younger, Wm.	200/- BW	1100		5.97%			

It takes two tables to cover all the sugars.

Scotch Ale grists: sugars								
Year	**Brewer**	**Beer**	**OG**	**CME**	**lactose**	**malt extract**	**caramel**	**other sugar**
1948	Drybrough	Burns	1070			2.08%		3.51%
1956	Drybrough	Burns	1073	1.67%		1.67%		2.22%
1960	Drybrough	Burns	1073	1.74%		1.74%	1.74%	
1951	Maclay	SA	1075				0.24%	4.44%
1957	Maclay	SA	1077			1.88%	0.47%	5.13%
1962	Thomas Usher	GSA	1077			2.20%		2.56%
1960	Younger, Robert	SA	1070			0.88%		
1949	Younger, Wm.	No. 3 Pale	1044					
1949	Younger, Wm.	No. 1	1074		3.77%			
1949	Younger, Wm.	Double Century	1057		4.88%			
1958	Younger, Wm.	No. 3L	1044					
1958	Younger, Wm.	Double Century	1057		3.28%		1.64%	
1958	Younger, Wm.	No. 3N	1045					12.70%
1958	Younger, Wm.	No. 1	1089					
1958	Younger, Wm.	200/- BW	1100					

Invert of some kind is easily the most popular. Followed by malt extract, which in beers from every brewery, except William Younger. Then there are all those proprietary sugars: Hydrol, Avona, CME. I've little idea about what the hell they were.

It's fascinating how lactose keeps popping up in unexpected places. As it does here in a couple of William Younger's beers.

There's more caramel than might appear from the tables. All the William Younger's beers must have been colour corrected with caramel at racking time. You can't get the colours in the analyses of the finished beers from the ingredients listed in the brewing record.

Celebration Beers

The Coronation of Queen Elizabeth II in 1953 prompted many brewers to produce a special brew to celebrate the event. Surprisingly, these weren't all Barley Wine or Old Ale type beers, though many were. Some were specifically called Coronation Ale, others had names with some sort of royal connection, like Kings Ale.

At least one brewery – Barclay Perkins – produced a beer to commemorate the Festival of Britain in 1951. The beer must have been a success, as it was still being brewed years later, even after Barclay's brewery had closed.

Audit Ales were strong beers which had originally been brewed in Oxford and Cambridge colleges. After their own breweries closed, colleges contracted the brewing out to commercial breweries.

Celebration beers 1951 - 1959								
Year	**Brewer**	**Beer**	**Price per pint d**	**OG**	**FG**	**ABV**	**App. Atten-uation**	**colour**
1955	Dales (Brewed by Wells & Winch)	Audit Ale	36	1062.2	1023.5	5.00	62.22%	115
1955	Wells & Winch	Audit Ale	36	1062.2	1023.3	5.03	62.54%	115
1958	Lacons	Audit Ale	54	1095	1017.8	9.65	81.26%	90
1955	Greene King	Audit Ale	36	1083.2	1017.7	8.59	78.73%	100
1951	Friary Holroyd	Audit Strong Ale	46.5	1084.6	1022.1	8.17	73.88%	52
1953	Morrell	College Ale	45	1069.2	1026	5.59	62.43%	52
1952	Barclay Perkins	Festival Ale	55.5	1070.5	1016.5	7.05	76.60%	27
1958	Courage, Barclay	Festival Ale	54	1077.9	1023.3	7.10	70.09%	25
1953	Taylor Walker	Coronation Ale	48	1075.1	1029.5	5.89	60.72%	56
1953	McMullen	Coronation Ale	63	1089.1	1034.7	7.04	61.05%	130
1953	Beasley	Coronation Ale	28	1043.1	1008.6	4.49	80.05%	130
1953	Benskin	Jubilee Beer	30	1054	1017.7	4.70	67.22%	86
1953	Masseys	Kings Ale	31.5	1065.5	1010.8	7.16	83.51%	140
1953	Catterall & Swarbrick	Royal Ale	48	1070.4	1021.4	6.37	69.60%	44
1959	Charrington	Royal Toby		1077.8	1018.9	7.70	75.71%	45
1955	Young & Co	Celebration Ale	36	1076.2	1015.8	7.91	79.27%	
1953	Rose	Kings Ale	45	1070.3	1014.3	7.32	79.66%	39
1953	Russells & Wrangham	Prince Ale	45	1073.4	1020.3	6.92	72.34%	79
1953	Raggetts	Kings Ale	48	1065.1	1010.4	7.17	84.02%	260
Source: Whitbread Gravity book held at the London Metropolitan Archives, document number LMA/4453/D/02/002.								

Festival Ale is the odd one out, being the only really pale beer in the table above.

Brown Ale

Only revived around 1900, Brown Ale became wildly popular in the middle of the century. It was one of the beers that boosted the popularity of bottled beer, especially in pubs.

Yet it varied immensely in nature. The distinction is often made between Northern and Southern Brown Ales. But it was more complex than that. Really what's really meant is standard-strength and strong Brown Ales. I'd prefer to classify them and Single Brown Ale and Double Brown Ale. Because there are plenty of examples of weak versions being brewed in the North and strong ones in the South.

Brown Ale doesn't appear at all in the brewing records of many breweries. For the simple reason that it wasn't brewed as a distinct beer, but was just a bottled version of Dark Mild. With perhaps some tweaking in the primings.

The stronger type of Brown Ale was brewed as its own beer. Though the most famous – Newcastle Brown Ale – was a blend of two beers. One of the best Southern examples of a stronger Brown Ale, Whitbread Double Brown was sadly discontinued in the mid-1950s.

The importance of Brown Ale in the London market is highlighted by just how many analyses there are of it in the Whitbread Gravity Book.

London Brown Ale <1038° 1946 - 1952

Year	Brewer	Beer	Price per pint d	OG	FG	ABV	App. Atten-uation	colour
1946	Barclay Perkins	Doctor Brown Ale	13.5	1034.1	1011.3	2.95	66.86%	105
1952	Barclay Perkins	Doctor Brown Ale	19	1034	1010.5	3.04	69.12%	98
1947	Beasley	Brown Ale	12	1030	1007.7	2.89	74.33%	83
1947	Charrington	Brown Ale	15	1027.7	1012	2.02	56.68%	91
1952	Charrington	Brown Ale	9d	1031.1	1008.5	2.93	72.67%	120
1950	Courage	Brown Ale	15	1029.7	1007.6	2.86	74.41%	83
1952	Courage	Nut Brown Ale	19	1032.4	1008.2	3.14	74.69%	87
1946	Hammerton	Nut Brown Ale	24	1026.5	1003.8	2.95	85.66%	79
1950	Hammerton	Nut Brown Ale	17	1029.8	1006.9	2.97	76.85%	83
1950	Ind Coope	Nut Brown Ale		1029	1009.5	2.52	67.24%	75
1952	Ind Coope	Nut Brown Ale	19	1030.9	1011.7	2.48	62.14%	83
1946	Mann Crossman	Brown Ale	14	1034.4	1008.8	3.32	74.42%	84
1950	Mann Crossman	Brown Ale	18	1035.8	1013.3	2.91	62.85%	98
1952	Meux	Nut Brown Ale	19	1029.8	1009.1	2.68	69.46%	106
1948	South London Brewery	SLB Brown Ale	16	1028	1011.1	2.18	60.36%	83
1946	Taylor Walker	Nut Brown Ale	17	1030.1	1007.6	2.92	74.75%	83
1952	Taylor Walker	Nut Brown Ale	19	1032.6	1011.7	2.70	64.11%	83
1946	Truman	Trubrown	12.5	1033.2	1011.8	2.76	64.46%	105
1951	Truman	Trubrown	19	1035.4	1012.8	2.92	63.84%	105
1946	Watney	Brown Ale	12	1029.6	1008.5	2.73	71.28%	87
1952	Watney	Brown Ale	18	1032	1010.8	2.74	66.25%	105
1950	Wenlock	Nut Brown Ale	15	1030.7	1012.5	2.35	59.28%	87
1952	Wenlock	Nut Brown Ale	19	1032.5	1012.5	2.58	61.54%	83
1947	Whitbread	Forest Brown	12	1028.9	1006.5	2.91	77.51%	83
1952	Whitbread	Forest Brown	21	1032.6	1012.1	2.65	62.88%	95
	Average		***16.7***	***1031.2***	***1009.9***	***2.76***	***68.55%***	***91.0***

Source:
Whitbread Gravity book held at the London Metropolitan Archives, document number LMA/4453/D/02/002.

A combination of low gravity and poor attenuation leaves only a couple over 3% ABV. The strongest is the granddaddy of all Brown Ales, Manns. Though it's quite a bit weaker than pre-war, when it had an OG in the low 1040°s and was almost 4% ABV.

There was a slight increase in gravity at the beginning of the 1950s. Where I have two analyses for the same brewery, you can see that the gravity of the later one is a point or two higher.

There seems to be a similar trend as amongst Mild Ales, where the London examples are darker and less well-attenuated than those from elsewhere.

Midlands Brown Ale <1038° 1948 - 1952								
Year	Brewer	Beer	Price per pint d	OG	FG	ABV	App. Atten-uation	colour
1952	Ansell	Nut Brown Ale	16	1036.2	1005.8	3.96	83.98%	48
1949	Davenport	Brown Ale	13.5	1031	1004	3.51	87.10%	60
1951	East Anglian Brewery	Brown Ale	24	1032.6	1008.3	3.15	74.54%	98
1948	Everards	Nut Brown Ale	18	1030.8	1003.7	3.53	87.99%	61
1948	Lacons	Brown Ale	19	1031.2	1009.6	2.79	69.23%	79
1952	Morgans	Brown Ale	22	1034.7	1005.2	3.84	85.01%	71
1948	Northampton Brewery	Brown Ale	18	1032.4	1008.4	3.11	74.07%	150
1952	Shipstone	Nut Brown Ale	15	1033.3	1006.7	3.45	79.88%	61
1952	Steward & Patteson	Brown Ale	23	1032.5	1010.3	2.87	68.31%	67
	Average		***18.7***	***1032.7***	***1006.9***	***3.36***	***78.90%***	***77.2***

Even though the average OG is just a little higher than in London, the greater degree of attenuation leaves more than 0.5% ABV higher.

Northern Brown Ale <1038° 1948 - 1952								
Year	Brewer	Beer	Price per pint d	OG	FG	ABV	App. Atten-uation	colour
1952	Birkenhead	Nut Brown Ale	16	1031.4	1005.8	3.33	81.53%	91
1952	Duttons	Nut Brown Ale	20	1029.9	1005.8	3.13	80.60%	55
1952	Hammonds	Brown Jack Ale	18	1029.5	1005.8	3.08	80.34%	105
1948	Samuel Smith	Taddy Brown Ale	18	1032.5	1013.8	2.41	57.54%	95
1952	Samuel Smith	Taddy Ale	18	1035.5	1009.7	3.34	72.68%	125
1948	Tennant Bros.	Brown Ale	18	1031.8	1010.2	2.79	67.92%	67
1952	Tennant Bros.	Brown Ale	20	1032.5	1012.2	2.62	62.46%	98
1952	Tetley	Family Ale	15	1035.5	1009	3.44	74.65%	53
1950	Vaux & Co	Maxim Ale	14	1033.5	1009.7	3.08	71.04%	105
	Average		***17.4***	***1032.5***	***1009.1***	***3.02***	***72.08%***	***88.2***
Source: Whitbread Gravity book held at the London Metropolitan Archives, document number LMA/4453/D/02/002.								

Northern versions seem to fall somewhere between the London and Midlands versions in terms of attenuation and colour. At least most examples are over 3% ABV.

Southern Brown Ale <1038° 1946 - 1952								
Year	**Brewer**	**Beer**	**Price per pint d**	**OG**	**FG**	**ABV**	**App. Atten-uation**	**colour**
1951	Benskin	Nut Brown Ale	16	1032.9	1008.1	3.22	75.38%	83
1952	Brickwoods	Brown Brew	18	1032.2	1008.9	3.02	72.36%	79
1952	Cobb & Co	Brown Ale	18	1034.3	1007.5	3.48	78.13%	79
1948	Devenish	Brown Ale	18	1030.5	1005.8	3.21	80.98%	67
1952	McMullen	Nut Brown Ale	18	1035.5	1012.6	2.96	64.51%	106
1948	Plymouth Breweries	Double Brown Ale	18	1035	1010.8	3.13	69.14%	63
1952	Plymouth Breweries	Double Brown Ale	18	1035.3	1008.3	3.50	76.49%	57
1948	Simonds	Brown Ale	18	1025.6	1006.3	2.50	75.39%	105
1952	Simonds	Berry Brown Ale	19	1032	1005.5	3.44	82.81%	60
1952	St. Anne's Well	Brown Ale	19	1034.1	1005.1	3.77	85.04%	98
1948	Tamplin	No. 1 Brown Ale	19	1033.6	1008.5	3.25	74.70%	87
1952	Tamplin	No.1 Ale	20	1034.1	1009.7	3.16	71.55%	79
1946	Tollemache	Golden Brown	13	1029.2	1006.1	3.00	79.11%	83
1952	Tollemache	Brown Ale	20	1032.5	1007.7	3.22	76.31%	79
1952	Ushers	Brown Ale	17	1033.6	1007.7	3.36	77.08%	79
1947	Wethered	Golden Brown Ale	12	1025.6	1004	2.81	84.37%	48
	Average		***17.6***	***1032.3***	***1007.7***	***3.19***	***76.46%***	***78.3***
Source: Whitbread Gravity book held at the London Metropolitan Archives, document number LMA/4453/D/02/002.								

The Southern averages are very similar to those for the Midlands. Once again, only a couple of examples dip below 3% ABV and those that do, only dip a little.

There are rather fewer stronger Brown Ales, but they come from a diverse set of locations, not just the Northeast.

Brown Ale >1038° 1946 - 1952								
Year	**Brewer**	**Beer**	**Price per pint d**	**OG**	**FG**	**ABV**	**App. Atten-uation**	**colour**
1952	Greenhall Whitley	Wilderspool Brown Ale	20	1038.7	1008.5	3.92	78.04%	79
1951	Hancocks	Nut Brown Ale	19	1039.3	1010.2	3.77	74.05%	33.5
1952	Hey & Son	White Rose Ale	20	1040.7	1007.9	4.27	80.59%	60
1952	J Bernard Ltd	Double Brown Ale	30	1047.5	1009.9	4.89	79.16%	42
1952	McMullen	Olde Time Ale	45	1060.6	1015	5.94	75.25%	105
1950	Murray	Brown Ale	24	1057.1	1013.4	5.69	76.53%	83
1949	Newcastle Breweries	Newcastle Brown Ale	22	1051.6	1012.2	5.12	76.36%	45
1952	Newcastle Breweries	Brown Ale	26	1052	1009.9	5.49	80.96%	45
1952	Northampton	Brown Ale	18	1038	1013	3.23	65.79%	210
1951	Peter Walker	Brown Peter Ale	20	1039.2	1008.3	4.02	78.83%	91
1948	Portsmouth United	Brown Ale	17	1038.2	1005.4	4.27	85.86%	56
1952	Vaux & Co	Double Maxim Ale	23	1049	1009.8	5.10	80.00%	48
1947	Whitbread	Double Brown	17	1043	1010.1	4.27	76.51%	100
1952	Whitbread	Double Brown	30	1053.8				
	Average		***23.6***	***1046.3***	***1010.3***	***4.61***	***77.53%***	***76.7***
Source: Whitbread Gravity book held at the London Metropolitan Archives, document number LMA/4453/D/02/002.								

Of course, there are the two classic Northeast examples, Newcastle Brown and Vaux Double Maxim. But also a couple from Scotland (Bernard and Murray), one from Wales (Hancocks) and three from the South of England (McMullen, Portsmouth United and Whitbread).

Some examples are quite pale and barely even brown at all, particularly those from the Northeast.

Moving on to the new Elizabethan Age, London Brown Ales still look different.

London Brown Ale <1038° 1953 - 1964								
Year	**Brewer**		**Price per pint d**	**OG**	**FG**	**ABV**	**App. Atten-uation**	**colour**
1956	Barclay Perkins	Doctor Brown Ale	20	1032.9	1009.9	2.98	69.91%	100
1954	Charrington	Brown Ale	19	1033.1	1009.1	3.11	72.51%	120
1963	Charrington	Brown Ale	22	1034	1011	2.97	67.65%	75
1956	Courage	Nut Brown Ale	20	1032.2	1011.9	2.62	63.04%	100
1962	Courage, Barclay	Berry Brown Ale	24	1032.9	1016.1	2.16	51.06%	120
1960	Friary Meux	Brown Ale	20	1030.2	1011.6	2.40	61.59%	
1956	Fullers	Brown Ale	20	1031.7	1009.4	2.89	70.35%	90
1955	Ind Coope	Nut Brown Ale	22	1033.6	1011.2	2.90	66.67%	105
1956	Mann Crossman	Brown Ale	22	1035.5	1013.2	2.88	62.82%	115

London Brown Ale <1038° 1953 - 1964

Year	Brewer		Price per pint d	OG	FG	ABV	App. Atten-uation	colour
1964	Mann Crossman	Brown Ale	25	1036.2	1013	3.00	64.09%	
1956	Meux	Nut Brown Ale	20	1030.9	1012.6	2.36	59.22%	120
1956	Taylor Walker	Nut Brown Ale	20	1032.4	1009.9	2.91	69.44%	95
1953	Truman	Trubrown	19	1034.1	1009.2	3.23	73.02%	110
1964	Truman	Trubrown	22	1035.4	1016.9	2.38	52.26%	100
1953	Watney	Brown Ale	19	1032.1	1009.9	2.87	69.16%	110
1964	Watney	Brown Ale	22	1033.4	1012.4	2.71	62.87%	135
1956	Wenlock	Brown Ale	20	1033	1013.6	2.50	58.79%	95
1954	Whitbread	Forest Brown	23	1034.8	1012.2	2.92	64.94%	95
1964	Whitbread	Forest Brown	22	1035.6	1011.2	3.16	68.54%	90
	Average		***21.1***	***1033.4***	***1011.8***	***2.79***	***64.63%***	***104.4***

Source:
Which Beer Report, 1960, pages 171 - 173.
Whitbread Gravity book held at the London Metropolitan Archives, document number LMA/4453/D/02/002.

The average OG has increased a little, but the rate of attenuation is even lower, leaving a very similar ABV. Only four of the nineteen examples manage to reach 3% ABV. The colour is still very dark. 1963 Charrington Brown Ale, the palest, is still the colour of Dark Mild.

Let's look at what was going on elsewhere in the UK.

Midlands Brown Ale <1038° 1953 - 1960

Year	Brewer		Price per pint d	OG	FG	ABV	App. Atten-uation	colour
1955	Alton Court	Brown Ale	26	1033.3	1008.4	3.23	74.77%	80
1955	Ansell	Nut Brown	19	1036	1004.3	4.13	88.06%	35
1959	Ansell	Bruno Sweet Brown Ale	23	1034.4	1013.6	2.68	60.47%	90
1960	Ansell	Nut Brown Ale	17	1032.9	1010.5	2.90	68.09%	
1959	Atkinson's	Brown Ale	26	1037	1016.5	2.64	55.41%	95
1955	Everards	Burton Brown	22	1033.1	1006.6	3.44	80.06%	75
1955	Mitchell & Butler	Sam Brown	23	1036.9	1011.2	3.33	69.65%	85
1955	Offilers	Nut Brown	19	1034.6	1010.1	3.17	70.81%	75
1955	Ruddle	Nut Brown Ale	19	1033.1	1008.2	3.23	75.23%	95
1955	Worthington	Nut Brown Ale	22	1036	1008.6	3.56	76.11%	80
	Average		***21.6***	***1034.7***	***1009.8***	***3.23***	***71.86%***	***78.9***

Source:
Which Beer Report, 1960, pages 171 - 173.
Whitbread Gravity book held at the London Metropolitan Archives, document number LMA/4453/D/02/002.

Still stronger, more attenuated and paler than in London. Though, surprisingly, no cheaper. The size of the Brown Ale market is demonstrated by the fact that Ansell produced two, quite different, versions. Atkinson, another Birmingham brewery, produced a similar beer to the sweet Ansell Brown Ale: dark and poorly attenuated.

Northern Brown Ale <1038º 1953 - 1964

Year	Brewer		Price per pint d	OG	FG	ABV	App. Atten-uation	colour
1964	Birkenhead	Nut Brown Ale	17	1033.1	1005.1	3.50	84.59%	110
1964	Camerons	Nut Brown	18	1031.6	1008.9	2.84	71.84%	95
1953	Duttons	Nut Brown Ale	18	1031	1006.1	3.23	80.32%	52
1964	Greenall Whitley	Bulls Eye Brown Ale	22	1036.2	1012.6	2.95	65.19%	120
1959	Hammonds	Brown Jack Ale	20	1034.7	1009.3	3.18	73.20%	70
1964	Hammonds	Brown Jack	20	1034.2	1013.7	2.56	59.94%	65
1964	Hey	White Rose Ale	24	1037.9	1010.9	3.38	71.24%	75
1964	Higsons	Brown Ale	19	1033.9	1009.3	3.08	72.57%	70
1955	Samuel Smith	Taddy Nut Brown	20	1035.2	1010.5	3.20	70.17%	100
1964	Samuel Smith	Taddy Nut Brown Ale	23	1035.8	1013.4	2.80	62.57%	95
1955	Samuel Webster	Sam Brown Ale	19	1035.7	1013	2.93	63.59%	95
1955	Tennant Bros.	Family Brown Ale	18	1031.9	1007.5	3.16	76.49%	50
1959	Tennant Bros.	Lion Brown Ale	23	1035.1	1009.2	3.24	73.79%	75
1964	Tetley	Family Ale	20	1033.4	1005.5	3.49	83.53%	60
1964	Vaux	Light Brown Ale	18	1032.9	1007.6	3.16	76.90%	40
1959	Websters	Sam Brown Ale	18	1036.8	1011.1	3.33	69.84%	95
1964	Websters	Sam Brown Ale	20	1036	1009.6	3.30	73.33%	95
	Average		***19.8***	***1034.4***	***1009.6***	***3.14***	***72.30%***	***80.1***

Source:
Whitbread Gravity book held at the London Metropolitan Archives, document number LMA/4453/D/02/002.

These look pretty similar to the Midlands set on average. Though again the rate of attenuation varies enormously. Clearly there was a market for very sweet, weak Brown Ales. While some of the paler versions are quite highly attenuated.

Southern Brown Ale <1038º 1953 - 1960

Year	Brewer		Price per pint d	OG	FG	ABV	App. Atten-uation	colour
1956	Cobbold	Cobnut Brown Ale	23	1035.7	1011.8	3.09	66.95%	75
1955	Flowers	Poacher Ale	22	1034.9	1014.2	2.67	59.31%	115
1960	Fremlins	Double Elephant	23	1033.4	1011	2.90	67.07%	
1956	Greene King	Harvest Brown Ale	22	1035.2	1013.9	2.75	60.51%	105
1956	Simonds	Berry Brown Ale	32	1031.9	1011.9	2.58	62.70%	85
1953	Tamplin	Baby Browm	24	1034.3	1007.9	3.43	76.97%	79
1954	Tollemache	Country Brown Ale	19	1032.5	1011.2	2.75	65.54%	90
1954	Tollemache	London Brown Ale	20	1036	1011.6	3.16	67.78%	80
1959	Tomson & Wotton	Tom Brown Ale		1033.5	1014	2.51	58.21%	110
	Average		***23.1***	***1034.2***	***1011.9***	***2.87***	***65.00%***	***92.4***

Source:
Which Beer Report, 1960, pages 171 - 173.
Whitbread Gravity book held at the London Metropolitan Archives, document number LMA/4453/D/02/002.

These look very like London Brown Ales: dark and poorly attenuated. Only two examples manage to crawl over 3% ABV.

Now West as well as South,

Southwestern Brown Ale <1038° 1954 - 1961								
Year	**Brewer**		**Price per pint d**	**OG**	**FG**	**ABV**	**App. Atten-uation**	**colour**
1960	Georges	Brown Ale	22	1035.1	1011.9	3.00	66.10%	
1956	Georges	Brown Ale	24	1035.2	1010.8	3.16	69.32%	90
1954	Gibbs Mew	Moonraker Brown Ale	16	1034.8	1009.5	3.28	72.70%	135
1958	Hall & Woodhouse	Nut Brown Ale	19	1034.4	1013.9	2.56	59.59%	95
1958	Hall & Woodhouse	"John Brown" Ale	19	1036.3	1011.8	3.06	67.49%	100
1961	Strong	Rumsey Brown	23	1032.3	1010	2.79	69.04%	140
1956	Stroud Brewery Ltd	Cotswold Brown Ale	22	1037.1	1010.1	3.50	72.78%	90
1960	Ushers	Brown Ale	18	1032.3	1010.65	2.80	67.03%	
1955	Wadworth	Middy Brown Ale	22	1034.5	1012.9	2.79	62.61%	95
1965	Wrekin	Nut Brown	25	1033.2	1009.9	2.91	70.18%	90
	Average		***21.0***	***1034.5***	***1011.1***	***2.98***	***67.68%***	***106.4***

Sources:
Which Beer Report, 1960, pages 171 - 173.
Whitbread Gravity book held at the London Metropolitan Archives, document number LMA/4453/D/02/002.

Another set of mostly quite sweet and weak Brown Ales.

Welsh Brown Ale <1038° 1957 - 1960								
Year	**Brewer**		**Price per pint d**	**OG**	**FG**	**ABV**	**App. Atten-uation**	**colour**
1957	Buckleys	Brown Brew	26	1035.9	1008.6	3.54	76.04%	120
1956	Felinfoel	John Brown Ale	22	1037.7	1010.5	3.52	72.15%	120
1960	Hancock	Nut Brown		1033				
	Average		***24.0***	***1035.5***	***1009.6***	***3.53***	***74.10%***	***120.0***

Source:
"Cardiff Pubs and Breweries" by Brian Glover, 2005. pages 97-101
Whitbread Gravity book held at the London Metropolitan Archives, document number LMA/4453/D/02/002.

It's difficult to draw too many conclusions from such a small sample, but they look more along the lines of Norther Brown Ales.

Scottish Brown Ale <1038° 1956 - 1958								
Year	Brewer		Price per pint d	OG	FG	ABV	App. Atten-uation	colour
1958	Blair	Brown Ale	32	1034.1	1011.7	2.80	65.69%	125
1956	Younger, Wm.	"Wee Willie"	24	1033.5	1009.6	3.10	71.34%	70
	Average		***28***	***1033.8***	***1010.7***	***2.95***	***68.52%***	***97.5***
Source: Whitbread Gravity book held at the London Metropolitan Archives, document number LMA/4453/D/02/002.								

An even smaller sample size for Scotland. The Blair Brown Ale looks like a sweet , dark one. The Younger beer not so much.

Finally strong Brown Ales. These are usually classified as "Northern" type Brown Ale, though the tables show that it was also brewed in other parts of the country.

Northern Brown Ale >1038° 1953 - 1964								
Year	Brewer	Beer	Price per pint d	OG	FG	ABV	App. Atten-uation	colour
1955	Alnwick	Brown Ale	26	1062.5	1020.6	5.43	67.04%	110
1955	Bass	Brown Ale	24	1054.7	1015.6	5.07	71.48%	85
1959	Bass	Brown Ale	36	1052.9	1015.6	4.84	70.51%	105
1960	Carlisle State Management	Nut Brown Ale	20	1040.6	1012.75	3.60	68.60%	
1955	Darley	Barley Brown	26	1040.1	1012.3	3.60	69.33%	250
1957	Glassons, Penrith	Beacon Brown Ale	28	1039.1	1009.6	3.83	75.45%	60
1964	John Smith	Double Brown	24	1047.3	1016.7	3.82	64.69%	80
1954	Newcastle Breweries	Brown Ale	26	1048.9	1010	5.06	79.55%	51
1959	Newcastle Breweries	Brown Ale	32	1052.2	1012.1	5.22	76.82%	50
1961	Newcastle Breweries	Brown Ale	30	1051.4	1008.2	5.40	84.05%	50
1964	Newcastle Breweries	Brown Ale	26	1049.2	1009.2	5.00	81.30%	50
1964	Nimmo	Brown Ale	25	1043.8	1011.7	4.01	73.29%	70
1955	Northern Clubs Federation	High Level Brown Ale	26	1053.6	1016.5	4.81	69.22%	75
1960	Northern Clubs Federation	Federation Brown Ale	22	1051.4	1010.4	5.13	79.77%	70
1953	Vale of Neath	Nut Brown Ale	30	1070.6	1019.3	6.68	72.66%	34
1955	Vaux	Double Maxim	24	1048.5	1012.8	4.63	73.61%	110
1960	Vaux	Double Maxim	24	1047.4	1009.75	4.90	79.43%	
1964	Vaux	Double Maxim	26	1047	1012.4	4.33	73.62%	60
1959	Websters	Old Brown	46.5	1071.4	1023.1	6.27	67.65%	110
	Average		***27.0***	***1051.2***	***1013.6***	***4.82***	***73.58%***	***83.5***
Source: Which Beer Report, 1960, pages 171 - 173. Whitbread Gravity book held at the London Metropolitan Archives, document number LMA/4453/D/02/002.								

This set contains the three classic examples of strong Brown Ale from the Northeast:

Newcastle Brown, Double Maxim and Federation Brown Ale. Nimmo, also from the Northeast, is represented by a slightly weaker version.

Southern Brown Ale >1038° 1953 - 1965								
Year	Brewer	Beer	Price per pint d	OG	FG	ABV	App. Atten-uation	colour
1959	Brickwoods	Brown Ale	24	1041.1	1013.9	3.52	66.18%	19
1956	Bullard	Brown Ale	24	1039.6	1004.4	4.59	88.89%	85
1955	Ind Coope	Double Brown Ale	25	1047.8	1012.6	4.57	73.64%	45
1956	Kemp Town	Double Dolphin Ale	28	1043.6	1013.8	3.86	68.35%	100
1953	Ushers Wiltshire	Triple Brown	38	1063.4	1013.6	6.50	78.55%	85
1955	Whitbread	Double Brown		1051.0	1013.5	4.96	73.53%	130
1953	Young & Son Portsmouth	Chestnut Brown Ale	26	1055.1	1016.5	5.01	70.05%	205
	Average		***27.5***	***1048.8***	***1012.6***	***4.71***	***74.17%***	***95.6***

Source:
Whitbread brewing record held at the London Metropolitan Archives, document number LMA/4453/D/01/123.
Whitbread Gravity book held at the London Metropolitan Archives, document number LMA/4453/D/02/002.

The Southern examples are a little bit weaker and rather darker, but are generally similar in terms of attenuation. Notice that some are specifically called Double Brown and in once case Triple Brown. The Brickwoods beer can hardly really be called brown its colour is so pale. 19 is pale even for a Bitter.

Scottish Brown Ale >1038° 1953 - 1965								
Year	Brewer	Beer	Price per pint d	OG	FG	ABV	App. Atten-uation	colour
1956	Aitchison	Gold Seal Brown Ale	21	1041.6	1013.9	3.58	66.59%	50
1958	Bernard	Double Brown Ale		1043	1013	3.89	69.77%	
1957	Ushers	Brown Export Ale	30	1044.4	1017.3	3.50	61.04%	130
1954	Younger, Wm.	Double Century Ale	36	1056.6	1023.3	4.29	58.83%	80
1957	Younger, Wm.	Edinburgh Brown Ale	28	1046.6	1013.1	4.34	71.89%	55
	Average		***28.8***	***1046.4***	***1016.1***	***3.92***	***65.62%***	***78.8***

Sources:
Which Beer Report, 1960, pages 171 - 173.
Whitbread Gravity book held at the London Metropolitan Archives, document number LMA/4453/D/02/002.

The Scottish examples are noticeably less well attenuated that the ones from other parts of the country. I suspect that some or all of these were beers specifically intended for the Northeast of England, where many Scottish breweries did a lot of business.

Brown Ale Grists

It's no shock to discover that Brown Ale grists were quite diverse. There's not a single ingredient that all the examples below have in common. They're quite diverse in terms of strength, too.

Brown Ale grists 1948 - 1965: malts

Year	Brewer	Beer	OG	pale malt	black malt	choc. malt	crystal malt	mild malt
1962	Clarke	1/5 Nobby BA	1035.5	71.52%				
1956	Shepherd Neame	Br	1026.3	72.24%				
1948	Whitbread	Double Brown	1047	81.27%		1.73%		
1954	Whitbread	Forest Brown	1032.4				6.91%	79.93%
1954	Whitbread	Double Brown	1053.3	82.02%		1.12%		
1961	Whitbread	Forest Brown	1033				7.70%	78.97%
1965	Whitbread	Forest Brown	1032.2				7.41%	72.84%
1952	Strong	BA	1033.5	28.30%				56.60%
1955	Flowers	BX	1030.4	81.25%			3.75%	
1959	Ushers	Watney Brown Ale	1030.7				4.97%	79.45%
1958	Bernard	DBA	1043	75.20%	0.82%			
1958	Younger, Wm.	BA	1031	57.35%				
1964	Eldridge Pope	Dorset Brown Ale	1025.5	71.68%			13.94%	
1955	Fuller	Old Harry	1051.1	76.59%				
1959	Fuller	SBA	1027	79.11%				
1969	Truman	BA	1030.7	65.43%			9.35%	
1965	Beasley	BA	1030			5.27%	10.54%	60.58%

Sources:
Clarke brewing record held at Manchester Central Library, document number M693/405/137.
Shepherd Neame brewing record held at the brewery.
Whitbread brewing records held at the London Metropolitan Archives, document numbers LMA/4453/D/01/116, LMA/4453/D/01/121, LMA/4453/D/01/122, LMA/4453/D/01/128 and LMA/4453/D/01/132.
79A01-A3-3-27
Ref Shakespeare Birthplace Trust DR227/215 Brewing Record Book No2
1075-275-6 Wiltshire archives at Chippenham
T & J Bernard brewing record held at the Scottish Brewing Archive, document number TJB6/1/1/1.
William Younger brewing record held at the Scottish Brewing Archive, document number WY/6/1/3/112.
Fullers brewing records held at the brewery
Derek's 1969 Ale book
Beasley brewing record held at the London Metropolitan Archives, document number ACC/2305/26/115.

It's clear from the paucity of roast malts – three beers with chocolate and one with black – that most of the colour was coming from some form of sugar. As some of these beers were parti-gyled with Mild, it's no surprise that mild malt was fairly popular as the base. I would have expected to see crystal malt in more examples.

Note that there's one malt that totally absent: brown malt.

Brown Ale grists 1948 - 1965: adjuncts								
Year	**Brewer**	**Beer**	**OG**	**flaked maize**	**wheat malt**	**roast barley**	**flaked barley**	**barley meal**
1962	Clarke	1/5 Nobby BA	1035.5	5.30%				
1956	Shepherd Neame	Br	1026.3		3.80%			
1948	Whitbread	Double Brown	1047					
1954	Whitbread	Forest Brown	1032.4					
1954	Whitbread	Double Brown	1053.3					
1961	Whitbread	Forest Brown	1033					
1965	Whitbread	Forest Brown	1032.2				16.67%	
1952	Strong	BA	1033.5					
1955	Flowers	BX	1030.4					
1959	Ushers	Watney Brown Ale	1030.7	5.79%		4.14%		
1958	Bernard	DBA	1043	13.08%				
1958	Younger, Wm.	BA	1031	30.88%				
1964	Eldridge Pope	Dorset Brown Ale	1025.5		4.65%			
1955	Fuller	Old Harry	1051.1	8.92%				
1959	Fuller	SBA	1027	9.49%				
1969	Truman	BA	1030.7			4.38%	5.26%	5.26%
1965	Beasley	BA	1030	5.27%				

I'd have put money on everyone but Whitbread having flaked maize (or flaked barley, depending on the year) in their Brown Ales.

Brown Ale grists 1948 - 1965: sugars									
Year	**Brewer**	**Beer**	**no. 2 sugar**	**no. 3 sugar**	**invert**	**lac-tose**	**cara-mel**	**malt extract**	**other sugar**
1962	Clarke	1/5 Nobby BA					2.65%	2.65%	15.89%
1956	Shepherd Neame	Br		12.67%			0.71%	0.63%	9.94%
1948	Whitbread	Double Brown		16.14%					0.86%
1954	Whitbread	Forest Brown		11.18%					1.97%
1954	Whitbread	Double Brown		15.73%					1.12%
1961	Whitbread	Forest Brown		10.91%					2.41%
1965	Whitbread	Forest Brown							3.09%
1952	Strong	BA		3.77%				3.77%	7.55%
1955	Flowers	BX				6.67%		1.67%	6.67%
1959	Ushers	Watney Brown Ale			3.86%		1.79%		
1958	Bernard	DBA			6.54%				4.36%
1958	Younger, Wm.	BA							11.76%
1964	Eldridge Pope	Dorset Brown Ale						3.54%	6.19%
1955	Fuller	Old Harry	10.41%				2.09%		1.98%
1959	Fuller	SBA	6.33%						5.07%
1969	Truman	BA							10.32%
1965	Beasley	BA		14.05%				3.51%	0.78%

There's a lot of invert sugar again, most of it in the form of No. 3. But there are also plenty of proprietary sugars and, presumably, some of those provide colour, too.

Light Ale

Another huge seller was the bottled equivalent of Ordinary Bitter, Light Ale. And as with Brown Ale, it was often drunk mixed with its draught brother.

You may wonder why I'm splitting apart Pale Ale and Light Ale, but not Pale Ale and IPA. There's a very short answer to that question. This is my book, self-published and I'll do what the heel I like. Also, Light Ale is quite a well-defined thing: a watery bottled Pale Ale. IPA was just too vague a term.

Its popularity owed as much to the shortcomings of draught Bitter as its own particular attributes. With the quality of draught dodgy and the bottled alternative pricey, many drinkers compromised on a mixture: Light and Bitter. A dull and lifeless half of Bitter could be perked up with a bottle of sparkling, fizzy Light Ale.

As with Brown Ale, many brewers didn't bother making Light Ale as its own particular brew. They just bottled their Ordinary Bitter. Though it does pop up in brewing records – with brewhouse names like LBA – a little more often.

Light Ale 1946 - 1961

Year	Brewer	Beer	Price per pint d	OG	FG	ABV	App. Atten-uation	colour
1960	Ansell	Triple Gold Light Ale	22	1039.1	1008.1	3.87	79.28%	24
1955	Ballingall	Angus Ale	22	1028.1	1008	2.60	71.53%	55
1950	Brickwoods	Light Bitter Ale	13.5	1027.7	1006.9	2.70	75.09%	24
1959	Camerons	Ebor Light Ale	24	1036.8	1011.9	3.11	67.66%	24
1948	Carlisle State Brewery	Dinner Ale	16	1034.3	1005	3.81	85.42%	34.5
1957	Charrington	Export Light Ale	30	1035.4	1008.3	3.52	76.55%	18
1961	Davenport	Continental Light Ale	30	1034	1005.3	3.59	84.41%	8
1959	Devenish	Light Ale	18	1030.6	1010.7	2.49	65.03%	23
1956	Dunmow	Family Ale	20	1031.6	1010.9	2.68	65.51%	25
1953	Duttons	Green Label Light Ale	18	1032	1006.8	3.27	78.75%	24
1956	Flowers	Light Ale	20	1030.1	1005.3	3.22	82.39%	17
1960	Fremlin	Elephant Light Ale	21	1031.5	1005.8	3.21	81.59%	23
1960	Friary Meux	Friary Ale	20	1030.6	1009.7	2.70	68.30%	
1959	Georges	Light Ale	24	1033	1008.7	3.15	73.64%	18
1952	Hammond	Prize Medal Ale	22	1033.8	1006.9	3.49	79.59%	21
1951	Harrods	Light Ale	17	1031.1	1008	2.99	74.28%	25
1949	John Smith	Light Ale	12	1029.2	1007.3	2.84	75.00%	29.5
1964	John Smith	Light Ale	21	1031.9	1009.6	2.79	69.91%	29
1949	Melbourne	Light Ale	20	1029	1005.9	3.00	79.66%	27.5
1952	Meux	Light Ale	18	1030.7	1007.9	2.95	74.27%	22.5
1951	Mitchell & Butler	Cape Ale	15	1034.8	1007.3	3.57	79.02%	19
1956	Mitchell & Butler	Cape Ale	30	1032.7	1008.5	3.14	74.01%	31
1960	Morland	Light Ale	19	1033.6	1009.5	3.01	71.73%	27
1953	Norman & Pring	Light Ale	6d	1031	1011	2.58	64.52%	17

Light Ale 1946 - 1961								
Year	Brewer	Beer	Price per pint d	OG	FG	ABV	App. Atten-uation	colour
1956	Rayments	Pelham Ale	19	1031.7	1006.9	3.22	78.23%	23
1960	Simonds	SB. Light Ale	20	1034.2	1009.5	3.20	72.22%	
1960	Strong	Golden Ale	20	1030.7	1006.1	3.20	80.29%	
1950	Style & Winch	Farmer Ale	17	1031.3	1008.4	2.97	73.16%	17
1955	Tennant Bros.	Light Dinner Ale	18	1030.8	1006.9	3.10	77.60%	23
1954	Tetley	Family Ale	24	1035.1	1007.2	3.62	79.49%	57
1960	Tollemache & Cobblold	Tolly Extra Quality Light Ale	24	1035.3	1010.6	3.20	69.97%	
1958	Ushers	Light Ale	30	1033.3	1007.2	3.26	78.38%	16
1959	W. Butler	Light Ale	24	1034.7	1009.6	3.14	72.33%	19
1946	Worthington	Dinner Ale	15	1037.1	1006.7	3.95	81.94%	20
1955	Worthington	Dinner Ale	18	1036.1	1007.8	3.68	78.39%	20
1950	Young & Son	Light Victory Ale	13.5	1029.3	1003.3	3.38	88.74%	25
1953	Young & Son	Light Victory Ale	17	1032.1	1007.6	3.18	76.32%	30.5
1949	Younger, Wm.	Sparkling Ale	20	1030.9	1004.8	3.39	84.47%	25.5
1960	Younger, Wm.	Younger's Pale Ale	22	1032.3	1006.2	3.40	80.96%	

Sources:
Whitbread Gravity book held at the London Metropolitan Archives, document number LMA/4453/D/02/002.
Which Beer Report, 1960, pages 171 - 173.

Light Ale Grists

Light Ale was really just a bottled version of the weakest kind of Bitter. At many breweries there's nothing specifically called Light Ale in the brewing records. It's just one of a draught Bitter packaged differently.

Light Ale grists: malts							
Year	Brewer	Beer	OG	pale malt	mild malt	crystal malt	wheat malt
1946	Shepherd Neame	LDA	1027.1	75.97%			
1956	Shepherd Neame	LDA	1029.4	76.51%			4.03%
1956	Adnams	LBA	1031.0	89.19%			
1955	Flowers	PX	1030.3	81.25%			3.75%
1959	Ushers Trowbridge	LB	1030.7	91.70%			
1964	Eldridge Pope	BK	1030.2	68.58%		7.22%	
1965	Beasley	Courage Light Ale	1032.0	47.16%	25.94%	4.72%	

Sources:
Shepherd Neame brewing record held at the brewery.
Adnams brewing record held at the brewery.
Ref Shakespeare Birthplace Trust DR227/215 Brewing Record Book No2
1075-275-6 Wiltshire archives at Chippenham
Beasley brewing record held at the London Metropolitan Archives, document number ACC/2305/26/115.

Not much to see there. Mostly it's just base malt, with wheat and crystal malt in a couple of examples. I'm assuming the wheat is for head retention rather than flavour.

Light Ale grists: adjuncts and sugars								
Year	Brewer	Beer	OG	wheat flour	flaked maize	flaked barley	malt extract	no. 1 sugar
1946	Shepherd Neame	LDA	1027.1			8.94%	0.74%	
1956	Shepherd Neame	LDA	1029.4				0.67%	
1956	Adnams	LBA	1031.0					10.81%
1955	Flowers	PX	1030.3				1.67%	
1959	Ushers Trowbridge	LB	1030.7				1.82%	
1964	Eldridge Pope	BK	1030.2	9.64%			6.02%	
1965	Beasley	Courage LA	1032.0		9.43%		1.57%	

There are surprisingly few adjuncts. I would have expected to see flaked maize in most of them.

Light Ale grists: sugars								
Year	Brewer	Beer	no. 3 sugar	invert	CWA	Wortex	caramel	other sugar
1946	Shepherd Neame	LDA	11.92%				2.43%	
1956	Shepherd Neame	LDA	13.42%			5.37%		
1956	Adnams	LBA						
1955	Flowers	PX		3.33%	10.00%			
1959	Ushers Trowbridge	LB		6.39%			0.09%	
1964	Eldridge Pope	BK		8.42%				0.13%
1965	Beasley	Courage LA	11.01%					0.17%

More No. 1 invert and less No. 3 would have been my guess. Though what's described as simply "invert" could have been No. 1. Caramel is a bit of a surprise, too, as these were pretty pale beers.

Lager

Bottom-fermenting beer first arrived in the UK in the 1860s (other than a brief experiment in Edinburgh in the 1840s). Initially, either Vienna or Munich style beers imported from the Continent. By the end of the 19th century Lager-brewing had gained a permanent foothold in the UK. Albeit in just a handful of breweries.

UK-brewed Lager

As Lager gained popularity in the 1950s, many regional breweries wanted to get in on the act. Previously the market had been totally supplied either by continental imports of by a handful of specialists. Before WW II only half a dozen UK brewers produced Lager: Wrexham Lager brewery, Red Tower, Alloa Brewery, Tennant, Jeffrey and Barclay Perkins. Now everyone was at it.

As most lacked the necessary equipment, they weren't very authentic. Fermented warm with a top-fermenting yeast and undergoing no lagering, they were really just golden Ales masquerading as Lager.

Lager brewed in England and Wales 1947 - 1965								
Year	**Brewer**	**Beer**	**Price per pint d**	**OG**	**FG**	**ABV**	**App. Atten-uation**	**colour**
1947	Barclay	Draught Lager	26	1033	1006.4	3.46	80.61%	8
1950	Barclay	Lager	31	1036.1	1008	3.65	77.84%	11
1957	Barclay	Pilsner Lager		1035	1006.3	3.73	82.00%	9
1961	Barclay	Pilsner Lager	36	1035.3	1007.5	3.61	78.75%	6
1952	Carling	Black Label	32	1042.3	1009.9	4.21	76.60%	10
1959	Carling	Black Label		1036.5	1004.4	4.18	87.95%	80
1963	Carling	Black Label	36	1035.3	1006.4	3.61	81.87%	5.5
1957	Charrington	Pilsner Lager	42	1036	1005.8	3.93	83.89%	5
1961	Charrington	Pilsner Lager	32	1036.3	1008.1	3.66	77.69%	8
1961	Eldridge Pope	König Pilsener Lager	36	1038.6	1007.3	3.91	81.09%	8
1949	Fayredael	"Sir Bell" Light Lager		1033.5	1010	3.04	70.15%	
1956	Flowers	Lager	36	1040.4	1014	3.41	65.35%	9
1956	Flowers	Lager	42	1045.3	1014	4.05	69.09%	9
1957	Flowers	Lager		1050	1017.5	4.20	65.00%	14
1961	Flowers	Lager	30	1044	1011.3	4.09	74.32%	12
1960	Greene King	Lager		1034.9	1006.4	3.56	81.66%	9.5
1961	Hall & Woodhouse	Brock Lager	36	1033.9	1004.1	3.73	87.91%	10
1957	Ind Coope	Pilsener Lager	40	1035.6	1007.2	3.69	79.78%	9
1961	Ind Coope	Grahams Skol	40	1033.6	1007.2	3.43	78.57%	9.5
1962	Ind Coope	Skol Export	48	1035.4	1008.3	3.52	76.55%	8
1962	Ind Coope	Skol Pilsener	38	1033.9	1006.4	3.57	81.12%	7
1965	Ind Coope	Skol International 2000 Lager	24	1044.2	1006.9	4.66	84.39%	7
1961	Lacons	Lager	34	1034.9	1007.1	3.48	79.66%	8
1959	Lees	Lager		1037.0				
1960	M & B	Export Lager	32	1039.7	1010	3.71	74.81%	7.5
1961	Phipps	Stein Lager	36	1034.8	1005.5	3.66	84.20%	7.5
1950	Red Tower	Lager	30	1035.8	1008.2	3.58	77.09%	13
1956	Red Tower	Pilsner Lager	30	1031.2	1005.9	3.29	81.09%	10
1960	Tennant Bros.	Lager	32	1035.2	1006.8	3.55	80.68%	8.5
1961	Tolly Cobbold	Kroner Lager	36	1033.1	1005.7	3.42	82.78%	9.5
1945	Wrexham	Pilsner Lager		1037	1011.8	3.26	68.11%	14.5

Sources:
Whitbread Gravity book held at the London Metropolitan Archives, document number LMA/4453/D/02/002.
Thomas Usher Gravity Book document TU/6/11 held at the Scottish Brewing Archive.
Lees brewing records held at the brewery.

The Scots, of course, had been early to the game and still brewed a large percentage of UK Lager. The style also gained a mass following in Scotland earlier than south of the border.

Lager brewed in Scotland 1950 - 1963								
Year	**Brewer**	**Beer**	**Price per pint d**	**OG**	**FG**	**ABV**	**App. Atten-uation**	**colour**
1950	Alloa Brewery	Light Lager		1043.4	1009.1	4.46	79.03%	7
1950	Alloa Brewery	Graham's Golden Lager	30	1040.6	1010.6	3.89	73.89%	9
1952	Alloa Brewery	Graham's Golden Lager	30	1039.2	1014.3	3.22	63.52%	15
1957	McEwan & Younger	Export Lager	30	1033.6	1006.3	3.55	81.25%	13
1957	McEwan & Younger	Export Lager		1035.2	1007.3	3.62	79.26%	13
1957	McEwan & Younger	Export Lager	42	1033.8	1010.9	2.96	67.75%	13
1958	McEwan & Younger	Export Lager	25	1034.3	1010.5	2.97	69.39%	9
1961	McEwan & Younger	Export Lager	42	1032.9	1010.1	2.85	69.30%	10
1954	Steel Coulson	Lager Beer	30	1032	1004.3	3.60	86.56%	11
1955	Tennent	Lager	30	1036.1	1007.7	3.69	78.67%	9
1957	Tennent	Lager Beer	33.33	1040.6	1008.6	4.16	78.82%	11
1960	Tennent	Lager	36	1036.3	1008.6	3.60	76.45%	
1963	Tennent	Lager	33.75	1036.9	1007.8	3.64	78.86%	7.5

Sources:
Whitbread Gravity book held at the London Metropolitan Archives, document number LMA/4453/D/02/002.
Which Beer Report, 1960, pages 171 - 173.

Imported Lager

A considerable quantity of Lager was imported, mostly from Denmark, The Netherlands and to a lesser extent Belgium and Germany. The first two countries had been supplying the UK market for decades. Germany, for obvious political reasons, had been imported more patchily, while Belgium had only recently got into the Lager game.

Denmark

Denmark was easily the biggest source of Lager, accounting for around 75% of imports from continental Europe. This was mostly in the form of Carlsberg and Tuborg, the country's two largest brewers.[7] And those imports rose during the 1950s: from 36,410 barrels in 1953, 209,244 barrels in 1959.[8]

As the table below shows, both Tuborg and Carlsberg sold beers of different strengths in the UK market. One at the puny strength expected by UK consumers and the other at something more like a continental Strength.

[7] 1962 Brewers' Almnack, page 58.
[8] 1962 Brewers' Almnack, page 58.

Lager brewed in Denmark 1947 - 1963								
Year	**Brewer**	**Beer**	**Price per pint d**	**OG**	**FG**	**ABV**	**App. Atten-uation**	**colour**
1947	Carlsberg	Lager		1033	1008	3.24	75.76%	
1947	Carlsberg	Pilsner		1035.6	1008.5	3.52	76.12%	13.5
1950	Carlsberg	Lager		1031.8	1010.9	2.70	65.72%	13
1952	Carlsberg	Pilsner Lager	32	1031.3	1011.2	2.60	64.22%	10
1957	Carlsberg	Danish Pilsner		1030.9	1009.7	2.74	68.61%	10
1957	Carlsberg	Danish Pilsner	40	1031.5	1008.4	2.99	73.33%	9
1959	Carlsberg	Pilsener	42	1031.2	1009.1	2.76	70.83%	15
1961	Carlsberg	Danish Pilsner	40	1030.5	1007.2	2.91	76.39%	7.5
1962	Carlsberg	Lager de Luxe	48	1052.8	1008.3	5.56	84.28%	8
1962	Carlsberg	Danish Pilsner	38	1030.4	1008	2.80	73.68%	8
1963	Carlsberg	Lager de Luxe	54	1052.1	1009.5	5.32	81.77%	8
1963	Carlsberg	Pilsner	38	1030.2	1005.4	3.10	82.12%	8
1963	Carlsberg	Pilsner	42	1029.9	1005.2	3.09	82.61%	7.5
1947	Tuborg	Pilsner		1036.6	1009.1	3.57	75.14%	11.5
1950	Tuborg	Lager		1032.9	1006.1	3.48	81.46%	11.5
1957	Tuborg	Export Beer	40	1052.3	1011.5	5.31	78.01%	7
1957	Tuborg	Lager	40	1030.7	1005.8	3.23	81.11%	10
1957	Tuborg	Export Tuborg Beer		1052.4	1006.9	5.95	86.83%	7
1957	Tuborg	Tuborg Lager		1031.2	1007.4	3.09	76.28%	13
1959	Tuborg	Tuborg Lager	42	1030.7	1005.8	3.23	81.11%	13
1961	Tuborg	Pilsner	40	1030.2	1005.6	3.08	81.46%	12
1963	Tuborg	Export Gold Lager		1052.7	1007.2	5.69	86.34%	8
1963	Tuborg	Pilsner	42	1031.5	1007	3.06	77.78%	12

Sources:
Whitbread Gravity book held at the London Metropolitan Archives, document number LMA/4453/D/02/002.
Thomas Usher Gravity Book document TU/6/11 held at the Scottish Brewing Archive.

It's interesting that both the Carlsberg and Tuborg watery Lager was stronger in 1947 than in the 1950s. This against the general trend in beer gravity in the UK over this period.

The Netherlands

Now for some beers from another great source of Lager in the UK, The Netherland:

Dutch-brewed Lager in the UK 1950 - 1963								
Year	**Brewer**	**Beer**	**Price per pint d**	**OG**	**FG**	**ABV**	**App. Atten-uation**	**colour**
1950	Amstel	Lager		1033.6	1008.1	3.31	75.89%	15.5
1957	Amstel	Lager	42	1030.8	1007.2	3.06	76.62%	9.5
1961	Amstel	Amstel Lager	36	1030.9	1006.1	3.10	80.26%	9.5
1957	Amstel	Amstel Lager		1031.9	1006.9	3.24	78.37%	12
1957	Bierbrouwerij De Wereld	Piraat Lager Beer	30	1032.8	1005.7	3.52	82.62%	9
1959	Bierbrouwerij De Wereld	Piraat King Size Ale	27.5	1031.1	1005.6	3.31	81.99%	10

Dutch-brewed Lager in the UK 1950 - 1963								
Year	**Brewer**	**Beer**	**Price per pint d**	**OG**	**FG**	**ABV**	**App. Atten-uation**	**colour**
1950	Breda	Lager (light)		1036.9	1007.8	3.78	78.86%	13.5
1961	Heineken	Lager Beer	36	1030.6	1006.3	3.04	79.41%	4.5
1963	Heineken	Lager	40	1030	1008.4	2.70	72.00%	6
1957	Heineken	Lager	42	1038.7	1009	3.86	76.74%	5
1961	Oranjeboom	Dutch Pilsner	36	1031.1	1006.9	3.02	77.81%	9.5
1963	Oranjeboom	Pilsner Lager	42	1031.6	1005.9	3.21	81.33%	7.5
1957	Oranjeboom	Dutch Lager		1035.4	1007.5	3.62	78.81%	10
1957	Oranjeboom	Dutch Pilsener	42	1033.3	1007.8	3.31	76.58%	9
1947	Z.H.B.	Z.H.B. Lager	30	1032.4	1008.2	3.14	74.07%	11.5
1950	Z.H.B.	Lager		1033.7	1008.4	3.28	75.07%	12
1957	Z.H.B.	Export Pilsner Lager		1032.3	1005.8	3.44	82.04%	13
1957	Z.H.B.	Export Pilsner Lager	42	1031.6	1006.2	3.30	80.38%	10
1961	Z.H.B.	Export Pilsner Lager	37	1032	1005.9	3.26	81.56%	8
	Average		***37.1***	***1032.7***	***1007.0***	***3.3***	***78.44%***	***9.6***

Source:
Whitbread Gravity book held at the London Metropolitan Archives, document number LMA/4453/D/02/002.

One thing is immediately obvious: all these beers were brewed specifically for the UK market. How do I know that? Because they're all way too weak to have been sold in Holland, where Pils is always a standard 5% ABV. They have the typical OG of British Lagers of the period: somewhere in the low 1030°s.

The names are pretty much as you would expect. Heineken, Amstel, Oranjeboom, ZHB. You might not have heard of the last one. It stands for Zuidhollandse Bierbrouwerij, which was a decent-sized brewery in The Hague. It closed in the early 1970s.

Bierbrouwerij De Wereld I'd never heard of. It was located in the village of Raamsdonk in Noord Brabant. The beers in the table can't have been brewed there because the brewery was bought and closed by Oranjeboom in 1948.

The one simply called Breda, must be Drie Hoefijzers. Which in 1968 formed Verenigde Nederlandse Brouwerijen Breda-Rotterdam with Oranjeboom. And which was later taken over by the UK's Allied Breweries.

Germany

Germany was another important source of imported Lager. Holsten would grow into an important UK Lager brand in the 1980s.

German-brewed Lager in the UK 1952 - 1963								
Year	Brewer	Beer	Price per pint d	OG	FG	ABV	App. Atten-uation	colour
1957	Dortmunder Union	Pilsener	47	1042.8	1007.4	4.61	82.71%	8
1963	Dortmunder Union	Pilsner	44	1042	1006.7	4.41	84.05%	9
1952	Dressler	Lager		1051.8	1009.4	5.53	81.85%	6.5
1963	Elbschloss	Ratsherrn Lager	48	1030.5	1006.3	3.03	79.34%	13
1961	Hackerbräu	Hackerbräu Light	66	1051.7	1014.5	4.65	71.95%	8
1957	Holsten	Holsten Pilsner		1044.7	1007.4	4.86	83.45%	8
1957	Holsten	Holsten Pilsner	42	1044.7	1008.2	4.75	81.66%	8
1961	Holsten	Holsten Lager	40	1044.1	1008.1	4.50	81.63%	7
1961	Holsten	Pilsner Lager	40	1045.5	1000.8	5.59	98.24%	7
1963	Holsten	Pilsner	44	1046.1	1006.7	4.92	85.47%	6
1957	Löwenbräu	Pale Bock	51	1061.9	1014.3	6.20	76.90%	6
1961	Patzenhofer	Patz Lager	42	1041	1007.5	4.36	81.71%	7.5
1959	St. Pauli	B.B. Lager		1030.7	1010.3	2.64	66.45%	7
1950	Tucher	Tucher Pils Lager		1055.1	1014.4	5.29	73.87%	15
	Average		***46.4***	***1045.2***	***1008.7***	***4.67***	***80.66%***	***8.3***
Source: Whitbread Gravity book held at the London Metropolitan Archives, document number LMA/4453/D/02/002.								

Norway and Sweden

One surprising name on the source countries for Lager imports was Norway. Though that's perhaps not quite as odd as it might first appear. Norway was very early to the Lager party, being one of the first places outside Central Europe to bottom ferment. There was a very simple reason why: they had endless supplies of natural ice.

Norwegian- and Swedish-brewed Lager in the UK 1955 - 1963								
Year	Brewer	Beer	Price per pint d	OG	FG	ABV	App. Atten-uation	colour
1956	Frydenlund	Peak Lager	30	1034.3	1005.7	3.72	83.38%	12
1959	Frydenlund	Peak Lager		1036.6	1007.5	3.78	79.51%	17
1955	Ringnes	Export Pilsener	48	1053.8	1010.9	5.59	79.74%	11
1957	Ringnes	Export Lager Beer		1052.5	1006.9	5.96	86.86%	13
1957	Ringnes	Export Lager	48	1054.5	1008.8	5.97	83.85%	9.5
1957	Schou	Norwegian Beer		1042.2	1006.6	4.64	84.36%	12
1959	Schou	Norwegian Beer	36	1041.2	1005.5	4.66	86.65%	8.5
1963	Schou	Export Lager	34	1030.4	1003	3.43	90.13%	6
1955	Swedish Beer Export	Three Towns Beer	30	1052.9	1008.7	5.77	83.55%	9
	Average		***37.7***	***1044.3***	***1007.1***	***4.84***	***84.23%***	***11.1***
Source: Whitbread Gravity book held at the London Metropolitan Archives, document number LMA/4453/D/02/002.								

In the days before artificial refrigeration, a supply of natural ice was essential when brewing Lager. The lagering process wasn't possible without it. Which is one of the reasons brewing Lager in earnest didn't kick off in the UK until the 1870s.

Ringnes Export, with an OG of over 1050°, doesn't look like a beer especially brewed for the UK. It's far too strong. Frydenlund Peak Lager, on the other hand, does look like a beer designed to fit the UK market. I'm not sure about the Schou Norwegian Beer. It's somewhere inbetween UK and Continental Lager strength.

Lager Grists

This is fun. I've grist details not just for some British Lagers, but also a couple brewed in The Netherlands for the UK market.

Lager grists 1953 - 1969: malts

Year	Brewer	Beer	OG	lager malt	crystal malt	black malt	amber malt	enzymic malt
1953	Barclay Perkins	Export	1045	72.22%				
1953	Barclay Perkins	Sparkling Beer	1045	70.27%	16.22%			
1953	Barclay Perkins	Dark	1047.8	78.43%	19.61%			
1953	Barclay Perkins	Draught	1034.4	96.55%			3.45%	
1962	Barclay Perkins	Export	1045.5	79.96%				
1962	Barclay Perkins	Harp Lager	1035.5	82.02%				
1962	Barclay Perkins	Sparkling Beer	1045.5	78.06%	10.77%			
1969	Elgood	Lager	1034.3	85.71%				
1959	Lees	Lager	1037	84.96%				
1963	Lees	Lager	1037	72.73%				9.09%
1964	Eldridge Pope	König Lager	1033.5	88.68%				
1969	Truman	LL	1034.6	82.76%				
1956	Amstel	PL	1031.6	87.09%				
1958	Heineken	P Eng	1030.8	94.94%	4.87%	0.19%		

Sources:
Whitbread brewing records held at the London Metropolitan Archives, document numbers ACC/2305/1/648 and ACC/2305/08/276.
Lees brewing record held at the brewery
Derek's 1969 Ale book
Amstel brewing record, document number 1506-555
Heineken brewing record held at the Amsterdamse Stadsarchief, document number 834-1770.

Now there's a shock – the base is always Lager malt. The carahell and kleurmout (in the table as crystal malt and black malt, respectively) in Heineken are more of a surprise. As is the amber malt in Barclay Perkins Draught.

Why can I be so sure that the Amstel and Heineken were for the UK market? Because they're so piss weak. Nowhere else in the world was Pils so weak.

Lager grists 1953 - 1969: adjuncts								
Year	Brewer	Beer	OG	flaked maize	grits	roast barley	flaked barley	flaked rice
1953	Barclay Perkins	Export	1045	5.56%	22.22%			
1953	Barclay Perkins	Sparkling Beer	1045	2.70%	10.81%			
1953	Barclay Perkins	Dark	1047.8			1.96%		
1953	Barclay Perkins	Draught	1034.4					
1962	Barclay Perkins	Export	1045.5		19.99%			
1962	Barclay Perkins	Harp Lager	1035.5	17.83%				
1962	Barclay Perkins	Sparkling Beer	1045.5	10.77%				
1969	Elgood	Lager	1034.3					9.52%
1959	Lees	Lager	1037					5.31%
1963	Lees	Lager	1037					9.09%
1964	Eldridge Pope	König Lager	1033.5					7.55%
1969	Truman	LL	1034.6				10.34%	
1956	Amstel	PL	1031.6					
1958	Heineken	P Eng	1030.8					

All of the UK-brewed Lagers, except for Barclay Perkins Draught, contained an adjunct of some sort. In variety of forms, though most of it was flaked. Though Barclay Perkins used grits in some of theirs.

Lager grists 1953 - 1969: sugars									
Year	Brewer	Beer	no. 1 sugar	Sol-prima	P.S. crystals	cane	malt extract	cara-mel	other sugar
1953	Barclay Perkins	Export							
1953	Barclay Perkins	Sparkling Beer							
1953	Barclay Perkins	Dark							
1953	Barclay Perkins	Draught							
1962	Barclay Perkins	Export						0.05%	
1962	Barclay Perkins	Harp Lager						0.15%	
1962	Barclay Perkins	Sparkling Beer						0.40%	
1969	Elgood	Lager		3.17%			1.59%		
1959	Lees	Lager	7.08%	2.65%					
1963	Lees	Lager		3.03%	6.06%				
1964	Eldridge Pope	König Lager							3.77%
1969	Truman	LL				6.90%			
1956	Amstel	PL							12.91%
1958	Heineken	P Eng							

The Barclay Perkins beers from 1953 and Heineken are the only examples to contain no sugar of any kind. Heineken, weirdly enough, is the only Reinheitsgebot compliant beer. I've no idea what Solprima is, but it only seems to turn up in Lager.

IV Recipes

Introduction to recipes

A couple of remarks before you dive into the recipes.

These recipes have been written using original brewing records as the source. The level of detail on old brewing logs varies greatly. Some are a bit vague. Many miss out completely vital pieces of information.

How have I coped with missing information? I'll be honest: I've guessed. Not just random guesses, but ones based on other sources, such as brewing manuals. Or later brewing records from the same brewery. It's not perfect, but it's the best that can be done.

Virtually no logs have any record of the hop additions. With the exception of some 20th-century Barclay Perkins logs. All the other hop additions listed in these recipes are a guesstimate. Feel free to tinker with them as suits you.

The ingredients, mashing details, OG and FG are always taken from the original brewing records.

Care should be taken with the quantity of hops used. I've reduces original quantities, to take into account the age of the hops. I've used a slightly rough and ready method – rounding down a bit, or in cases with really old hops, a lot.

In 20th-century recipes, the sugars are a problem. Brewers used a whole range of different sugars, many of them proprietary brands. I'm not sure if exact equivalents are available at all today, let alone to home brewers.

Hops are rather simpler. Where it says EK or MK, you can't go far wrong with Goldings and Fuggles, respectively. Cluster is best for anything called American, Oregon, Californian or Pacific.

All the recipes are for 6 US, 5 Imperial, gallons. Or 23 litres, if you're all modern. And 72% efficiency.

1946 Adnams XX Mild

1948 wasn't a great year for Mild drinkers. Most of those available were pretty watery. Gravities under 1030° were common.

Adnams XX is a good example of these very low-gravity beers. On the other hand, it does at least have an interesting grist. Containing both crystal and amber malt. There's only a small amount of adjuncts in the form of flaked barley (that's a wartime thing) plus some No. 3 invert. For once, I haven't had to make any substitutions. Well other, than caramel 1000 SRM for Tintose. But that's obviously a type of caramel as the quantity used is so small.

The hops are English. The log has no further details. I've plumped for the good old Fuggles and Goldings combination.

The original mashing scheme includes an underlet, which raised the temperature to 150° F.

1946 Adnams XX		
mild malt	4.25 lb	73.15%
amber malt	0.33 lb	5.68%
crystal malt 60 L	0.33 lb	5.68%
flaked barley	0.33 lb	5.68%
No. 3 invert sugar	0.50 lb	8.61%
Caramel 1000 SRM	0.07 lb	1.20%
Fuggles 120 mins	0.75 oz	
Goldings 30 min	0.25 oz	
OG	1027	
FG	1005.5	
ABV	2.84	
Apparent attenuation	79.63%	
IBU	15	
SRM	13	
Mash at	148° F	
Sparge at	170° F	
Boil time	120 minutes	
pitching temp	59° F	
Yeast	WLP025 Southwold	

1946 Adnams PA

Times were happier for Bitter drinkers, who at least got something over 3% ABV.

The recipe is just about as simple as they got: base malt with a little bit of sugar and flaked barley. It doesn't leave a great deal to discuss.

The hops were exactly the same as in XX. I've guessed that it was dry hopped as most Bitters were. The logs, sadly, make no mention of dry hopping.

An underlet raised the temperature of the mash to 151° F.

1946 Adnams PA		
pale malt	3.25 lb	40.63%
mild malt	3.75 lb	46.88%
flaked barley	0.50 lb	6.25%
No. 1 invert sugar	0.50 lb	6.25%
Fuggles 120 mins	1.75 oz	
Goldings 30 mins	0.50 oz	
Goldings dry hops	0.25 oz	
OG	1036	
FG	1009	
ABV	3.57	
Apparent attenuation	75.00%	
IBU	32	
SRM	4.5	
Mash at	149° F	
Sparge at	170° F	
Boil time	120 minutes	
pitching temp	58.5° F	
Yeast	WLP025 Southwold	

1946 Adnams DS

Most breweries still produced their own Stout after WW II. They varied in style. Many were of the sweet, lactose-ridden type. Others were more like traditional Stouts, just lower in gravity. DS is an example of the latter.

The grist is reasonably complex, with chocolate and crystal malt in addition to black malt. Plus some No.3 invert and caramel.

The hops are identical to the other beers, but split 50-50 this time.

An underlet raised the mash temperature to 150° F.

1946 Adnams DS		
mild malt	7.00 lb	75.68%
black malt	0.50 lb	5.41%
chocolate malt	0.50 lb	5.41%
crystal malt 60 L	0.50 lb	5.41%
No. 3 invert sugar	0.50 lb	5.41%
caramel 1000 SRM	0.25 lb	2.70%
Fuggles 120 mins	1.00 oz	
Goldings 30 mins	1.00 oz	
OG	1039	
FG	1012.5	
ABV	3.51	
Apparent attenuation	67.95%	
IBU	26	
SRM	32	
Mash at	148° F	
Sparge at	170° F	
Boil time	120 minutes	
pitching temp	58.5° F	
Yeast	WLP025 Southwold	

1951 Adnams XXXX

One of my favourite types of beer is a good old Southern Old Ale. Which is basically just a strong Mild.

The details might have changed a little, but Adnams still brew an Old Ale similar to this. Simply a beefed up version of their Mild. The grist is much the same a XX Mild. Just with a little more of everything.

Adnams have continued to brew a draught beer in this style right up until the present. The OG is a bit lower, but it's definitely still along these lines.

1951 Adnams XXXX		
mild malt	9.75 lb	84.20%
amber malt	0.50 lb	4.32%
crystal malt 80 L	0.50 lb	4.32%
No. 3 invert sugar	0.75 lb	6.48%
caramel 1000 SRM	0.08 lb	0.69%
Fuggles 120 min	2.00 oz	
Goldings 30 min	0.75 oz	
OG	1053	
FG	1017.5	
ABV	4.70	
Apparent attenuation	66.98%	
IBU	35	
SRM	16	
Mash at	148º F	
Sparge at	170º F	
Boil time	120 minutes	
pitching temp	59º F	
Yeast	WLP025 Southwold	

1953 Adnams Tally Ho

Named beers – ones without generic names like Bloggs Bitter – are mostly aa fairly recent phenomenon. Tally Ho, which dates back to at least 1879, is a notable exception.

It's also a beer that is still around today. There's real longevity. It hasn't even changed all that much in terms of strength, which also makes it an oddity. Another odd thing about Tally Ho is that it sometimes appeared on draught. Mostly beers of this strength were only available in bottled form

It's basically a beefed up version of their XX Mild Ale and XXXX Old Ale. The grist contains all the same ingredients: medium malt (which I've interpreted as mild malt), amber malt, crystal malt, No. 3 invert sugar and a bit of caramel.

As always, the hop varieties are a guess, A pretty conservative one and Fuggles and Golding accounted for around 75% of UK-grown hops at the time.

1953 Adnams Tally Ho		
mild malt	13.00 lb	75.76%
amber malt	1.25 lb	7.28%
crystal malt 80 L	1.25 lb	7.28%
no. 3 invert sugar	1.50 lb	8.74%
caramel	0.16 lb	0.93%
Fuggles 120 min	1.50 oz	
Fuggles 60 min	1.50 oz	
Goldings 30 min	1.50 oz	
Goldings dry hops	0.25 oz	
OG	1080	
FG	1016.1	
ABV	8.45	
Apparent attenuation	79.88%	
IBU	47	
SRM	32	
Mash at	150º F	
Sparge at	170º F	
Boil time	120 minutes	
pitching temp	58º F	
Yeast	WLP025 Southwold	

1958 Adnams LBA

Every brewery had a bottled Light Ale in the 1950s. It wasn't just a standard beer behind the bar, it was an essential one.

Important for breweries, because bottled beer was in vogue. And it was more profitable. Yes, it cost more to produce, but drinkers were prepared to pay quite a premium for it. That's why breweries were mad keen on promoting bottled beer. They made more money on it. And they had far more control about what condition it reached the consumer in.

A light simple Pale Ale. Intended for slurping, rather than sipping.

1958 Adnams LBA		
pale malt	5.75 lb	85.19%
No. 1 invert sugar	1.00 lb	14.81%
Fuggles 120 min	0.50 oz	
Fuggles 60 min	0.50 oz	
Goldings 30 min	0.50 oz	
OG	1032	
FG	1008	
ABV	3.18	
Apparent attenuation	75.00%	
IBU	20	
SRM	4.5	
Mash at	143° F	
Sparge at	170° F	
Boil time	120 minutes	
pitching temp	60° F	
Yeast	WLP025 Southwold	

1959 Adnams PA

Adnams draught Bitter hasn't changed a great deal since 1950. It's recognisably the same beer.

It has dropped two gravity points. And there's a touch of mild malt in addition to the pale malt. But the grist is still the very simple combination of base malt and sugar. I've simplified the sugar a little, the original also contained 124 lbs of Hydrol and 2.5 lbs of sucramel. Not having the faintest idea what either of those are, I've just bumped up the quantity of No. 1 invert.

The hops were English (1957, 1958) and Styrian (1958). Not exactly complicated a lot of these old Bitter recipes.

1959 Adnams PA		
pale malt	5.00 lb	71.43%
mild malt	0.75 lb	10.71%
No. 1 invert sugar	1.25 lb	17.86%
Styrian Goldings 95 mins	0.75 oz	
Fuggles 60 mins	0.75 oz	
Goldings 30 mins	0.75 oz	
Goldings dry hops	0.25 oz	
OG	1034	
FG	1011	
ABV	3.04	
Apparent attenuation	67.65%	
IBU	33	
SRM	5	
Mash at	151° F	
Sparge at	179° F	
Boil time	95 minutes	
pitching temp	60.5° F	
Yeast	WLP025 Southwold	

1959 Adnams XXX

It's May, the weather is wonderful – what could be more appealing than a nice watery 1950's Mild?

And this version of Adnams XXX Mild, at under 3% ABV, is certainly pretty watery. Though perhaps not quite as watery as it looks. I have a Whitbread Gravity Book analysis for Adnams Mild from 1967 and that lists the OG as 1033.5°. Yet a brewing record from the same year gives the OG as 1031°.

Why the discrepancy? Probably because of primings. Most breweries don't bother listing them in the brewing record. When they do, 2° or 3° is typical for the gravity boost primings give to a beer of this gravity. Primings probably account for the difference between the calculated colour and the one given in the analysis, which is around 20 SRM.

To simulate this, you could add another 0.5 lb of No. 3 invert at racking time. That should get you somewhere near the colour and effective OG.

It's surprising how different this recipe is from 1950 XX. The earlier beer contained amber malt and caramel, but no pale malt.

I know little about the hops, other than that they were English and from the 1957 and 1958 harvests.

1959 Adnams XXX		
mild malt	3.75 lb	57.69%
pale malt	0.75 lb	11.54%
crystal malt 80L	0.75 lb	11.54%
No. 3 invert sugar	1.25 lb	19.23%
Fuggles 95 mins	0.50 oz	
Fuggles 60 mins	0.50 oz	
Goldings 30 mins	0.25 oz	
OG	1030	
FG	1008	
ABV	2.91	
Apparent attenuation	73.33%	
IBU	20	
SRM	13	
Mash at	150° F	
Sparge at	170° F	
Boil time	95 minutes	
pitching temp	60.5° F	
Yeast	WLP025 Southwold	

1959 Adnams XXXX

There's a tradition in the South of England of having draught Old Ale as a winter special. But a specific type of Old Ale. One that's really a type of strong Mild.

The recipe for XXXX is certainly very similar to that of XXX. The only real differences are that XXXX has all mild malt as base and has 1 cwt. of something called Hydrol. No idea what that is, so I've just bumped up the amount of No. 3 invert.

The recipe has changed a little since 1949. The amber malt has been dropped and the gravity is 7 points lower.

The hops were all English from the 1957 and 1958 crops.

Adnams still brew an Old Ale which is very similar to this beer. I had a few pints of it in the Lord Nelson on my only visit to Southwold. Lovely stuff, when on form.

1959 Adnams XXXX		
mild malt	6.75 lb	69.23%
crystal malt 80L	1.75 lb	17.95%
No. 3 invert sugar	1.25 lb	12.82%
Fuggles 125 mins	1.00 oz	
Goldings 30 mins	1.00 oz	
OG	1046	
FG	1014.5	
ABV	4.17	
Apparent attenuation	68.48%	
IBU	27	
SRM	18	
Mash at	150° F	
Sparge at	170° F	
Boil time	125 minutes	
pitching temp	60° F	
Yeast	WLP025 Southwold	

1959 Adnams DS Stout

There have been considerable changes to DS since 1950. Both in terms of recipe and strength.

The biggest change to the grist is the dropping of amber malt and replacing black malt with chocolate malt. Also dropped is the caramel. Which explains why this version is a good bit paler in colour.

The gravity is three points lower than in 1950. Can you really call a beer of just 1037° a Stout? I guess you must, as there were plenty of beers like this in the 1950s.

Not much to report about the hops, except that they were all English.

1959 Adnams DS Stout		
pale malt	1.25 lb	15.15%
mild malt	4.25 lb	51.52%
chocolate malt	0.75 lb	9.09%
crystal malt 80 L	1.25 lb	15.15%
No. 3 invert sugar	0.75 lb	9.09%
Fuggles 110 mins	0.75 oz	
Fuggles 60 mins	0.50 oz	
Goldings 30 mins	0.50 oz	
OG	1037	
FG	1011.5	
ABV	3.37	
Apparent attenuation	68.92%	
IBU	25	
SRM	27	
Mash at	148° F	
Sparge at	170° F	
Boil time	110 minutes	
pitching temp	60° F	
Yeast	WLP025 Southwold	

1965 Adnams XXX

Judging by the number of entries in the brewing book, Adnams Mild was still a popular beer in 1965. Though it may already have been overtaken by Bitter in terms of sales.

The recipe hasn't changed a huge amount. There's rather more base malt and less crystal and sugar, but it's not an enormous difference. And there's been a change in the proprietary sugar, from Hydrol to Laevuline. Not that that helps you much as I'm pretty sure neither of those is available commercially.

The OG is a tiny bit higher and the attenuation better, leaving a beer that just scrapes over 3% ABV.

1965 Adnams XXX		
mild malt	5.00 lb	76.92%
crystal malt 80L	0.50 lb	7.69%
No. 3 invert sugar	1.00 lb	15.38%
Fuggles 90 mins	0.75 oz	
Fuggles 60 mins	0.50 oz	
Goldings 30 mins	0.25 oz	
OG	1031	
FG	1008	
ABV	3.04	
Apparent attenuation	74.19%	
IBU	24	
SRM	11	
Mash at	140° F	
Sparge at	170° F	
Boil time	90 minutes	
pitching temp	59° F	
Yeast	WLP025 Southwold	

1965 Adnams BB

I'm assuming BB stands for Best Bitter. That's how it usually works. Oh. And I have an analysis from the Daily Mirror in 1970 for Adnams Best Bitter at about the same OG.

Not much to discuss with the grist. It really was that simple. There was a small amount of something called sucramel, but the vast bulk really was No. invert sugar.

As so often, I've had to guess the hop varieties, knowing nothing more than that they. I've plumped for the classics. Other English hop varieties of the period are available.

1965 Adnams BB		
pale malt	6.75 lb	85.71%
enzymic malt	0.125 lb	1.59%
No. 1 invert sugar	1.00 lb	12.70%
Fuggles 60 mins	1.25 oz	
Goldings 30 mins	1.00 oz	
Goldings dry hops	0.25 oz	
OG	1037	
FG	1009.5	
ABV	3.64	
Apparent attenuation	74.32%	
IBU	29	
SRM	5	
Mash at	141° F	
Sparge at	170° F	
Boil time	60 minutes	
pitching temp	59° F	
Yeast	WLP025 Southwold	

1966 Adnams LBA

In 1965, Adnams appear to have only brewed five beers: Mild, Bitter, Stout, Tally Ho! and LBA. That's a bit of a guess about Tally Ho!, as I managed to miss it when I was photographing their 1960s records. Easily done when a beer is only brewed occasionally. Though, presumably, they bottled the Mild as Brown Ale.

Just has a look at some analyse of Adnams beers. It looks like they continued to brew their Old ale, XXXX, both in bottled and draught form. Must have missed that one, too.

As their Light Ale, LBA would have been only available bottled. It's really just a weaker, bottled version of their Best Bitter.

1966 Adnams LBA		
pale malt	5.75 lb	83.64%
enzymic malt	0.125 lb	1.82%
No. 1 invert sugar	1.00 lb	14.55%
Fuggles 60 mins	1.00 oz	
Goldings 30 mins	0.75 oz	
OG	1033	
FG	1008	
ABV	3.31	
Apparent attenuation	75.76%	
IBU	24	
SRM	5	
Mash at	142° F	
Sparge at	170° F	
Boil time	90 minutes	
pitching temp	61° F	
Yeast	WLP025 Southwold	

1965 Adnams DS Stout

Adnams not only continued to brew a Stout as a non piss-weak gravity, the OG even increased a little. One point, admittedly. But better than nothing

I know from the good old Whitbread Gravity Book that there was no lactose in the 1961 version. I'm assuming there was none added here, too. There's a decent level of bitterness and the degree of attenuation isn't too crazily low. Not stupidly sweet. And, at a touch over 3% ABV, just about intoxicating.

It's not the darkest of Stouts so there may have been some caramel colour correction. I'll leave that up to you.

1965 Adnams DS Stout		
mild malt	5.50 lb	64.71%
chocolate malt	0.75 lb	8.82%
crystal malt 80 L	1.25 lb	14.71%
No. 3 invert sugar	1.00 lb	11.76%
Fuggles 125 mins	1.25 oz	
Goldings 30 mins	1.00 oz	
OG	1038	
FG	1015	
ABV	3.04	
Apparent attenuation	60.53%	
IBU	32	
SRM	28	
Mash at	140° F	
Sparge at	170° F	
Boil time	125 minutes	
pitching temp	59° F	
Yeast	WLP025 Southwold	

1946 Barclay Perkins IPA

Bored of watery Milds? Here's a watery IPA to balance things out.

Not that Barclay's IPA had ever been that strong. Even in the 1920's it only had an OG of around 1045º, which, at the time, was only very slightly above average OG.

The effect of the war is clear to see in the grist. Like most UK breweries, Barclays had used flaked maize in their beers after this became legal in 1880. The only times they didn't, was when it wasn't possible. Basically, at certain points during the two World Wars.

Maize wasn't available for most of WW II and breweries were instructed to replace it with flaked barley. In addition to that, there's pale malt and crystal malt, as you might expect, but also No. 3 invert sugar. That's usually reserved for dark beers. Things like Mild Ale and Stout. Pale Ales usually contained either No. 1 or No. 2 invert.

There are four different copper hops: Mid-Kent Fuggles (1943, 1944 CS), Mid-Kent Goldings (1945), Mid-Kent Colgates (1944), plus East Kent Goldings (1945) dry hops. Though the Colgates are a guess. It just says "C's" in the brewing record. One of the things I really like about Barclays brewing records is that they can be bothered to say what the hop variety was, not just where they were grown.

As with Whitbread's, this IPA was an exclusively bottled beer.

1946 Barclay Perkins IPA		
pale malt	5.55 lb	78.72%
crystal malt 60 L	0.50 lb	7.09%
flaked barley	0.25 lb	3.55%
No. 3 invert sugar	0.75 lb	10.64%
Fuggles 90 min	0.75 oz	
Fuggles 60 min	0.75 oz	
Goldings 30 min	0.75 oz	
Goldings dry hops	0.50 oz	
OG	1031.5	
FG	1009	
ABV	2.98	
Apparent attenuation	71.43%	
IBU	31	
SRM	9	
Mash at	151º F	
Sparge at	165º F	
Boil time	90 minutes	
pitching temp	61º F	
Yeast	Wyeast 1099 Whitbread Ale	

1946 Barclay Perkins XLK

Ever since the 1880s, XLK had been Barclay Perkins Ordinary Bitter. Though, obviously, the gravity had dropped a bit over the year. Quite a lot, actually.

The initial version had the impressive OG of 1053°. Though to put that into context, their weakest Mild Ale was 1055° at the time.

The grist is relatively simple: base malt, crystal malt and sugar. Whit's listed below as mild malt was actually SA malt. I'm quite surprised at the type of sugar used: No. 3. I'd have expected No. 1 or No. 2. No. 3 was usually reserved for dark beers.

Some of the hops are just described as "Bs". I've interpreted this as Bramling Cross. I could be wrong. I suppose they could be Brewers' Gold, too. The other hops, described as "Fs", I'm pretty certain are Fuggles.

1946 Barclay Perkins XLK		
pale malt	3.75 lb	54.82%
mild malt	1.75 lb	25.58%
crystal malt 60 L	0.67 lb	9.80%
No. 3 invert sugar	0.67 lb	9.80%
Bramling Cross 90 mins	0.50 oz	
Bramling Cross 75 mins	0.50 oz	
Fuggles 60 mins	0.50 oz	
Fuggles 30 mins	0.50 oz	
Goldings dry hops	0.50 oz	
OG	1031.5	
FG	1008	
ABV	3.11	
Apparent attenuation	74.60%	
IBU	33	
SRM	9	
Mash at	151° F	
Sparge at	165° F	
Boil time	90 minutes	
pitching temp	60.5° F	
Yeast	Wyeast 1099 Whitbread Ale	

1947 Barclay Perkins PA (bottling)

I've a strong suspicion that this was a replacement for or a renaming of IPA. The two beers have similar gravities and were both available exclusively in bottled form.

Whether that's true or not, both beers occupied the same style slot: Light Ale. Though that's a term that seems to have been rarely used inside breweries. Most of the beers that would have been ordered as Light Ale in the pub were called something else in the brewhouse.

There are a couple of significant differences with the grist of IPA: there's no crystal malt and the No. 3 invert has been replaced by No. 1 invert. Unsurprisingly, given the recipe changes, bottling PA is a good bit paler.

Another change is in the level of hopping, which was a good bit higher in IPA. That's reflected in the lower IBU number here. The hops were all reasonably fresh, being EK Goldings (1945), Styrian (1945) and Worcester Goldings (1945). As this brew was in early January 1947, the hops weren't as old as they might appear on first glance.

Bottling PA also wasn't dry hopped as IPA had been. Overall, it must have been a much less hop-accented beer.

1947 Barclay Perkins PA (bottling)			
pale malt		6.25 lb	86.21%
flaked maize		0.50 lb	6.90%
No. 1 invert sugar		0.50 lb	6.90%
Styrian Goldings 90 mins		0.50 oz	
Goldings 60 mins		0.50 oz	
Goldings 30 mins		0.50 oz	
OG		1032.5	
FG		1006.5	
ABV		3.44	
Apparent attenuation		80.00%	
IBU		23	
SRM		4	
Mash at		150° F	
Sparge at		165° F	
Boil time		90 minutes	
pitching temp		60.5° F	
Yeast	Wyeast 1099 Whitbread Ale		

1947 Barclay Perkins PA export

A real surprise is finding a pretty much full-strength Pale Ale at the height of austerity. Such a shame that none of it was going to be drunk in Britain.

Because this is surely a beer destined for foreign markets. The name sort of gives that away. Plus it was brewed in a tiny batch. A mere 20 barrels and not parti-gyled. Obviously, it was brewed on their small kit.

1947 Barclay Perkins PA export		
pale malt	11.50 lb	92.00%
No. 1 invert sugar	1.00 lb	8.00%
Bramling Cross 90 mins	1.50 oz	
Goldings 60 mins	1.50 oz	
Goldings 30 mins	1.50 oz	
Goldings dry hops	0.50 oz	
OG	1055.5	
FG	1021.5	
ABV	4.50	
Apparent attenuation	61.26%	
IBU	63	
SRM	6	
Mash at	150º F	
Sparge at	165º F	
Boil time	150 minutes	
pitching temp	58º F	
Yeast	Wyeast 1099 Whitbread Ale	

1946 Barclay Perkins KK (trade)

If you're wondering what "trade" is all about, it means that this is the draught version of KK, known as Burton down the pub. There was also a bottling version, which was sold as Southwarke Olde Ale.

If you flick forward a couple of recipes, you'll see that the recipe is almost identical to that of XX Mild. The only difference is that while that has its base malt split between mild malt and SA malt, while KK used pale malt and SA malt, interpreted here as mild malt.

It looks like a beer that I'd like to drink myself: a sort of strong, hoppy Dark Mild. Yum.

1946 Barclay Perkins KK (trade)		
pale malt	3.25 lb	35.93%
mild malt	3.00 lb	33.17%
amber malt	0.50 lb	5.53%
crystal malt 60 L	0.67 lb	7.41%
flaked barley	0.50 lb	5.53%
No. 3 invert sugar	1.00 lb	11.06%
caramel 1000 SRM	0.125 lb	1.38%
Bramling Cross 90 mins	0.75 oz	
Fuggles 75 mins	0.75 oz	
Goldings 60 mins	0.75 oz	
Goldings 30 mins	0.75 oz	
Goldings dry hops	0.50 oz	
OG	1042.5	
FG	1014	
ABV	3.77	
Apparent attenuation	67.06%	
IBU	44	
SRM	18	
Mash at	150° F	
Sparge at	165° F	
Boil time	90 minutes	
pitching temp	60° F	
Yeast	Wyeast 1099 Whitbread Ale	

1946 Barclay Perkins KK (bottling)

Here's the bottling version of KK which I just mentioned. Considering it bears the same name, it's surprisingly different. It wasn't branded as Burton, however, being sold under the name of Southwark Olde Ale.

The grist contains no amber malt and the sugar in No. 1 rather than No. 3. Though the brewing record does have "3" crossed out, replaced with a red "1". Was that a mistake or a recipe change? The other photos I have of this beer aren't much help. One lists No. 3, the other No. 1.

Another big difference with the draught version is the lack of dry hops. This isn't unusual. Bottled beers often lacked the draught version's dry hops. There are more copper hops, however. 8.85 lbs per quarter of malt as opposed to 8.35 lbs. Not a massive difference, but I'm sure it's no mistake.

It may look modest today, but 1047.5° was a pretty huge OG in 1946.

1946 Barclay Perkins KK (bottling)		
pale malt	7.75 lb	74.70%
crystal malt	0.50 lb	4.82%
flaked barley	0.50 lb	4.82%
No. 1 invert sugar	1.50 lb	14.46%
caramel 1000 SRM	0.125 lb	1.20%
Bramling Cross 90 mins	1.00 oz	
Fuggles 75 mins	1.00 oz	
Fuggles 60 mins	1.00 oz	
Goldings 30 mins	1.00 oz	
OG	1047.5	
FG	1018	
ABV	3.90	
Apparent attenuation	62.11%	
IBU	55	
SRM	15	
Mash at	152° F	
Sparge at	165° F	
Boil time	90 minutes	
pitching temp	60° F	
Yeast	Wyeast 1099 Whitbread Ale	

1946 Barclay Perkins IBS (Scotland)

A great example of how austerity affected beer styles is this rather watery version of Russian Stout. Especially brewed for the Scottish market.

A combination of a puny OG and very poor rate of attenuation leave under 3.5% ABV. Not exactly powerful for an Imperial Stout. Though the true FG was almost certainly lower. What's shown in the recipe is the racking gravity and there was probably some secondary conditioning after that.

The very high percentage of dark grains – almost a third of the grist – probably didn't help with the attenuation. But must have resulted in quite a rich beer, which probably drank above its strength. Though I doubt it would have fooled anyone into thinking it was a full-strength Imperial Stout.

I've increased the quantity of No. 3 Invert sugar to allow for the primings added at racking time.

1946 Barclay Perkins IBS (Scotland)			
pale malt		2.75 lb	28.71%
mild malt		2.75 lb	28.71%
brown malt		1.00 lb	10.44%
amber malt		1.00 lb	10.44%
roast barley		1.00 lb	10.44%
No. 3 invert sugar		0.75 lb	7.83%
caramel 1000 SRM		0.33 lb	3.44%
Bramling Cross 90 mins		1.50 oz	
Goldings 30 mins		1.50 oz	
OG		1045.5	
FG		1019	
ABV		3.51	
Apparent attenuation		58.24%	
IBU		43	
SRM		38	
Mash at		150° F	
Sparge at		165° F	
Boil time		90 minutes	
pitching temp		60.5° F	
Yeast	Wyeast 1099 Whitbread Ale		

1946 Barclay Perkins BS

It's surprising just how many Stouts Barclay Perkins were still churning out in 1947. None of them particularly stout.

One thing they all have in common is a very high percentage of roast grains. In this case 25% of the grist. The amount of roast barley is particularly large at 11%. I'm going to go out on a limb here and say that BS must have been pretty roasty.

Very heavy priming – I gallon per barrel – raises the effective OG by three points. I've increased the quantity of No. 3 Invert sugar to account for this.

The hops aren't the freshest, so I've knocked down the rate a little. MK Fuggles (1945), MK Goldings (1944) and EK Goldings (1945) with EKG dry hops (1946).

1946 Barclay Perkins BS		
mild malt	5.25 lb	59.46%
brown malt	0.75 lb	8.49%
amber malt	0.50 lb	5.66%
crystal malt 60 L	0.50 lb	5.66%
roast barley	1.00 lb	11.33%
No. 3 invert sugar	0.50 lb	5.66%
caramel 1000 SRM	0.33 lb	3.74%
Fuggles 90 mins	0.50 oz	
Fuggles 75 mins	0.50 oz	
Goldings 60 mins	0.50 oz	
Goldings 30 mins	0.50 oz	
Goldings dry hops	1.00 oz	
OG	1041	
FG	1015	
ABV	3.44	
Apparent attenuation	63.41%	
IBU	28	
SRM	39	
Mash at	149° F	
Sparge at	165° F	
Boil time	90 minutes	
pitching temp	60° F	
Yeast	Wyeast 1099 Whitbread Ale	

1946 Barclay Perkins LS

Even less stout than BS was the LS (London Stout) parti-gyled with it. It doesn't even break 3% ABV.

London Stout was Barclay's draught Stout, something that was still reasonably common at this point in London pubs. It would look even punier, were it not for the gallon of primings per cask. They bump up the effective OG by three points.

1946 Barclay Perkins LS			
mild malt		4.00 lb	55.17%
brown malt		0.67 lb	9.24%
amber malt		0.33 lb	4.55%
crystal malt 60 L		0.25 lb	3.45%
roast barley		0.75 lb	10.34%
No. 3 invert sugar		1.00 lb	13.79%
caramel 1000 SRM		0.25 lb	3.45%
Fuggles 90 mins		0.33 oz	
Fuggles 75 mins		0.33 oz	
Goldings 60 mins		0.33 oz	
Goldings 30 mins		0.33 oz	
Goldings dry hops		1.00 oz	
OG		1032.5	
FG		1010	
ABV		2.98	
Apparent attenuation		69.23%	
IBU		20	
SRM		35	
Mash at		149° F	
Sparge at		165° F	
Boil time		90 minutes	
pitching temp		60° F	
Yeast	Wyeast 1099 Whitbread Ale		

1947 Barclay Perkins Victory Stout

1947 wasn't a great year for British brewing. Gravities were still falling, despite the war being over.

Which explains why Barclay Perkins had a Stout that was under 3% ABV. How ironic that such a feeble beer was called Victory Stout. Though the primings would have raised the effective OG to 1037°

Though, with all dark malts it probably drank heavier than it really was. The grist is anything but simple, with five different grains. I'm slightly disturbed by the low percentage of base malt, not much more than a third of the grist. In the original, it's three-quarters SA malt, a quarter mild malt. As I doubt you'll be able to buy SA malt, I've specified all mild malt. It's probably about the closest equivalent.

The hops were all from Kent, Mid-Kent Fuggles (1946), East Kent Tolhursts (1946), Mid-Kent BG (1946) and Kent Fuggles (1945). All pretty fresh then, leaving quite a bitter beer. All that roast barley would have made it taste even more bitter.

I'm really intrigued as to how this beer would taste. Loads of dark malt, quite heavily hopped, but with quite a lot of residual sugar, too. Weak and bitter. Probably how a lot of Britons were feeling in 1947.

1947 Barclay Perkins Victory Stout		
mild malt	2.75 lb	37.52%
brown malt	0.75 lb	10.23%
amber malt	0.50 lb	6.82%
crystal malt 60 L	0.50 lb	6.82%
roast barley	1.00 lb	13.64%
No. 3 invert sugar	1.50 lb	20.46%
caramel 1000 SRM	0.33 lb	4.50%
Fuggles 90 min	1.00 oz	
Fuggles 60 min	1.00 oz	
Goldings 30 min	1.00 oz	
OG	1034	
FG	1014	
ABV	2.65	
Apparent attenuation	58.82%	
IBU	43	
SRM	39	
Mash at	147° F	
Sparge at	165° F	
Boil time	90 minutes	
pitching temp	61° F	
Yeast	Wyeast 1099 Whitbread Ale	

1947 Barclay Perkins XX

The late 1940s weren't the best time to be a Mild drinker. At least if you wanted to get pissed. Watery was the key word.

Though there are some rather interesting recipes. Like XX, for example. Rather than being coloured up solely with sugar, there are two coloured malt: crystal and amber. The real grist was even more complicated than it appears in the recipe, as two-thirds of what is listed as mild malt was really SA malt.

The hops were a combination of Mid-Kent Fuggles from the 1945 and 1946 crop and Mid-Kent Tolhursts from 1944.

To account for the primings, which raised the effective OG by three points at racking time, I've added more No. 3 Invert sugar.

1947 Barclay Perkins XX			
mild malt		5.00 lb	68.97%
amber malt		0.33 lb	4.55%
crystal malt 60 L		0.50 lb	6.90%
flaked barley		0.33 lb	4.55%
No. 3 invert sugar		1.00 lb	13.79%
caramel 1000 SRM		0.09 lb	1.24%
Fuggles 75 min		0.50 oz	
Fuggles 60 min		0.50 oz	
Fuggles 30 min		0.50 oz	
OG		1033.5	
FG		1009	
ABV		3.24	
Apparent attenuation		73.13%	
IBU		21	
SRM		15	
Mash at		149° F	
Sparge at		165° F	
Boil time		75 minutes	
pitching temp		60.5° F	
Yeast	Wyeast 1099 Whitbread Ale		

1954 Barclay Perkins Sparkling Beer

Barclay Perkins took the plunge into Lager brewing immediately after the end of WW I. In the interwar years, it was one of only six UK breweries that produced Lager. The others were the Alloa Brewery, Jeffreys, Red Tower, Tennant and the Wrexham Lager Brewery. Of those, only Red Tower was in England (Manchester).

Of the several Lagers that Barclay Perkins brewed, Sparkling Beer was the oddest. Introduced just before WW II, it seems to have been exclusively brewed for export. Much seems to have been consumed either by the military or aboard ships. It was also one of the first beers to be canned.

It's difficult to say what style it's meant to be. The label makes no mention of the fact it's a Lager. Based on its amber colour, I guess you could call it a Vienna Lager.

Barclay Perkins certainly went the whole hog when brewing Lager, employing a complicated mashing scheme with multiple rests. Interestingly, their Lagers were their only beers to contain grits. They usually used flaked maize. The grist is pretty simple with, in addition to the grits, just pilsner malt and crystal malt.

East Kent Goldings may seem an odd choice of hops for a Lager. They did sometimes use a mixture of Goldings and Saaz, but I know from earlier brewing records that Saaz were double the price of Goldings.

In addition to the main mash, there was also a cereal mash for the grits:

mash in	122° F	stand 20 minutes
raise to	154° F	stand 20 minutes
boil	212° F	for 5 minutes

Main mash:

mash in	122° F	
raise to	154° F	stand 30 minutes
raise with grits to	168° F	
hold at	168° F	45 minutes
Sparge at	165° F	

1954 Barclay Perkins Sparkling Beer		
pilsner malt	7.50 lb	71.29%
crystal malt 60 L	1.50 lb	14.26%
grits	1.50 lb	14.26%
caramel 1000 SRM	0.02 lb	0.19%
Goldings 120 mins	1.00 oz	
Goldings 30 mins	0.75 oz	
OG	1046	
FG	1008	
ABV	5.03	
Apparent attenuation	82.61%	
IBU	24	
SRM	11	
Mash at	154° F	
Sparge at	165° F	
Boil time	120 minutes	
pitching temp	47.5° F	
Yeast	Wyeast 2042 Danish lager	

1955 Barclay Perkins Export

One of the initial set of Lagers brewed by Barclay Perkins was Export, a pale and reasonably strong beer.

The original version had an OG of 1050°, not that much higher than 30 years later. Export had fared better in the war than most beers. I suppose that's because it was a fancy pants Lager that drinkers expected to pay a premium price for.

Initially, all Barclay's Lagers were only available in bottles. But by WW II some, including Export, were available on draught, packaged in 11 and 5.5 gallon casks. They were obviously continental casks as that's 50 and 25 litres in metric.

The recipe is incredibly simple: just pilsener malt and grits. Along with Saaz and East Kent Goldings as hops.

A high degree of attenuation leaves Export with a continental Lager like strength, over 5% ABV.

There was also a cereal mash for the grits in addition to the main mash:

mash in	122° F	stand 20 minutes
raise to	154° F	stand 20 minutes
boil	212° F	for 5 minutes

Main mash:

mash in	122° F	
raise with grits to	154° F	stand 30 minutes
hold at	168° F	stand 35 minutes
Sparge at	165° F	

1955 Barclay Perkins Export		
pilsner malt	7.25 lb	70.73%
grits	3.00 lb	29.27%
Goldings 120 mins	0.75 oz	
Saaz 30 mins	0.75 oz	
OG	1046	
FG	1007	
ABV	5.16	
Apparent attenuation	84.78%	
IBU	18	
SRM	3	
Mash at	154° F	
Sparge at	165° F	
Boil time	120 minutes	
pitching temp	47° F	
Yeast	Wyeast 2042 Danish lager	

1955 Barclay Perkins Draught Lager

Draught Lager was the weakest of Barclay Perkins' bottom-fermenting beers. And looks more like the type of modern British Lager that everyone loves than the others.

In contrast to the previous two Barclay's Lagers, Draught doesn't have any grits in the recipe. Instead there's flaked maize. I've no idea why that should be. It does make the process simpler as there's no need for a cereal mash.

I'm slightly surprised by the presence of amber malt in the grist. Is that for colour or flavour? It's not a huge amount so I can't imagine it has much impact on the finished beer.

The hops are all East Kent Goldings from the 1953 crop.

Here's the full mashing scheme:

mash in	121° F	
raise to	156° F	stand 20 minutes
raise to	170° F	
hold at	170° F	stand 35 minutes
Sparge at	165° F	

1955 Barclay Perkins Draught Lager			
pilsner malt		6.50 lb	83.87%
amber malt		0.25 lb	3.23%
flaked maize		1.00 lb	12.90%
Goldings 120 mins		0.50 oz	
Goldings 30 mins		0.50 oz	
OG		1035	
FG		1008	
ABV		3.57	
Apparent attenuation		77.14%	
IBU		13	
SRM		2.5	
Mash at		156° F	
Sparge at		165° F	
Boil time		120 minutes	
pitching temp		47° F	
Yeast	Wyeast 2042 Danish lager		

1962 Barclay Perkins Export

By this point, Export was the only one of Barclay's original set of Lagers that was still in production.

Not much has happened to the recipe since 1955. The percentage of grits has come down from 29% to 20%. And there's been the addition of a small amount of caramel. Over with the hops, Hallertau have replaced East Kent Goldings.

There has been a significant change in the mashing scheme. The mash is now held at three temperatures: 147° F, 158° F and 168° F. Instead of 154° F and 168° F.

First, the cereal mash, where 2 quarters of malt accompanied the 7 quarters of grits:

mash in	122° F	stand 20 minutes
raise to	150° F	stand 20 minutes
boil	212° F	for 15 minutes

Now the main mash:

mash in	122° F	
raise with grits to	147° F	stand 20 minutes
raise to	158° F	stand 15 minutes
raise to	168° F	stand 35 minutes
Sparge at	165° F	

1962 Barclay Perkins Export		
pilsner malt	8.25 lb	80.41%
grits	2.00 lb	19.49%
caramel 1000 SRM	0.01 lb	0.10%
Hallertau 120 mins	0.75 oz	
Saaz 30 mins	0.75 oz	
OG	1045.5	
FG	1008	
ABV	4.96	
Apparent attenuation	82.42%	
IBU	18	
SRM	4	
Mash at	147° F	
Sparge at	165° F	
Boil time	120 minutes	
pitching temp	45.5° F	
Yeast	Wyeast 2042 Danish lager	

1962 Harp Lager

It's always nice to have recipes for beers people might actually have heard of. Like Harp Lager.

The brand originated with Guinness – hence the name Harp – but was taken over by a consortium of brewers, including Guinness. One of the other brewers was the Courage group. The obvious place for them to brew it was Barclay Perkins Lager brewery on Park Street.

Guinness sent very detailed instructions on exactly how it should be brewed. Which, initially at least, was in a very traditional German way. Including a decoction mash, proper lagering and natural carbonation. Not really surprising, as it was developed by a German brewer.

When they signed up for Harp, Courage seems to have dropped some of the Barclay's Lagers. In particular, Draught Lager. To which Harp does bear an uncanny resemblance, in terms of strength and ingredients.

This was the decoction mash with 8 quarters of malt:

mash in	129° F	stand 15 minutes
raise to	147° F	stand 10 minutes
raise to	158° F	stand 10 minutes
boil	212° F	for 20 minutes

This was added to the main mash which was running in parallel:

mash in	122° F	
raise with decoction to	147° F	stand 20 minutes
raise to	167° F	stand 30 minutes
Sparge at	165° F	

1962 Harp Lager		
pilsner malt	6.25 lb	80.54%
flaked maize	1.50 lb	19.33%
caramel 1000 SRM	0.01 lb	0.13%
Hallertau 120 mins	0.50 oz	
Saaz 30 mins	0.50 oz	
OG	1035.5	
FG	1010	
ABV	3.37	
Apparent attenuation	71.83%	
IBU	13	
SRM	3.4	
Mash at	147° F	
Sparge at	165° F	
Boil time	120 minutes	
pitching temp	45.5° F	
Yeast	Wyeast 2042 Danish lager	

1962 Barclay Perkins Sparkling Beer

Courage did continue to brew Barclay's Lager intended for export, Sparkling Beer.

Though there have been some changes. The grits have been replaced by flaked maize, meaning there was no need for a cereal mash. Unlike with Harp Lager, there wasn't a decoction mash instead. Just the main step mash.

The fermentation was very cool, hitting a maximum of just 49° F.

This is the full mashing scheme:

mash in	121° F	
raise to	147° F	stand 30 minutes
raise to	158° F	stand 15 minutes
raise to	168° F	stand 15 minutes
Sparge at	165° F	

1962 Barclay Perkins Sparkling Beer		
pilsner malt	8.00 lb	75.76%
crystal malt 60 L	1.25 lb	11.84%
flaked maize	1.25 lb	11.84%
caramel 1000 SRM	0.06 lb	0.57%
Hallertau 120 mins	0.75 oz	
Saaz 30 mins	0.75 oz	
OG	1046	
FG	1009	
ABV	4.89	
Apparent attenuation	80.43%	
IBU	18	
SRM	12	
Mash at	147° F	
Sparge at	165° F	
Boil time	120 minutes	
pitching temp	46° F	
Yeast	Wyeast 2042 Danish lager	

1947 Boddington IP

IP, the beer known as Boddington's Bitter, had started life as the strongest of the brewery's Pale Ales. In 1914, it had an OG of 1053°.

By 1947, two World Wars had knocked that down to 1037°, the level of an Ordinary Bitter. Though the high degree of attenuation meant that it was almost 4% ABV.

The influence of the war is plain to see in the presence of flaked barley, which brewers were forced to use. At breweries like Boddington who'd used adjuncts before the war, it replaced flaked maize. The invert sugar is my approximation for three proprietary sugars: 2 cwt DMS, 1.5 cwt Fla, 2 cwt. B.

There were two copper hops, about which all I know is that they were English and from the 1945 season. There were also 3 lbs of hopulon, a preparation of hops. According to a Whitbread brewing record, 1 lb hopulon is the equivalent of 7 lbs of hops. So I've bumped up the hop quantity by 21 lbs.

Oddly, given the vagueness of the hop descriptions, which usually just list the grower, the dry hops are specifically listed as Brewer's Gold.

1947 Boddington IP		
pale malt	6.25 lb	75.76%
enzymic malt	0.25 lb	3.03%
flaked barley	0.50 lb	6.06%
malt extract	0.25 lb	3.03%
No. 2 invert sugar	1.00 lb	12.12%
Fuggles 110 mins	1.00 oz	
Goldings 30 mins	0.75 oz	
Brewer's Gold dry hops	0.50 oz	
OG	1037	
FG	1007	
ABV	3.97	
Apparent attenuation	81.08%	
IBU	23	
SRM	6	
Mash at	146.5° F	
Sparge at	162° F	
Boil time	110 minutes	
pitching temp	61° F	
Yeast	Wyeast 1318 London ale III (Boddingtons)	

1947 Boddington XX

I can remember Boddie's Mild quite well. It was one of the semi-dark kind. Though compared to their straw-coloured Bitter, it looked pretty dark. I assume that the version I drank was the direct successor to this beer.

With an OG of just 1028°, it's not exactly high-gravity. Though, thanks to a high degree of attenuation, it is just about 3% ABV. So just about intoxicating.

The grist is fairly simple: pale malt, crystal malt, flaked barley and sugar. Two different types of sugar: Fla. and invert. I've substituted No. 3 invert for them. Hopefully it's somewhere close to what was in the original. The black malt appears to have been added to the copper along with the caramel.

The hops were English (1945), Styrian (1945), Czech (1945) and 3 lbs hopulon. I've bumped up the hops by 21 lbs to account for the latter. The quantity of Styrian hops is so small – 2 lbs out of 105 lbs, I've left them out.

1947 Boddington XX			
pale malt		3.75 lb	24.63%
crystal malt 80 L		0.50 lb	3.28%
black malt		0.06 lb	0.39%
enzymic malt		0.125 lb	0.82%
flaked barley		0.75 lb	4.93%
malt extract		9.25 lb	60.76%
No. 3 invert sugar		0.75 lb	4.93%
caramel 1000 SRM		0.04 lb	0.26%
Fuggles 115 mins		0.75 oz	
Saaz 30 mins		0.75 oz	
OG		1028	
FG		1005.5	
ABV		2.98	
Apparent attenuation		80.36%	
IBU		21	
SRM		14	
Mash at		154° F	
Sparge at		162° F	
Boil time		115 minutes	
pitching temp		62° F	
Yeast	Wyeast 1318 London ale III (Boddingtons)		

1951 Boddington IP

A few years on, and Boddies' Bitter has changed a bit. Proof that commercial recipes are often in a permanent state of flux.

For a start, the gravity has increased by three points. And the rate of attenuation has gone up, leaving a beer over 4.5% ABV. Hopulon, the hop preparation has been dropped.

The other big change is the lack of an adjunct. I was quite surprised to see that. Because I know Boddington included flaked maize in the 1960's and 1970's. Pretty much in all their IP recipes, really, other than in war years. It's a surprise to see them brewing with just malt and sugar.

The hopping rate has been reduced. Another surprise. I'd expected it to be much more bitter, given the beer's reputation. 19 calculated IBUs is bugger all. Though as the beer is extremely dry, maybe it comes across as more.

The recipe shows a clear paranoia about diastatic power, including both enzymic and diastatic malt extract. It really is a bit odd how many brewers worked in the 1950s.

One nice thing. The description of the base malt is just one word: Newark.

1951 Boddington IP		
pale malt	7.50 lb	83.33%
enzymic malt	0.25 lb	2.78%
malt extract	0.25 lb	2.78%
No. 2 invert sugar	1.00 lb	11.11%
Fuggles 90 mins	0.75 oz	
Goldings 30 mins	0.75 oz	
Brewer's Gold dry hops	0.125 oz	
Goldings dry hops	0.25 oz	
OG	1040	
FG	1005	
ABV	4.63	
Apparent attenuation	87.50%	
IBU	19	
SRM	6	
Mash at	153° F	
Sparge at	160° F	
Boil time	110 minutes	
pitching temp	61° F	
Yeast	Wyeast 1318 London ale III (Boddingtons)	

1951 Boddington XX

Boddington's Mild has changed a bit since 1947. Mostly for the better.

For a start the gravity has increased by four points. And there are no longer any adjuncts in the grist, the flaked barley having been dropped.

The small amounts of black malt and caramel have a big impact on the colour, boosting it around 5 points. Both were added in the copper. They get the colour to what's listed in the brewing record: 62 EBC.

1951 Boddington XX			
pale malt		5.25 lb	73.68%
crystal malt 80 L		0.67 lb	9.40%
black malt		0.05 lb	0.70%
enzymic malt		0.125 lb	1.75%
No. 3 invert sugar		1.00 lb	14.04%
caramel 1000 SRM		0.03 lb	0.42%
Fuggles 75 mins		0.75 oz	
Fuggles 45 mins		0.75 oz	
Fuggles dry hops		0.05 oz	
OG		1032	
FG		1005	
ABV		3.57	
Apparent attenuation		84.38%	
IBU		21	
SRM		15	
Mash at		153° F	
Sparge at		162° F	
Boil time		75 minutes	
pitching temp		63° F	
Yeast	Wyeast 1318 London ale III (Boddingtons)		

1951 Boddington Stout

Here's proof that not all English Stouts were sweet after WW II. With the level of hopping and rate of attenuation, there's no way this would have come across as sweet.

The grist is quite interesting, too, with four different malts: pale amber, crystal and black. There's a surprisingly large amount of amber malt, almost a third of the grist. So much, in fact, that I'm wondering whether it was diastatic or not. Malt, as with XX, seems to have been added in the copper.

At least Boddington brewed their Stout properly. And didn't parti-gyle it with Bitter, as some other breweries did.

It's hopped at a rate of 6.5 lbs per quarter of malt, which is quite high. Higher than their Bitter. That's reflected in the IBU count.

1951 Boddington Stout		
pale malt	4.25 lb	44.00%
crystal malt 80 L	1.25 lb	12.94%
amber malt	3.00 lb	31.06%
black malt	0.50 lb	5.18%
No. 3 invert sugar	0.33 lb	3.42%
caramel 1000 SRM	0.33 lb	3.42%
Fuggles 95 mins	1.00 oz	
Fuggles 45 mins	1.00 oz	
OG	1040	
FG	1012	
ABV	3.70	
Apparent attenuation	70.00%	
IBU	27	
SRM	38	
Mash at	153° F	
Sparge at	162° F	
Boil time	95 minutes	
pitching temp	61° F	
Yeast	Wyeast 1318 London ale III (Boddingtons)	

1951 Boddington CC

CC, Boddington's Strong Ale, was dropped during WW II and didn't resurface until 1951, when UK brewing was finally starting to pick up.

Surprisingly, it's almost as strong as it was in 1939, when the OG was 1056°. The relatively modest strength and the fact that it was dry hopped has me wondering whether CC was sometimes sold on draught.

For some reason there's no enzymic malt in CC. No idea why that is. It does, however, contain diastatic malt extract. Just like all their other beers.

Also like most of their other beers, the rate of attenuation was quite high, squeezing the ABV to almost 6%.

1951 Boddington CC			
pale malt		9.75 lb	78.79%
crystal malt 80 L		1.50 lb	12.12%
No. 3 invert sugar		1.00 lb	8.08%
caramel 1000 SRM		0.125 lb	1.01%
Fuggles 120 mins		1.75 oz	
Brewers Gold 120 mins		0.25 oz	
Fuggles 30 mins		2.00 oz	
Brewers Gold dry hops		0.25 oz	
Fuggles dry hops		0.25 oz	
OG		1055	
FG		1011	
ABV		5.82	
Apparent attenuation		80.00%	
IBU		52	
SRM		22	
Mash at		153° F	
Sparge at		162° F	
Boil time		120 minutes	
pitching temp		63° F	
Yeast	Wyeast 1318 London ale III (Boddingtons)		

1966 Boddington IP

I'm intrigued to see how Boddington's Bitter developed in recent times. So another recipe, this time from a few years later.

The most obvious difference with the 1951 version is the gravity, which is 1.5 points lower. There are two new ingredients: wheat and flaked maize.. Otherwise, the grist is very similar: pale malt, enzymic malt, wheat, flaked maize and sugar. The same three proprietary sugars, DMS, Fla. And Br. DMS is probably Diastatic Malt Syrup. That's the malt extract in the recipe below.

The hops are very vague again. I all know is that they were English. And there were slightly fewer than in 1951.

The rate of attenuation is very high, just a tad under 90%, which must have left a very dry beer.

1966 Boddington IP		
pale malt	6.75 lb	76.44%
enzymic malt	0.25 lb	2.83%
wheat	0.25 lb	2.83%
flaked maize	0.25 lb	2.83%
malt extract	0.33 lb	3.74%
No. 2 invert sugar	1.00 lb	11.33%
Fuggles 90 min	1.00 oz	
Goldings 30 min	0.75 oz	
Goldings dry hops	0.25 oz	
OG	1038.5	
FG	1004	
ABV	4.56	
Apparent attenuation	89.61%	
IBU	23	
SRM	6	
Mash at	146° F	
Sparge at	162° F	
Boil time	90 minutes	
pitching temp	62.5° F	
Yeast	Wyeast 1318 London ale III (Boddingtons)	

1966 Boddington XX

There's been very little change to XX since 1951. The gravity has fallen by half a point, but otherwise it's much the same.

Though it looks like quite a complicated recipe, many of the ingredients are only used in tiny quantities.

As is so often the case, I have no information about the hops other than that they were English and there were two different types.

1966 Boddington XX		
pale malt	4.75 lb	69.80%
crystal malt 80 L	0.75 lb	11.02%
black malt	0.05 lb	0.73%
enzymic malt	0.125 lb	1.84%
malt extract	0.33 lb	4.85%
No. 3 invert sugar	0.75 lb	11.02%
caramel 1000 SRM	0.05 lb	0.73%
Fuggles 120 min	0.75 oz	
Goldings 30 min	0.75 oz	
OG	1031.5	
FG	1003.5	
ABV	3.70	
Apparent attenuation	88.89%	
IBU	22	
SRM	15	
Mash at	146° F	
Sparge at	162° F	
Boil time	120 minutes	
pitching temp	62.5° F	
Yeast	Wyeast 1318 London ale III (Boddingtons)	

1966 Boddington Best Mild

Now here's a big change: another Mild has appeared. Which is slightly odd. My guess would be that it happened in the middle of the 1950s.

The recipe is near identical to XX. There's just a little more pale malt, a little less caramel and no black malt in Best Mild. Unsurprisingly, it's a paler beer.

I can remember Boddington Mild not really being dark, but half dark. Though, compared to their pale Bitter, it did appear dark. Now I can see what's happened. They brewed a Dark Mild then when they introduced a Best Mild made it pale. Which was usually the way it worked: Ordinary Mild dark, Best Mild pale. Then at some point, probably in the 1970s, Boddington dropped their Ordinary Mild.

1966 Boddington Best Mild		
pale malt	5.25 lb	71.33%
crystal malt 80 L	0.75 lb	10.19%
enzymic malt	0.25 lb	3.40%
malt extract	0.33 lb	4.48%
No. 3 invert sugar	0.75 lb	10.19%
caramel 1000 SRM	0.03 lb	0.41%
Fuggles 120 min	0.75 oz	
Goldings 30 min	0.75 oz	
OG	1033.5	
FG	1003.5	
ABV	3.97	
Apparent attenuation	89.55%	
IBU	22	
SRM	13	
Mash at	147° F	
Sparge at	162° F	
Boil time	90 minutes	
pitching temp	62° F	
Yeast	Wyeast 1318 London ale III (Boddingtons)	

1966 Boddington Strong Ale

At some point in the 1950s or early 1960s, Boddington dropped their Strong Ale CC. And replaced it with a new, stronger beer simply called Strong Ale.

At 7.5 % ABV, it's a Strong Ale in anyone's book. That was achieved by a very high degree of attenuation for a beer of such a hefty gravity. I's an odd feature of British beer that, while most of it became quite watery, some strong and very strong beers were almost always knocking about.

There's nothing very exciting about the recipe. It's much like their other beers, save for the lack of enzymic malt.

1966 Boddington Strong Ale		
pale malt	11.25 lb	75.86%
crystal malt 80 L	1.75 lb	11.80%
wheat malt	0.33 lb	2.23%
malt extract	0.50 lb	3.37%
No. 3 invert sugar	1.00 lb	6.74%
Fuggles 90 min	1.25 oz	
Goldings 30 min	1.25 oz	
Goldings dry hops	0.25 oz	
OG	1065.5	
FG	1008.5	
ABV	7.54	
Apparent attenuation	87.02%	
IBU	29	
SRM	17	
Mash at	146° F	
Sparge at	162° F	
Boil time	90 minutes	
pitching temp	62.5° F	
Yeast	Wyeast 1318 London ale III (Boddingtons)	

1966 Boddington Stout

Boddington continued to brew a rather unusual Stout. Unusual, because it wasn't piss-weak or ridiculously sweet.

There hasn't been a huge change to the grist since 1951. The same malts – pale, amber, crystal and black are still there – with only a small alteration to their proportions.

I like the look of this Stout. Plenty of coloured malts and a reasonable degree of bitterness. Plus, unlike most other English Stouts, it was well-attenuated.

1966 Boddington Stout		
pale malt	2.00 lb	27.62%
crystal malt 80 L	1.25 lb	17.27%
amber malt	2.25 lb	31.08%
black malt	0.50 lb	6.91%
wheat malt	0.33 lb	4.56%
malt extract	0.25 lb	3.45%
No. 3 invert sugar	0.33 lb	4.56%
caramel 1000 SRM	0.33 lb	4.56%
Fuggles 120 min	1.00 oz	
Fuggles 30 min	1.00 oz	
OG	1038.5	
FG	1008	
ABV	4.03	
Apparent attenuation	79.22%	
IBU	26	
SRM	37	
Mash at	147° F	
Sparge at	163° F	
Boil time	95 minutes	
pitching temp	62° F	
Yeast	Wyeast 1318 London ale III (Boddingtons)	

1961 Clarke 1/2 MB

Clarke is a bonus brewery. I came across a brewing book of theirs totally by chance. Because it's mixed in with Boddington's ones.

A mis-cataloguing, I'm sure. There are other Clarke's brewing records archived in Stockport, where the brewery was based. They were bought and closed by Boddington, presumably to get hold of their pubs. That's just how things worked, if you wanted to expand your business.

According to the ever handy "Century of British Brewers plus plus" (by Norman Barber 2013, page 107) Richard Clarke & Co. Ltd. was founded in 1865 and bought by Boddington in 1963.

The log I found looks like the last. A bit sad that.

MB must mean Mild Beer. Dark, by the look of the recipe. Quite possibly darkened more with primings. A lot of that went on.

The grist has the bizarrely-fashionable and probably pointless enzymic malt, along with base malt, flaked maize and sugar. So pretty standard stuff. The log just says "invert". No.3 is my guess.

Slightly unusually for a Mild, MB is dry hopped. Not a huge amount, but about the as much as a Bitter of the same strength. Talking of hops, they were Kent (1960 harvest), Sussex (1960), Worcester (1960) plus Worcester (1960) dry hops I've interpreted the Kent and Sussex hops as Fuggles, the Worcester hops as Goldings.

1961 Clarke 1/2 MB		
pale malt	5.75 lb	79.31%
enzymic malt	0.125 lb	1.72%
flaked maize	0.25 lb	3.45%
caramel 1000 SRM	0.125 lb	1.72%
glucose	0.25 lb	3.45%
No. 3 invert sugar	0.50 lb	6.90%
malt extract	0.25 lb	3.45%
Fuggles 90 min	0.50 oz	
Goldings 30 min	0.50 oz	
Goldings dry hops	0.125 oz	
OG	1033	
FG	1012.5	
ABV	2.71	
Apparent attenuation	62.12%	
IBU	13.4	
SRM	14	
Mash at	154° F	
Sparge at	170° F	
Boil time	90 minutes	
pitching temp	62° F	
Yeast	Wyeast 1318 London ale III (Boddingtons)	

1962 Clarke 1/5 Nobby BA

Clarke didn't have a huge range of beers. The brewing record has page after page of Mild and Bitter. Then look . . . here's a Brown Ale. Yippee!

They're a rare breed to start with. This set was the last place I'd expect to find one. The 1/5, if you're wondering, is the price per pint. 1 shilling and 5 pence. The same price as their Bitter, which is coming up next.

That price has me wondering about how Nobby was packaged. They couldn't have sold it at that price bottled. It's the same price as their Bitter of about the same gravity. Was this a draught beer, or did they just work out the price that it would be on draught? I've no idea and thinking about it is making my head hurt.

The recipe is much like the Mild, except there's no glucose here. The hopping rate is similar to that for their Bitter at 6.5 lbs per quarter of malt, while the Mild has just 4.5 lbs.

Now I think about it, BA could also stand for Best Ale. That is, Best Mild. That would make sense. I don't know. Make your own mind up.

1962 Clarke 1/5 Nobby BA		
pale malt	5.25 lb	68.85%
enzymic malt	0.125 lb	1.64%
flaked maize	0.50 lb	6.56%
caramel 1000 SRM	0.25 lb	3.28%
No. 3 invert sugar	1.25 lb	16.39%
malt extract	0.25 lb	3.28%
Fuggles 90 min	0.67 oz	
Goldings 30 min	0.67 oz	
Goldings dry hops	0.25 oz	
OG	1035.5	
FG	1014	
ABV	2.84	
Apparent attenuation	60.56%	
IBU	18	
SRM	22	
Mash at	154º F	
Sparge at	170º F	
Boil time	90 minutes	
pitching temp	63º F	
Yeast	Wyeast 1318 London ale III (Boddingtons)	

1961 Clarke 1/5 BB

In the 1950s and early 1950s, the bulk of a brewery's trade – especially smaller ones – was draught Bitter and Mild. They might not bother with such exotic items as Stout or other fancy bottled beers and just buy them in.

It's possible Clarke did produce bottled beers, spun out of their draught products. But it looks like they concentrated of Bitter and Mild. That's not so unusual. It was the bulk of the pub trade.

The recipe isn't that different from the Mild. My image of Mild and Bitter being to completely different things shattered long ago. At least there is one feature that distinguished them here: the Bitter is quite a bit more heavily hopped.

The rate of attenuation is rubbish. I assume it must have fallen from that. Especially as this would have been cask conditioned.

1961 Clarke 1/5 BB		
pale malt	6.50 lb	82.33%
enzymic malt	0.125 lb	1.58%
flaked maize	0.50 lb	6.33%
caramel 1000 SRM	0.02 lb	0.25%
glucose	0.25 lb	3.17%
No. 1 invert sugar	0.25 lb	3.17%
malt extract	0.25 lb	3.17%
Fuggles 90 min	1.00 oz	
Goldings 30 min	1.00 oz	
Goldings dry hops	0.125 oz	
OG	1036	
FG	1014.5	
ABV	2.84	
Apparent attenuation	59.72%	
IBU	26	
SRM	6	
Mash at	154° F	
Sparge at	170° F	
Boil time	90 minutes	
pitching temp	62° F	
Yeast	WLP013 London Ale (Worthington White Shield)	

1948 Drybrough 60/-

Scottish Light, one of the most confusingly-named styles of beer. Because it was often pretty dark.

Drybrough, taken over my Watney, didn't have the greatest reputation in their later years. When they became a Keg Heavy factory. With the odd drop of Keg Light, just to, er, lighten things up.

Enzymic malt features, as it did in many post-war beers. Though in much larger quantities here. The malt extract, on the other hand, is a typically minute quantity. As so often, there are loads of different sugars: 2 cwt Fison, 3 cwt CMM, 3 cwt Avona. And, as usual, I've refined them down to a single type of invert.

The presence of flaked barley is a hangover from the war years. Once restrictions were lifted and imports of maize were available again, brewers switch back to flaked maize.

Unusually, this batch was brewed single-gyle. Mostly 60/- was parti-gyled, either with Burns Ale of 54/- and XXP.

The hops were all English, from the 1946 and 1947 crop.

1948 Drybrough 60/-		
pale malt	5.25 lb	77.32%
flaked barley	0.75 lb	11.05%
malt extract	0.04 lb	0.59%
No. 2 invert sugar	0.75 lb	11.05%
Fuggles 90 min	0.50 oz	
Goldings 30 min	0.50 oz	
Goldings dry hops	0.50 oz	
OG	1030	
FG	1012	
ABV	2.38	
Apparent attenuation	60.00%	
IBU	14	
SRM	5	
Mash at	145° F	
Sparge at	165° F	
Boil time	90 minutes	
pitching temp	60° F	
Yeast	WLP028 Edinburgh Ale	

1948 Drybrough 54/-

If you though the 60/- was watery, wait until you see this baby.

It's the same as 60/- – well it was parti-gyled with it – but there's just a little bit less of everything. Unless they were knocking back a whisky with every pint, I can't see how any adult could get even vaguely pissed on beers like this. At barely more than 2% ABV, it's just about a temperance beer.

Introduced just after WW I, 54/- never had a very impressive OG. In the 1920s it was 1033° and in 1933 it was a mere 1030°. It was dropped in early 1954.

1948 Drybrough 54/-		
pale malt	4.50 lb	73.53%
enzymic malt	0.67 lb	10.95%
black malt	0.04 lb	0.65%
flaked barley	0.50 lb	8.17%
malt extract	0.08 lb	1.31%
No. 2 invert sugar	0.33 lb	5.39%
Fuggles 90 min	0.50 oz	
Goldings 30 min	0.50 oz	
Goldings dry hops	0.50 oz	
OG	1027	
FG	1011	
ABV	2.12	
Apparent attenuation	59.26%	
IBU	15	
SRM	6	
Mash at	144° F	
Sparge at	165° F	
Boil time	90 minutes	
pitching temp	60° F	
Yeast	WLP028 Edinburgh Ale	

1948 Drybrough XXP

The strongest of Drybrough's trio of Pale Ales was XXP. A designation Scottish brewers seemed to like. William Younger also brewed an XXP, though that was their equivalent of 60/-.

There's a weird feature of Scottish Pale Ales: as the gravity increases, so does the degree of attenuation. Whatever the OG, the FGs tend to be fairly similar. This must have been deliberate, as I've seen the same trait at multiple breweries.

Obviously, it's like 60/-, but scaled up a bit.

1948 Drybrough XXP		
pale malt	6.50 lb	69.56%
enzymic malt	1.00 lb	10.70%
black malt	0.05 lb	0.54%
flaked barley	1.00 lb	10.70%
malt extract	0.125 lb	1.34%
No. 2 invert sugar	0.67 lb	7.17%
Fuggles 90 min	0.75 oz	
Goldings 30 min	0.75 oz	
Goldings dry hops	0.67 oz	
OG	1041	
FG	1014	
ABV	3.57	
Apparent attenuation	65.85%	
IBU	19	
SRM	8	
Mash at	144° F	
Sparge at	165° F	
Boil time	90 minutes	
pitching temp	60° F	
Yeast	WLP028 Edinburgh Ale	

1948 Drybrough Burns Ale

In typical Scottish fashion, Drybrough only had the one recipe. From which they brewed three Pale Ales of varying degrees of wateriness and a Strong Ale, Burns. Named after the poet, not the facial hair.

There's a little more black malt in this one, but otherwise it's much the same recipe as the single-gyle 60/-. But with more oomph. Lot's more oomph. Enough oomph to get you intoxicating after fewer than a dozen pints.

Though due to the rubbish degree of attenuation, it's only a little over 5% ABV. You'd expect a beer of this gravity to be at least 6.5% ABV.

1948 Drybrough Burns Ale		
pale malt	11.25 lb	70.87%
enzymic malt	1.75 lb	11.02%
black malt	0.125 lb	0.79%
flaked barley	1.50 lb	9.45%
malt extract	0.25 lb	1.57%
No. 2 invert sugar	1.00 lb	6.30%
Fuggles 90 min	1.25 oz	
Goldings 30 min	1.25 oz	
Goldings dry hops	1.00 oz	
OG	1070	
FG	1031	
ABV	5.16	
Apparent attenuation	55.71%	
IBU	24	
SRM	12	
Mash at	145° F	
Sparge at	165° F	
Boil time	90 minutes	
pitching temp	60° F	
Yeast	WLP028 Edinburgh Ale	

1956 Drybrough 60/-

Not much has changed with Sixty Bob since 1948. But one development is quite important: it's crept over 3% ABV. They must have been dancing in the streets of Edinburgh.

The increased alcohol content is thanks to an increase in OG of two points and a higher degree of attenuation.

The grist is still pretty simple, though there's now a tiny amount of black malt, presumably for colour. Flaked maize has appeared to supplement the flaked barley. It's quite unusual to see flaked barley in a beer as late as this. Most brewers switched back to maize as soon as it was available again.

There's a whole cocktail of sugars: 1 cwt Fison, 2 cwt invert, 2 cwt Avona, 1 cwt Hydrol and 1 cwt CME. I've simplified that to just No. 2 invert.

1956 Drybrough 60/-		
pale malt	5.00 lb	71.79%
enzymic malt	0.25 lb	3.59%
black malt	0.01 lb	0.14%
flaked maize	0.33 lb	4.74%
flaked barley	0.50 lb	7.18%
malt extract	0.125 lb	1.79%
No. 2 invert sugar	0.75 lb	10.77%
Fuggles 90 min	0.75 oz	
Goldings 30 min	0.50 oz	
Goldings dry hops	0.50 oz	
OG	1032	
FG	1009	
ABV	3.04	
Apparent attenuation	71.88%	
IBU	18	
SRM	6	
Mash at	147º F	
Sparge at	165º F	
Boil time	90 minutes	
pitching temp	60º F	
Yeast	WLP028 Edinburgh Ale	

1956 Drybrough XXP

The stronger XXP has also seen its OG boosted by two gravity points to a very respectable 1043°.

However, XXP was brewed in far smaller quantities than 60/-, in batches of just 30 to 60 barrels compared to ones of 250 to 400 barrels. Clearly most drinkers had to content themselves with the weaker beer.

As it was parti-gyled with 60/-, the recipe is essentially identical, just a bit more of everything.

1956 Drybrough XXP		
pale malt	6.75 lb	71.92%
enzymic malt	0.25 lb	2.66%
black malt	0.01 lb	0.11%
flaked maize	0.50 lb	5.33%
flaked barley	0.75 lb	7.99%
malt extract	0.125 lb	1.33%
No. 2 invert sugar	1.00 lb	10.66%
Fuggles 90 min	0.75 oz	
Goldings 30 min	0.75 oz	
Goldings dry hops	0.50 oz	
OG	1043	
FG	1014	
ABV	3.84	
Apparent attenuation	67.44%	
IBU	20	
SRM	7	
Mash at	147° F	
Sparge at	165° F	
Boil time	90 minutes	
pitching temp	61.5° F	
Yeast	WLP028 Edinburgh Ale	

1956 Drybrough Export

Now here's a confusing beer. XXP looks very much like a beer filling the Export slot, that is the strongest Pale Ale in a Scottish brewery's range. Then they introduce a beer that's actually called Export.

Even more confusingly, it's only a little bit stronger than XXP. I find it hard to imagine where it fitted in. About the only way it would make any sense is if it was a bottled beer. Sure enough, I can find a label for something called Drybrough's Export Ale. One that looks like it's from the 1950s or early 1960s, as there's no mention of the volume of the contents.

Just like XXP, Export was parti-gyled with 60/-. Meaning all my comments about that recipe also apply here.

1956 Drybrough Export		
pale malt	7.50 lb	76.45%
enzymic malt	0.125 lb	1.27%
black malt	0.06 lb	0.61%
flaked maize	0.50 lb	5.10%
flaked barley	0.50 lb	5.10%
malt extract	0.125 lb	1.27%
No. 2 invert sugar	1.00 lb	10.19%
Fuggles 90 min	0.75 oz	
Goldings 30 min	0.75 oz	
Goldings dry hops	0.25 oz	
OG	1045	
FG	1013.5	
ABV	4.17	
Apparent attenuation	70.00%	
IBU	19	
SRM	9	
Mash at	147° F	
Sparge at	165° F	
Boil time	90 minutes	
pitching temp	61.5° F	
Yeast	WLP028 Edinburgh Ale	

1956 Drybrough Burns Ale

Drybrough's strongest beer has also had a gravity increase, this time by three points.

There is something to report about this recipe. It was still parti-gyled with 60/-, but it this brew there was considerably more black malt than usual, 160 lbs rather than 90 lbs. Presumably because they wanted a darker colour for Burn Ale.

The rate of attenuation is still rubbish. Even worse than in 1948 and barely over 50%. Perhaps it had a secondary conditioning in a tank that lowered the

1956 Drybrough Burns Ale		
pale malt	12.25 lb	75.38%
enzymic malt	0.25 lb	1.54%
black malt	0.25 lb	1.54%
flaked maize	1.00 lb	6.15%
flaked barley	0.75 lb	4.62%
malt extract	0.25 lb	1.54%
No. 2 invert sugar	1.50 lb	9.23%
Fuggles 90 min	1.50 oz	
Goldings 30 min	1.50 oz	
Goldings dry hops	0.25 oz	
OG	1073	
FG	1034.5	
ABV	5.09	
Apparent attenuation	52.74%	
IBU	32	
SRM	16	
Mash at	147° F	
Sparge at	165° F	
Boil time	90 minutes	
pitching temp	61° F	
Yeast	WLP028 Edinburgh Ale	

1965 Drybrough 60/-

Drybrough was still churning out considerable quantities of 60/-. Some of it in the form of Keg Light.

I can't imagine kegging did a beer as light as this any favours. Though there's no reason why it couldn't taste perfectly fine, if served on cask.

With the minimal bitterness, it's amazing to think that 60/- was technically a Pale Ale. The hopping looks feeble even for a Mild. But that's the Scots for you. They didn't care for many hops in their beer. At least in the 20th century.

1965 Drybrough 60/-		
pale malt	4.75 lb	72.96%
black malt	0.01 lb	0.15%
flaked maize	0.75 lb	11.52%
malt extract	0.25 lb	3.84%
No. 2 invert sugar	0.75 lb	11.52%
Fuggles 90 min	0.50 oz	
Goldings 30 min	0.25 oz	
Goldings dry hops	0.25 oz	
OG	1031	
FG	1011	
ABV	2.65	
Apparent attenuation	64.52%	
IBU	11	
SRM	6	
Mash at	146° F	
Sparge at	165° F	
Boil time	90 minutes	
pitching temp	61° F	
Yeast	WLP028 Edinburgh Ale	

1965 Drybrough Keg Heavy

There's a name to fill a drinker's heart with dread: Keg Heavy. Not a well-loved type of beer.

By 1965 it made up a large proportion of what Drybrough brewed, having overtaken 60/- as their most popular product. What was odd about their beer range in the 1950s was that it lacked a 70/-. Keg Heavy seems to have first appeared around June 1960, though there had been a beer of a similar gravity, B/XXP (presumably Bottling XXP), for a while before.

This looks very much like an English Ordinary Bitter. Except for the poor attenuation and the very low level of hopping. It must have been pretty sweet. All those residual sugars probably took on a lovely boiled sweet character after heavy pasteurisation. I'm sure it tasted great.

1965 Drybrough Keg Heavy		
pale malt	6.00 lb	74.91%
black malt	0.01 lb	0.12%
flaked maize	1.00 lb	12.48%
malt extract	0.25 lb	3.12%
No. 2 invert sugar	0.75 lb	9.36%
Fuggles 90 min	0.50 oz	
Goldings 30 min	0.50 oz	
OG	1037	
FG	1014	
ABV	3.04	
Apparent attenuation	62.16%	
IBU	14	
SRM	6	
Mash at	146° F	
Sparge at	165° F	
Boil time	90 minutes	
pitching temp	62° F	
Yeast	WLP028 Edinburgh Ale	

1966 Drybrough MBA Brown Ale

I've only just twigged what this beer is. I can be so dumb sometimes. The big clue is that Drybrough was taken over by Watney Mann in 1965. MBA obviously stands for Mann's Brown Ale.

Which explains why the recipe is so radically different from all their others. I say all their others. They only had the one recipe, from which they brewed Pale Ales of varying degrees of wateriness.

It must have been weird for Drybrough's brewers to suddenly have all these exotic ingredients: crystal malt, No. 3 invert and torrefied barley. The ingredients are so different from the ones they normally used that I can only assume that it's very similar to the London-brewed version.

With Brown Ale hugely popular at the time, Drybrough must have already had one in their portfolio. Which they doubtless constructed from 60/- plus priming sugars. With Mann's being a renowned national brand, I'm sure Drybrough's own Brown Ale was quickly dropped after the takeover.

1966 Drybrough MBA Brown Ale		
pale malt	4.25 lb	57.90%
black malt	0.09 lb	1.23%
crystal malt 60 L	1.75 lb	23.84%
torrefied barley	0.50 lb	6.81%
No. 3 invert sugar	0.50 lb	6.81%
caramel 500 SRM	0.25 lb	3.41%
Fuggles 90 min	0.50 oz	
Goldings 30 min	0.50 oz	
OG	1034	
FG	1012	
ABV	2.91	
Apparent attenuation	64.71%	
IBU	13	
SRM	21	
Mash at	145 / 158° F	
Sparge at	165° F	
Boil time	90 minutes	
pitching temp	62° F	
Yeast	WLP028 Edinburgh Ale	

1964 Eldridge Pope Dorset Special Ale

There's something rather Scottish about parti-gyling a strong, dark beer with standard-strength Pale Ales. Which is what Eldridge Pope did with Dorset Special Ale.

Their propensity for parti-gyling explains why Eldridge Pope had so many different products. It would all be rather confusing. If I didn't have labels and Whitbread Gravity Book entries to help me out. It's thanks to the Gravity Book that I know this was a dark beer.

What style is it? You could call it a Strong Ale or an Old Ale. It's a little too weak to be a Barley Wine.

How did they get it dark? It must have been through some sort of priming at racking time. Because you'll never get a beer dark enough with the ingredients listed in the brewing record. I've added the quantity needed to hit the right shade.

I'm not sure what purpose the wheat flour is serving. But they threw some of it in all their beers, other than the Stouts.

1964 Eldridge Pope Dorset Special Ale		
pale malt	12.50 lb	74.85%
crystal malt 60 L	1.00 lb	5.99%
wheat flour	0.75 lb	4.49%
malt extract	0.50 lb	2.99%
No. 2 invert sugar	1.75 lb	10.48%
caramel 1000 SRM	0.20 lb	1.20%
Styrian Goldings 90 mins	0.25 oz	
Fuggles 90 min	1.50 oz	
Goldings 30 min	1.50 oz	
OG	1075	
FG	1024	
ABV	6.75	
Apparent attenuation	68.00%	
IBU	33	
SRM	22.5	
Mash at	148° F	
Sparge at	160° F	
Boil time	90 minutes	
pitching temp	60° F	
Yeast	WLP099 Super High Gravity Thomas Hardy	

1964 Eldridge Pope Strong Old Ale

Eldridge Pope didn't just have a Strong Ale. They also had an Old Ale, which, despite the name, wasn't really all that strong.

It's another one where I'm pretty sure that the colour was darker than the ingredients implied. So I've added some caramel to the recipe to get the right colour. I know that this was available in bottles – I've seen the labels. But it might also have been sold on draught during the winter.

Eldridge Pope were also enthusiastic user of malt extract. Presumably because of the enzymes.

1964 Eldridge Pope Strong Old Ale			
pale malt		8.25 lb	73.14%
crystal malt 60 L		0.75 lb	6.65%
wheat flour		0.50 lb	4.43%
malt extract		0.33 lb	2.93%
No. 2 invert sugar		1.25 lb	11.08%
caramel 1000 SRM		0.20 lb	1.77%
Styrian Goldings 90 mins		0.25 oz	
Fuggles 90 min		1.00 oz	
Goldings 30 min		1.00 oz	
OG		1051	
FG		1013	
ABV		5.03	
Apparent attenuation		74.51%	
IBU		27	
SRM		20	
Mash at		148° F	
Sparge at		160° F	
Boil time		90 minutes	
pitching temp		59° F	
Yeast	WLP099 Super High Gravity Thomas Hardy		

1964 Eldridge Pope IPA

Eldridge Pope were big fans of parti-gyling. They squeeze two, three, four or even more different beers out of one brew. This batch of IPA was part of a five-way parti-gyle, along with the Dorset Special Ale and Special Old Ale above, the BAK that follows and another Pale Ale. Quite a set.

IPA fills the Best Bitter slot in Eldridge Pope's range. There was also a bottled version, which was identical save for the dry hops. Though I am only guessing that the draught version was dry hopped. As with most other breweries, they didn't bother recording the dry hops in the brewing record.

1964 Eldridge Pope IPA		
pale malt	7.00 lb	75.03%
crystal malt 60 L	0.50 lb	5.36%
wheat flour	0.50 lb	5.36%
malt extract	0.33 lb	3.54%
No. 2 invert sugar	1.00 lb	10.72%
Styrian Goldings 90 mins	0.25 oz	
Fuggles 90 min	0.75 oz	
Goldings 30 min	0.75 oz	
Goldings dry hops	0.25 oz	
OG	1043	
FG	1011.5	
ABV	4.17	
Apparent attenuation	73.26%	
IBU	23	
SRM	9	
Mash at	148° F	
Sparge at	160° F	
Boil time	90 minutes	
pitching temp	60° F	
Yeast	WLP099 Super High Gravity Thomas Hardy	

1964 Eldridge Pope BAK

At the bottom of the Pale Ale pile was BAK, which presumably stands for Bottling AK. Effectively, it was their Light Ale.

Light certainly describes BAK well. It's not quite 3% ABV and under 20 (calculated) IBUs.

1964 Eldridge Pope BAK		
pale malt	4.75 lb	73.08%
crystal malt 60 L	0.50 lb	7.69%
wheat flour	0.33 lb	5.08%
malt extract	0.25 lb	3.85%
No. 2 invert sugar	0.67 lb	10.31%
Styrian Goldings 90 mins	0.13 oz	
Fuggles 90 min	0.50 oz	
Goldings 30 min	0.50 oz	
OG	1030	
FG	1008	
ABV	2.91	
Apparent attenuation	73.33%	
IBU	16	
SRM	7	
Mash at	148° F	
Sparge at	160° F	
Boil time	90 minutes	
pitching temp	60° F	
Yeast	WLP099 Super High Gravity Thomas Hardy	

1964 Eldridge Pope Best Bitter

This is essentially the same beer as the BAK above. The only difference being that BAK was a bottled beer and Best Bitter a draught beer.

Though "Best" is a bit of a stretch as a description of a Bitter that's only just about 3% ABV. The dry hops area guess. Most draught Bitters were dry-hopped, so it's fair enough to assume that this was, too. It's strange that Eldridge Pope didn't have a beer in the Ordinary Bitter category, something 1035-1037°.

The recipe is the same as for all Eldridge Pope's Pale Ales: pale and crystal malt, wheat flour, malt extract and sugar. Quite an odd combination, but it obviously worked.

1964 Eldridge Pope BB		
pale malt	4.75 lb	70.37%
crystal malt 60 L	0.50 lb	7.41%
wheat flour	0.67 lb	9.93%
malt extract	0.33 lb	4.89%
No. 2 invert sugar	0.50 lb	7.41%
Fuggles 90 min	0.75 oz	
Goldings 30 min	0.75 oz	
Goldings dry hops	0.125 oz	
OG	1030	
FG	1007.5	
ABV	2.98	
Apparent attenuation	75.00%	
IBU	20	
SRM	7	
Mash at	148° F	
Sparge at	160° F	
Boil time	90 minutes	
pitching temp	61.5° F	
Yeast	WLP099 Super High Gravity Thomas Hardy	

1964 Eldridge Pope Special Mild

At least I think the S in the brew house name SM stands for Special. However inappropriate that might be, given this beer's puny OG.

I know from an entry in the Whitbread Gravity Book that the colour was way darker than BeerSmith calculated. So I've added caramel to correct it.

The percentage of sugar in this recipe is quite low for a Mild. 10% - 15% was more typical.

1964 Eldridge Pope Special Mild		
pale malt	4.50 lb	72.52%
crystal malt 60 L	0.75 lb	12.09%
wheat flour	0.25 lb	4.03%
malt extract	0.125 lb	2.01%
brown sugar	0.125 lb	2.01%
white sugar	0.125 lb	2.01%
caramel 1000 SRM	0.33 lb	5.32%
Fuggles 90 min	0.50 oz	
Goldings 30 min	0.50 oz	
OG	1026	
FG	1007	
ABV	2.51	
Apparent attenuation	73.08%	
IBU	14	
SRM	24	
Mash at	148° F	
Sparge at	160° F	
Boil time	90 minutes	
pitching temp	61.5° F	
Yeast	WLP099 Super High Gravity Thomas Hardy	

1964 Eldridge Pope Dorset Brown Ale

Essentially identical of the Mild was Eldridge pope's Brown Ale. It was often parti-gyled with it, though this particular example also had XXXX in the mix, too.

This is another beer that was darker than the recipe implies. I've added enough caramel to get the colour right.

The hopping is very similar in all Eldridge Pope's beers. In this case, it's Kent (1961), Worcester (1962) and Sussex (1962). Some of the others also contain a small amount of Styrian Goldings.

1964 Eldridge Pope Dorset Brown Ale		
pale malt	4.00 lb	66.67%
crystal malt 60 L	0.75 lb	12.50%
wheat flour	0.25 lb	4.17%
malt extract	0.25 lb	4.17%
brown sugar	0.25 lb	4.17%
white sugar	0.25 lb	4.17%
caramel 1000 SRM	0.25 lb	4.17%
Fuggles 90 min	0.50 oz	
Goldings 30 min	0.50 oz	
OG	1025.5	
FG	1006.5	
ABV	2.51	
Apparent attenuation	74.51%	
IBU	14	
SRM	20	
Mash at	148° F	
Sparge at	160° F	
Boil time	90 minutes	
pitching temp	61.5° F	
Yeast	WLP099 Super High Gravity Thomas Hardy	

1964 Eldridge Pope XXXX

Parti-gyled with the Brown Ale above, it was just about exactly its double. Making this, effectively, a double-strength Mild.

I mentioned earlier that the Strong Old Ale might have been sold on draught. I'm now thinking this was more likely the draught beer. It's very similar in strength to the Old Ale.

What's in the recipe as brown sugar is my interpretation of "Barb syrup". I'm guessing the Barb stands for Barbados.

1964 Eldridge Pope XXXX			
pale malt		8.25 lb	70.03%
crystal malt 60 L		1.50 lb	12.73%
wheat flour		0.50 lb	4.24%
malt extract		0.50 lb	4.24%
brown sugar		0.50 lb	4.24%
white sugar		0.33 lb	2.80%
caramel 1000 SRM		0.20 lb	1.70%
Fuggles 90 min		1.25 oz	
Goldings 30 min		1.25 oz	
OG		1053	
FG		1017	
ABV		4.76	
Apparent attenuation		67.92%	
IBU		29	
SRM		21	
Mash at		148° F	
Sparge at		160° F	
Boil time		90 minutes	
pitching temp		59° F	
Yeast	WLP099 Super High Gravity Thomas Hardy		

1964 Eldridge Pope Double Stout

Yet another Eldridge Pope recipe that I've had to fiddle with. Another reason to thank the Whitbread Gravity Book.

There's an entry from 1959 for something called Double Sweet Stout. The OG is a few points higher than in the brewing record, but what swung it for me was the FG. Which was also several points higher. That says one thing to me: lactose at racking time. Which is what I've assumed.

Elsewhere in the grist, there's chocolate and crystal malt, plus the usual sugar and malt extract. You may have noticed that the basic recipes for all a brewery's beers are usually pretty similar. It makes sense not to have too many different ingredients. And when you're parti-gyling, there's not much choice.

The recipe is an interesting mixture of bitterness and lactose sweetness. Looks like a winner to me.

1964 Eldridge Pope Double Stout		
pale malt	4.50 lb	46.97%
crystal malt 60 L	1.50 lb	15.66%
chocolate malt	1.25 lb	13.05%
malted oats	0.33 lb	3.44%
malt extract	0.33 lb	3.44%
lactose	0.50 lb	5.22%
brown sugar	0.67 lb	6.99%
white sugar	0.50 lb	5.22%
Fuggles 90 min	1.25 oz	
Goldings 30 min	1.25 oz	
OG	1043	
FG	1019	
ABV	3.18	
Apparent attenuation	55.81%	
IBU	32	
SRM	34	
Mash at	147° F	
Sparge at	165° F	
Boil time	90 minutes	
pitching temp	59° F	
Yeast	WLP099 Super High Gravity Thomas Hardy	

1964 Eldridge Pope Oat Malt Stout

Parti-gyled with the Double Stout above was a weaker beer, Oat Malt Stout. Which explains one thing: why there was Oat Malt in Double Stout.

Unfortunately, I've no Gravity Book analysis for this beer. So I've no idea if it included lactose or not. I've guessed no, but I could be wrong. Throw in a half pound of lactose if you fancy.

It's weird how quickly Oat Stouts disappeared. There were still quite a few about in the mid-1960s. By the end of the 1970s there were none.

1964 Eldridge Pope Oat Malt Stout		
pale malt	3.50 lb	54.90%
crystal malt 60 L	1.00 lb	15.69%
chocolate malt	1.00 lb	15.69%
malted oats	0.25 lb	3.92%
malt extract	0.25 lb	3.92%
brown sugar	0.25 lb	3.92%
white sugar	0.125 lb	1.96%
Fuggles 90 min	1.00 oz	
Goldings 30 min	1.00 oz	
OG	1030	
FG	1011.5	
ABV	2.45	
Apparent attenuation	61.67%	
IBU	29	
SRM	27	
Mash at	147° F	
Sparge at	165° F	
Boil time	90 minutes	
pitching temp	60° F	
Yeast	WLP099 Super High Gravity Thomas Hardy	

1967 Eldridge Pope Barley Wine

I've strayed slightly beyond the period to include this Barley Wine from Eldridge Pope. It's one of the paler types of barley Wine that popped up in reaction to the success of Gold Label.

There are a few interesting points about the recipe. It was brewed in a parti-gyle with three Pale Ales. But the way the parti-gyle was performed left the recipe for this quite different from the Pale Ales. Because the Barley Wine consisted of exclusively first wort. And the sugars all went in the later coppers. Meaning the Barley Wine contained no sugar while all the other beers did.

Then there's the presence of pilsner malt. It isn't in the other Pale Ale parti-gyles, meaning its purpose must be to keep down the colour of Barley Wine.

It's pretty heavily hopped and hits almost 50 (calculated IBUs).

1967 Eldridge Pope Barley Wine		
pale malt	10.75 lb	55.13%
pilsner malt	4.00 lb	20.51%
crystal malt 60 L	1.00 lb	5.13%
crystal malt 80 L	0.75 lb	3.85%
wheat flour	2.25 lb	11.54%
malt extract	0.75 lb	3.85%
Cluster 105 mins	1.00 oz	
Fuggles 90 mins	1.00 oz	
Fuggles 60 mins	1.00 oz	
Goldings 30 mins	0.50 oz	
Styrian Goldings 30 mins	0.50 oz	
OG	1085.5	
FG	1029.5	
ABV	7.41	
Apparent attenuation	65.50%	
IBU	47	
SRM	13	
Mash at	144° F	
Sparge at	165° F	
Boil time	105 minutes	
pitching temp	60.25° F	
Yeast	WLP099 Super High Gravity Thomas Hardy	

1949 Elgood XK

It's good to look at breweries of different sizes. As well as the big urban ones like Whitbread and Courage, small rural breweries like Elgood.

This is a good example of a Mild in times of austerity. 1949 was a difficult year. Average OG had increased a little since its nadir in 1947, but only by one point, hitting the dizzying heights of 1033.43°. Which meant there had to be plenty of beer below 1030°. You weren't going to get plastered on XK, not even with grim determination.

There aren't any real surprises in the grist, other than that it has a base of mild malt rather than pale malt. Their stronger Bitter, PA, had a base of mostly pale malt with a little mild malt. It's the classic English combination of malt, flaked maize and sugar. With a little malt extract on the side. That seems to be very common in 1950's recipes. I think it's for enzymes, but I'm not sure.

The sugar is described as simply "invert" and "Silcose". I've chosen to interpret that as all No. 1 invert. I know from other examples of XK that it was No. 1 invert that it contained..

I've no idea what the hops are, other than that they're English. Fuggles seems a fair enough guess, but Goldings would be equally valid. You can take your pick.

The original mashing scheme was 15 minutes at 147° F, followed by an underlet that raised the mash temperature to 155° F where it was held for 1.75 hours.

1949 Elgood XK		
mild malt	4.75 lb	83.92%
crystal malt 60 L	0.33 lb	5.83%
malt extract	0.25 lb	4.42%
No. 1 invert sugar	0.33 lb	5.83%
Fuggles 145 mins	0.75 oz	
Fuggles 60 mins	0.75 oz	
OG	1026.5	
FG	1006	
ABV	2.71	
Apparent attenuation	77.36%	
IBU	23	
SRM	6	
Mash at	147° F	
Sparge at	167° F	
Boil time	145 minutes	
pitching temp	62° F	
Yeast	WLP025 Southwold	

1949 Elgood PA

In contrast to their Mild, Elgood's Bitter had a reasonable gravity. Coupled with decent attenuation, it left a beer of over 4% ABV.

There isn't a huge difference in the grists. The base is mostly pale malt here, but there's still some mild malt. No crystal, either, but the malt extract and No. 1 invert are exactly the same.

There were three types of hops: Worcester (1947), Sussex (1947) and Kent (1947). I've interpreted that as Fuggles and Goldings. I've guessed that it was dry hopped, as almost all Bitters were at the time.

1949 Elgood PA		
pale malt	6.25 lb	78.13%
mild malt	0.75 lb	9.38%
malt extract	0.50 lb	6.25%
No. 1 invert sugar	0.50 lb	6.25%
Fuggles 105 mins	0.75 oz	
Fuggles 60 mins	0.75 oz	
Goldings 30 mins	0.50 oz	
Goldings dry hops	0.25 oz	
OG	1038	
FG	1007	
ABV	4.10	
Apparent attenuation	81.58%	
IBU	27	
SRM	6	
Mash at	149° F	
Sparge at	167° F	
Boil time	105 minutes	
pitching temp	62° F	
Yeast	WLP025 Southwold	

1953 Elgood BPA

One of the most popular styles of the 1950's was Light Ale, a low-gravity, bottled Pale ale. It was often mixed with draught Bitter, usually in the hope of livening up cask beer in poor condition.

At 1031°, BPA (presumably standing for Bottled Pale Ale) was pretty typical for a Light Ale of the time. Not exactly heady stuff.

The recipe isn't exactly what you'd call complicated. Just malt, a bit of sugar and a dash of malt extract. And a single, unspecified type of hop. Fuggles are just my guess. What isn't a guess this time are the hop additions, which are handily noted in the log. The vast majority were added at the start of the boil.

The original mashing scheme was 20 minutes at 149° F, followed by an underlet and 1 hour 40 minutes at 152° F.

1953 Elgood BPA		
pale malt	6.00 lb	88.89%
No. 2 invert sugar	0.50 lb	7.41%
malt extract	0.25 lb	3.70%
Fuggles 95 mins	1.50 oz	
Fuggles 30 mins	0.25 oz	
Fuggles hop back	0.125 oz	
OG	1031	
FG	1006.5	
ABV	3.24	
Apparent attenuation	79.03%	
IBU	27	
SRM	5	
Mash at	152° F	
Sparge at	167° F	
Boil time	95 minutes	
pitching temp	62° F	
Yeast	WLP025 Southwold	

1953 Elgood X

They certainly liked their Mild watery in the 1950s. Or rather, drinkers had no choice as that's just the way it came.

Elgood's Mild, X, makes their Light Ale look headily alcoholic. Which is quite an achievement. X was brewed at around the effective minimum gravity. No matter how watery your beer was, you paid the tax for a beer of 1027°. So there was no real economic point in brewing anything much weaker than that.

The grist is, er, interesting. I don't think I've ever seen flaked barley and flaked rice used in the same beer before. Obviously, there's the malt extract Elgood threw in all their beers. Then there's a sugar just described as invert. And another called carmose. I'll go out a limb here and guess that's some sort of caramel.

The hops were all English and all quite old. This beer was brewed in October 1953 and the hops were all from the 1950 harvest.

1953 Elgood X		
Mild malt	4.50 lb	76.14%
flaked rice	0.25 lb	4.23%
flaked barley	0.33 lb	5.58%
No. 3 invert sugar	0.33 lb	5.58%
malt extract	0.25 lb	4.23%
caramel 1000 SRM	0.25 lb	4.23%
Fuggles 95 mins	1.00 oz	
Fuggles 30 mins	0.25 oz	
OG	1026	
FG	1006.5	
ABV	2.58	
Apparent attenuation	75.00%	
IBU	20	
SRM	20	
Mash at	153° F	
Sparge at	176° F	
Boil time	95 minutes	
pitching temp	61° F	
Yeast	WLP025 Southwold	

1954 Elgood Strong Ale

I make a point of trying to collect new brewing records whenever I'm in the UK. On my last trip I managed to pick ones up from a couple of sources. One being Elgood.

I first asked the brewery if I could drop by a couple of years ago. The reason I hadn't made it there until now is purely a question of the practicalities. Wisbech has no train station. Even though it isn't that far from Newark, getting there by public transport is a nightmare. Luckily my mate Henry has a van and he drove me down.

Before we go any further, I'll point out the problems that I had with this recipe. Basically, the numbers don't add up. The grist consisted of 14 quarters, 93 barrels of water were used in mashing and sparging and there were 80 barrels of wort in the copper. But there were just 19.5 barrels in the fermenter. Where did the other 60 barrels of wort go? I can't imagine it was thrown away.

To take this discrepancy into account, I've divided the hopping rate by four. And then reduced them some more because they were from the 1950 season. I know nothing else about them, other than that they were English. 5 of the 85 lbs really were added in the hop back.

The grist is almost as simple as it appears. There really just is a single base malt. The sugar in the original, however, is half invert and half something called Muntona.

The mashing scheme is an infusion stood at 149° F for 20 minutes followed by an underlet held at 152° F for 100 minutes. Then sparging, obviously.

1953 Elgood Strong Ale		
pale malt	9.00 lb	90.00%
No. 2 invert sugar	1.00 lb	10.00%
Fuggles 95 mins	0.75 oz	
Fuggles 60 mins	0.75 oz	
Fuggles hop back	0.13 oz	
OG	1047	
FG	1017	
ABV	3.97	
Apparent attenuation	63.83%	
IBU	20	
SRM	7	
Mash at	152° F	
Sparge at	167° F	
Boil time	95 minutes	
pitching temp	61° F	
Yeast	WLP025 Southwold	

1964 Elgood Stout

The Stouts from regional breweries are an odd lot. Lots of them have the winning combination of very low OG and high FG.

Pretty sure what you get is a beer that's watery and sweet at the same time. This falls into that category. Though it isn't as insanely under-attenuated as some Scottish Sweet Stouts. The weakest as were under 2% ABV.

I wonder who drank Stouts like this? Grannies are what comes to my mind. But is that just because when I saw people drinking this type of stuff in the 1970s, they'd been drinking it for decades? Sweet Stout was trendy once. There wouldn't be so many examples, otherwise.

1964 Elgood Stout		
mild malt	2.00 lb	28.25%
pale malt	3.50 lb	49.44%
black malt	0.33 lb	4.66%
No. 3 invert sugar	0.50 lb	7.06%
caramel 1000 SRM	0.75 lb	10.59%
Fuggles 95 mins	0.75 oz	
Fuggles 30 mins	0.50 oz	
OG	1030	
FG	1013	
ABV	2.25	
Apparent attenuation	56.67%	
IBU	19	
SRM	44	
Mash at	150° F	
Sparge at	168° F	
Boil time	95 minutes	
pitching temp	60° F	
Yeast	WLP025 Southwold	

1949 Fullers X

1949 wasn't a great year for British brewing. Though average gravity was finally starting to creep up after a decade of decline. Though not for Fuller's mild. Its OG had fallen by two points since 1946.

Wartime restrictions can still be seen in the grist, which contains flaked barley. That was a government ordained replacement for flaked maize, English brewer's go-to adjunct. Other than that, there's just pale malt and sugar. Though the latter only made up around 5% of the total, surely another hangover from the war.

I've substituted No. 2 invert for a proprietary sugar called PEX and caramel for another one called intense.

I can't tell you much about the hops, other than that they were from the 1946, 1947 and 1948 harvests. I've guessed Fuggles. Other options are possible. I've reduced the quantity to take account of the hops' age.

The mashing heat I've given is for the initial infusion. An hour of mashing and 25 minutes standing there was an underlet that raised the temperature of the mash to 155°. It's a very typical mashing scheme of the period.

1949 Fullers X		
pale malt	5.25 lb	80.65%
flaked barley	1.00 lb	15.36%
glucose	0.125 lb	1.92%
No. 2 invert sugar	0.125 lb	1.92%
caramel 2000 SRM	0.01 lb	0.15%
Fuggles 90 min	0.50 oz	
Fuggles 30 min	0.50 oz	
OG	1028.5	
FG	1008	
ABV	2.71	
Apparent attenuation	71.93%	
IBU	13	
SRM	16	
Mash at	150° F	
Sparge at	168° F	
Boil time	90 minutes	
pitching temp	62.5° F	
Yeast	WLP002 English Ale	

1949 Fullers BO

Burton Old – in case you're wondering what BO stands for – was Fuller's, er, Burton Ale. The strong, dark Ale that was a common sight on London bars.

The war hadn't been kind to it, though it fared better than many Fullers beers. It only fell from 1055.5° to 1041.5°. That's good going, compared to what happened to PA.

If you're thinking that the recipe looks very much like that for X Ale, you'd be right. The two were parti-gyled together. Making this really just a souped-up Mild Ale. The comments on the recipe for the X Ale above also apply here.

1949 Fullers BO		
pale malt	7.50 lb	80.43%
flaked barley	1.50 lb	16.09%
glucose	0.05 lb	0.54%
No. 2 invert	0.125 lb	1.34%
caramel 1000 SRM	0.15 lb	1.61%
Fuggles 90 min	0.75 oz	
Fuggles 30 min	0.50 oz	
Goldings dry hops	0.50 oz	
OG	1041.5	
FG	1012.5	
ABV	3.84	
Apparent attenuation	69.88%	
IBU	17	
SRM	14.5	
Mash at	148° F	
Sparge at	168° F	
Boil time	90 minutes	
pitching temp	62° F	
Yeast	WLP002 English Ale	

1949 Fullers PA

How the might were fallen in the early years of austerity. Fullers PA, their top of the range Bitter, entered WW II with a very respectable OG of 1051°. By the autumn of 1946 it was down to just 1029.5°.

By 1949 it had lost another gravity point. Which left it the same as X Ale. Quite a comedown. In case you're wondering what eventually happened to PA, it's the direct ancestor of Chiswick Bitter.

The malt bill is extremely simple: pale malt. Though there were four different types: Sanders, Thompson, Guffer and Crisp. Well, at least the last one is still around. In addition to that there's quite a lot of flaked barley and just a hint of sugar. I've substituted more No. 2 invert for the proprietary sugar PEX.

The hops are exactly the same as in X, except the proportions are different. There's more of the 1947 and 1948 ones and less of the 1946.

As with X, there was an underlet after an hour of mashing and 25 minutes standing. It raised the temperature of the mash to 153°.

Fullers employed the dropping system of fermentation at this point. After around 12 hours in a narrow, cylindrical fermenter, the wort was dropped into a shallow square to complete fermentation.

1949 Fullers PA		
pale malt	5.25 lb	77.09%
flaked barley	1.25 lb	18.36%
No. 1 invert sugar	0.04 lb	0.59%
No. 2 invert sugar	0.25 lb	3.67%
caramel 1000 SRM	0.02 lb	0.29%
Fuggles 90 min	0.75 oz	
Fuggles 30 min	0.50 oz	
Goldings dry hops	0.25 oz	
OG	1028.5	
FG	1005.5	
ABV	3.04	
Apparent attenuation	80.70%	
IBU	18	
SRM	7	
Mash at	151° F	
Sparge at	168° F	
Boil time	90 minutes	
pitching temp	62° F	
Yeast	WLP002 English Ale	

1949 Fullers SPA

The introduction of a stronger Bitter, SPA, was a sign that things were finally starting to improve for British drinkers. Several breweries created similar beers around this time.

This is a beer that you might well have drunk yourself. Though not under the name SPA. In the 1950s it underwent a name change and became London Pride.

There's not much that can be said about the recipe as it's identical to that for PA, the two beers being parti-gyled together. There is one small difference, however. I've not specified any dry hops. There's no mention of dry-hopping in Fuller's records, but I know that currently London Pride isn't dry-hopped. I'm guessing that PA was. I could be wrong.

In terms of gravity, it's much like the current incarnation. The recipe, though, is quite different. Today there's some crystal in the grist and a tiny amount of chocolate malt for colour. And no sugar or adjuncts.

1949 Fullers SPA		
pale malt	8.00 lb	80.20%
flaked barley	1.50 lb	15.04%
No. 1 invert sugar	0.07 lb	0.70%
No. 2 invert sugar	0.38 lb	3.76%
caramel 1000 SRM	0.03 lb	0.30%
Fuggles 90 min	1.00 oz	
Fuggles 30 min	0.75 oz	
OG	1043	
FG	1012	
ABV	4.10	
Apparent attenuation	72.09%	
IBU	23	
SRM	7	
Mash at	151° F	
Sparge at	168° F	
Boil time	90 minutes	
pitching temp	62° F	
Yeast	WLP002 English Ale	

1949 Fullers P

I got all excited the first time I spotted P in a post-war Fuller's log. Was this the last London Porter, I asked myself? Well yes. And no.

Yes, because it is basically the same beer as their pre-war draught Porter. But also no, as this wasn't a draught beer and wasn't marketed as porter. It was a bottled beer called Nourishing Stout.

It's another minimum gravity beer at just 1027°. A crappy degree of attenuation leaves it at under 2.5% ABV. You weren't going to get pissed very quickly on this baby.

The grist contains just three malts: pale, crystal and black. Unusually for a London brewer, Fullers stopped using brown malt in the early 1920s. Unlike their other beers, which had only around 5% sugar, P contains loads, over 20% of the grist.

I've made some guesstitutions when it comes to the sugar. In the original, what I have as caramel was 50% London caramel, 50% Carmeline. As in the other recipes, I've substituted No. 2 invert for PEX. Special Dark I've interpreted as No. 4 invert.

The hops are the same 1946, 1947 and 1948 ones, in the same proportions as for X Ale.

Once again there was an underlet 1 hour and 25 minutes into the mash, which raised the temperature from 147° F to 150° F.

1949 Fullers P		
pale malt	3.50 lb	56.82%
black malt	0.50 lb	8.12%
crystal malt 60 L	0.50 lb	8.12%
flaked barley	0.33 lb	5.36%
caramel 1000 SRM	0.33 lb	5.36%
No. 2 invert	0.25 lb	4.06%
No. 4 invert	0.75 lb	12.18%
Fuggles 90 min	0.67 oz	
Fuggles 30 min	0.50 oz	
OG	1027	
FG	1009	
ABV	2.38	
Apparent attenuation	66.67%	
IBU		
SRM		
Mash at	146° F	
Sparge at	170° F	
Boil time	90 minutes	
pitching temp	62° F	
Yeast	WLP002 English Ale	

1959 Fullers X

At the end of the 1950s, X Ale, or Hock as it was also known, was still a big seller for Fullers. That's reflected in the batch sizes, which were usually 200-300 barrels.

The OG has bounced back a little since 1949, leaving a beer of just about 3% ABV. This being a cask beer, by the time it had come into condition that would undoubtedly have been a bit higher.

Some things haven't changed. There's still just a single malt. Though the adjunct element of the grist has changed from flaked barley to flaked maize. PEX I've again replaced with No. 2 invert. I've substituted No. 3 invert for the other proprietary sugar, CDM (Caramelized Dextro-Maltose).

The hops are mostly Kent Fuggles from the 1958 crop, with a small amount of Golding Varieties from the same year.

The temperature of the mash was raised from 146° F to 151° F by an underlet after 1.5 hours.

1959 Fullers X		
pale malt	5.50 lb	78.35%
flaked maize	0.67 lb	9.54%
No. 2 invert sugar	0.50 lb	7.12%
No. 3 invert sugar	0.25 lb	3.56%
caramel 2000 SRM	0.10 lb	1.42%
Fuggles 90 min	0.75 oz	
Fuggles 30 min	0.75 oz	
Goldings Varieties 30 min	0.125 oz	
OG	1031.5	
FG	1009.5	
ABV	2.91	
Apparent attenuation	69.84%	
IBU	19	
SRM	17	
Mash at	146° F	
Sparge at	166° F	
Boil time	90 minutes	
pitching temp	62° F	
Yeast	WLP002 English Ale	

1959 Fullers SBA

Brown Ale is a frustrating style. Because it so rarely turns up in brewing records. A few breweries did make a Brown Ale as its own beer, but often it was simply the draught Mild tweaked a little before bottling.

So I'm always overjoyed when I come across an example, like SBA. Which stands for Special Brown Ale. Though I'm not sure what's so special about a beer of just 2.7% ABV.

It is sort of just Fullers X Ale. It was parti-gyled with and is only a touch weaker.

For comments on recipe and process, see at the X Ale above.

1959 Fullers SBA		
pale malt	4.50 lb	80.00%
flaked maize	0.50 lb	8.89%
No. 2 invert sugar	0.50 lb	8.89%
No. 3 invert sugar	0.125 lb	2.22%
Fuggles 90 min	0.75 oz	
Fuggles 30 min	0.50 oz	
Goldings Varieties 30 min	0.125 oz	
OG	1027	
FG	1006.5	
ABV	2.71	
Apparent attenuation	75.93%	
IBU	24	
SRM	6	
Mash at	146° F	
Sparge at	166° F	
Boil time	90 minutes	
pitching temp	62° F	
Yeast	WLP002 English Ale	

1959 Fullers Old Burton Extra

Here's another beer that was parti-gyled with X, Old Burton Extra. Their draught Burton Ale.

Before WW II, Fullers brewed two draught Burtons: Burton Old and Old Burton Extra. The former was the standard strength for the style at the time, 1055.5°. While OBE was a good bit stronger at 1069°, which was very strong for a draught beer then. Though they brewed it in tiny quantities, usually fewer than 10 barrels.

Not that this was brewed in large batch. Just 9.75 barrels, along with 61 barrels of Strong Ale and 270 barrels of X Ale. That's the sort of thing you can only achieve with parti-gyling.

1959 Fullers Old Burton Extra		
pale malt	8.25 lb	78.57%
flaked maize	1.00 lb	9.52%
No. 2 invert sugar	1.00 lb	9.52%
No. 3 invert sugar	0.25 lb	2.38%
Fuggles 90 min	0.75 oz	
Fuggles 30 min	0.75 oz	
Goldings dry hops	0.50 oz	
OG	1049.5	
FG	1014.5	
ABV	4.63	
Apparent attenuation	70.71%	
IBU	18	
SRM	8	
Mash at	143° F	
Sparge at	166° F	
Boil time	90 minutes	
pitching temp	60° F	
Yeast	WLP002 English Ale	

1959 Fullers Strong Ale

You guessed it – yet another beer that was parti-gyled with X Ale. This time it's a strong bottled beer. Which looks remarkably similar to pre-WW II Old Burton Extra.

I can see from Whitbread Gravity Book entries that it was packaged in nip bottles. My guess is that punters would order a bottle as a night cap to end the evening. It was quite expensive 16d for a nip (third of a pint) in 1953, when a pint of draught London Pride only cost 20d.

Being parti-gyled with X Ale, it was really a super-strong Mild. Something along the lines of a pre-WW I XXX Ale. I wonder if they ever sneaked out a pin or two of it in the winter? Some breweries did have a pin of something very strong on the bar during the cold months.

1959 Fullers Strong Ale		
pale malt	12.00 lb	78.28%
flaked maize	1.50 lb	9.78%
No. 2 invert sugar	1.50 lb	9.78%
No. 3 invert sugar	0.33 lb	2.15%
Fuggles 90 min	1.25 oz	
Fuggles 30 min	1.00 oz	
Goldings dry hops	0.50 oz	
OG	1072.5	
FG	1021.5	
ABV	6.75	
Apparent attenuation	70.34%	
IBU	22	
SRM	10	
Mash at	143° F	
Sparge at	166° F	
Boil time	90 minutes	
pitching temp	61° F	
Yeast	WLP002 English Ale	

1960 Fullers PA

Fullers continued to brew considerable quantities of their Ordinary Bitter, PA. Though it was always parti-gyled with London Pride.

This particular parti-gyle consisted of 301 barrels of PA, 200 of London Pride and 61 of Export London Pride. Which show that, although London Pride has a strong following, it was still PA that sold most.

It's a bit too weak to really class as an Ordinary Bitter. I'd call it a Boy's Bitter, that is a Pale Ale with the gravity of Ordinary Mild.

The recipe is like all those from Fullers: pale malt flaked maize and sugar. The No. 2 invert and glucose are in the recipe. The No. 3 is my substitution for PEX and CDM.

For once, I really know what the hops were: Kent Goldings Varieties from the 1958 crop and Worcester Fuggles also from 1958. The dry hops are a total guess.

1960 Fullers PA		
pale malt	6.00 lb	82.93%
flaked maize	0.75 lb	10.37%
No. 2 invert sugar	0.33 lb	4.56%
No. 3 invert sugar	0.03 lb	0.41%
glucose	0.125 lb	1.73%
Fuggles 90 min	0.75 oz	
Goldings Varieties 30 min	0.75 oz	
Goldings dry hops	0.25 oz	
OG	1032	
FG	1009	
ABV	3.04	
Apparent attenuation	71.88%	
IBU	22	
SRM	4	
Mash at	144° F	
Sparge at	168° F	
Boil time	90 minutes	
pitching temp	61° F	
Yeast	WLP002 English Ale	

1960 Fullers London Pride

London Pride sold in decent quantities for what was quite a strong Bitter. I can understand why. It's a cracking beer when looked after properly.

This particular example was parti-gyled with the PA in the previous recipe. Which doesn't leave much to discuss about this recipe. Unless . . . I compare to today's version.

It intrigues me that London Pride always seems to have tasted pretty much the same, even though there was a big change of the recipe, I think in the 1990s, when Fullers went all malt. The current version is pale malt, crystal malt and a tiny amount of chocolate malt for colour.

1960 Fullers London Pride		
pale malt	8.00 lb	80.60%
flaked maize	1.25 lb	12.59%
No. 2 invert sugar	0.50 lb	5.04%
No. 3 invert sugar	0.05 lb	0.50%
glucose	0.125 lb	1.26%
Fuggles 90 min	1.00 oz	
Goldings Varieties 30 min	1.00 oz	
OG	1043.5	
FG	1011.5	
ABV	4.23	
Apparent attenuation	73.56%	
IBU	27	
SRM	5	
Mash at	144° F	
Sparge at	168° F	
Boil time	90 minutes	
pitching temp	60° F	
Yeast	WLP002 English Ale	

1960 Fullers Export London Pride

I'm not sure if at this point Fullers was really exporting London Pride. This could just have been the name for a stronger version. Though I know that today Export London Pride really is the stronger bottled version destined for export.

I'm not sure exactly when it was first brewed, but the first sighting I have of it is in 1959. Obviously, it being a parti-gyle with the standard version, the recipe is the same. Which in turn is the same as the PA recipe. They liked to keep things simple.

1960 Fullers Export London Pride		
pale malt	8.75 lb	81.97%
flaked maize	1.25 lb	11.71%
No. 2 invert sugar	0.50 lb	4.68%
No. 3 invert sugar	0.05 lb	0.47%
glucose	0.125 lb	1.17%
Fuggles 90 min	1.25 oz	
Goldings Varieties 30 min	1.00 oz	
OG	1048.5	
FG	1012.5	
ABV	4.76	
Apparent attenuation	74.23%	
IBU	29	
SRM	6	
Mash at	144° F	
Sparge at	168° F	
Boil time	90 minutes	
pitching temp	60° F	
Yeast	WLP002 English Ale	

1959 Fullers Nourishing Stout

It wasn't until the late 1950s that Fullers finally got around to changing P to NS in the brewhouse. Even though the beer had been marketed as Nourishing Stout for more than a decade.

It was unusual in being the only beer in Fullers range that wasn't parti-gyled. Which probably made it quite uneconomical to brew. It was produced in batches of a little over 100 barrels in a brewhouse with a normal brew length of 300-500 barrels. 100 barrels was probably about the minimum amount the equipment could cope with.

The recipe hasn't changed a great deal since 1949. There are still three malts: pale, black and crystal. The sugars remain PEX (for which I've substituted No. 2 invert), Special Dark (No. 4 invert) and two types of caramel: London caramel and Carmeline.

From Whitbread Gravity Book analyses for Nourishing Stout, I can see that it wasn't tinkered with after primary fermentation. Some breweries added lactose at racking time.

The hops were Worcester Fuggles from the 1958 crop and Goldings varieties from 1957.

1959 Fullers Nourishing Stout		
pale malt	3.00 lb	44.44%
black malt	0.75 lb	11.11%
crystal malt 60 L	0.50 lb	7.41%
flaked maize	0.50 lb	7.41%
No. 2 invert	0.250 lb	3.70%
No. 4 invert	1.250 lb	18.52%
caramel 2000 SRM	0.50 lb	7.41%
Fuggles 90 min	0.75 oz	
Fuggles 30 min	0.50 oz	
Goldings Varieties 30 min	0.25 oz	
OG	1031.5	
FG	1011.5	
ABV	2.65	
Apparent attenuation	63.49%	
IBU	22	
SRM	54	
Mash at	140° F	
Sparge at	170° F	
Boil time	90 minutes	
pitching temp	61° F	
Yeast	WLP002 English Ale	

1948 Lees Bitter

This iteration of Lees Bitter is notable for being very unremarkable. If you get what I mean.

If you've been paying attention, you might have noticed the lack of crystal malt in many Bitters, as is the case here. It's surprisingly recently that it became a standard element of Pale Ale grists.

Black malt is slightly unusual in a Bitter. The quantity is so small it's clearly just to add a little colour. The No.2 invert in the recipe is my substitution for invert and CWA.

As the hops were all English, I've guessed Fuggles and Goldings. The chances are they were that, or something similar.

An underlet raised the mashing temperature to 149° F.

1948 Lees Bitter		
pale malt	7.00 lb	86.63%
black malt	0.08 lb	0.99%
enzymic malt	0.125 lb	1.55%
glucose	0.125 lb	1.55%
No. 2 invert sugar	0.75 lb	9.28%
Fuggles 105 mins	1.00 oz	
Goldings 30 min	1.00 oz	
Goldings dry hops	0.25 oz	
OG	1038	
FG	1010	
ABV	3.70	
Apparent attenuation	73.68%	
IBU	26	
SRM	8	
Mash at	147° F	
Sparge at	170° F	
Boil time	105 minutes	
pitching temp	60° F	
Yeast	Wyeast 1318 London ale III (Boddingtons)	

1950 Lees K

This is actually Lees Ordinary Mild. I've no idea why they called it K. But it had been around for a long time – since at least 1884. It lasted until 1955, when the brewhouse name was changed to simply Mild.

As far as I can tell, K was always pale in colour. A trait that continued after its name was changed to Mild. Lees were unusual in having an Ordinary Mild that was pale and a Best Mild that was dark. Usually it was the other way around.

The sugars in the original were Invert and Proteinex, for which I've substituted No. 1 and No. 2 invert.

An underlet after 20 minutes raised the mash temperature to 150° F.

1950 Lees K		
pale malt	4.50 lb	75.38%
crystal malt 80 L	0.25 lb	4.19%
black malt	0.06 lb	1.01%
enzymic malt	0.080 lb	1.34%
glucose	0.250 lb	4.19%
No. 1 invert sugar	0.33 lb	5.53%
No. 2 invert sugar	0.50 lb	8.38%
Fuggles 105 min	0.50 oz	
Goldings 30 min	0.50 oz	
Goldings dry hops	0.125 lb	
OG	1028	
FG	1007	
ABV	2.78	
Apparent attenuation	75.00%	
IBU	15	
SRM	9	
Mash at	148° F	
Sparge at	170° F	
Boil time	105 minutes	
pitching temp	61° F	
Yeast	Wyeast 1318 London ale III (Boddingtons)	

1948 Lees Best Mild

The effect of the war in lowering gravities left Lees with a Best Mild that wasn't much over 1030°. Though Lees only introduced Best Mild in 1946, presumably to offer drinkers something with a bit more kick than their watery K Mild.

The recipe is quite different from K, mostly because Best Mild is much darker in colour. There's quite a lot more black malt and the sugars are different: Invert and PS crystals. I've substituted No. 3 invert.

Annoyingly, this period of Lees records doesn't include the FG. I've made a guess based on their beers from the 1930s.

An underlet raised the mash temperature to 149° F.

1948 Lees Best Mild		
pale malt	5.75 lb	69.70%
black malt	0.25 lb	3.03%
crystal malt 80 L	0.75 lb	9.09%
enzymic malt	0.25 lb	3.03%
No. 3 Invert	1.25 lb	15.15%
Fuggles 105 mins	0.75 oz	
Goldings 30 mins	0.75 oz	
Goldings dry hops	0.125 oz	
OG	1032	
FG	1006	
ABV	3.44	
Apparent attenuation	81.25%	
IBU	21	
SRM	19	
Mash at	147° F	
Sparge at	170° F	
Boil time	90 minutes	
pitching temp	60° F	
Yeast	Wyeast 1318 London ale III (Boddingtons)	

1948 Lees "C" Ale

I was so delighted when I came across this beer in the Lees records. Finally, I'd find out for certain what a "C" Ale was.

It must have been 10 years ago when I first stumbled across a reference to "C" Ale in the history of a Manchester brewery. What the hell was it and why did it have that name? It turned out that several breweries in the Manchester area brewed one at one time or another. It was obviously some sort of strong bottled beer. But as to what the name signifies, I've no idea.

Stylistically, it's much like a London Burton Ale, just bottled rather than draught.

The grist is surprisingly similar to Lees Bitter from the same year. Except here there's some crystal malt and rather more black malt. I've had to do some interpretation on the sugars, which are listed as simply Invert and CWA. No. 2 invert is my choice.

The hops are rather vaguely described in the log. I just know that they were English and from the 1947 crop.

The initial mashing heat of 150° F was raised to 152° F by an underlet.

1948 Lees "C" Ale		
pale malt	7.50 lb	75.34%
black malt	0.125 lb	1.26%
crystal malt 60 L	0.50 lb	5.02%
enzymic malt	0.25 lb	2.51%
glucose	0.33 lb	3.31%
No. 2 invert sugar	1.25 lb	12.56%
Fuggles 105 mins	0.75 oz	
Fuggles 60 mins	0.50 oz	
Goldings 30 mins	0.50 oz	
Goldings dry hops	0.25 oz	
OG	1050	
FG	1014	
ABV	4.76	
Apparent attenuation	72.00%	
IBU	21	
SRM	13	
Mash at	150° F	
Sparge at	170° F	
Boil time	105 minutes	
pitching temp	59° F	
Yeast	Wyeast 1318 London ale III (Boddingtons)	

1952 Lees Stout

I may as well complete the Lees set with their Stout. In case any of you feels like recreating a 1950's Manchester pub.

This would have been a purely bottled product. London brewers were still producing draught Stouts, but in most of the country they didn't make it past WW II. The change in packaging seems to have changed the type of Stouts being brewed. Ones with lower gravities and sometimes, but not always, rather sweet. And it was becoming a pensioners' drink.

London brewers stuck with relatively complicated Stout grists in the 20th century, going for a combination of pale, brown and black malt, plus sugar. Lees went even further, having five malts, oatmeal and sugar in their Stout. With around 15% roasted malt, this must have been quite a thick and tasty beer, despite the modest gravity.

As usual, the recipe employs some guesswork. There was no FG, which is particularly frustrating in the case of a 1950's Stout. Because the rates of attenuation were all over the shop, from 45% to 95% with everything inbetween. So when I say the FG is a guess, it's a big guess.

The hop variety is another guess. All I know for sure is that they were English. As 75% of the hops grown in England at the time were Fuggles, that seems a good enough choice. Plus you wouldn't waste classy Goldings in a Stout like this. No point with all that roast going on.

On the plus side, the logs do include the mashing heat, not just strike and tap heat. The initial mash temperature was 146° F, raised to 148° F by an underlet.

1952 Lees Stout		
pale malt	4.25 lb	54.84%
brown malt	0.25 lb	3.23%
black malt	0.25 lb	3.23%
chocolate malt	0.50 lb	6.45%
crystal malt	0.50 lb	6.45%
oatmeal	0.50 lb	6.45%
No. 3 invert sugar	1.50 lb	19.35%
Fuggles 90 min	1.00 oz	
Fuggles 30 min	1.00 oz	
OG	1038	
FG	1010	
ABV	3.70	
Apparent attenuation	73.68%	
IBU	27	
SRM	29	
Mash at	148° F	
Sparge at	170° F	
Boil time	90 minutes	
pitching temp	60° F	
Yeast	Wyeast 1318 London ale III (Boddingtons)	

1955 Lees Mild

Lees didn't go in for simple recipes when it came to their Milds.

The original contained no less than five types of sugar: 1 cwt Invert, 3 cwt C.M.E., 1 cwt C.W.E., 2 cwt Proteinex, 1 cwt P.S. Crystals. Don't ask me what they all are. I haven't the foggiest. So I've just gone for a combination of invert sugars.

The grist is notable for containing two base malt, pale and mild. Plus a bit of crystal and the obligatory enzymic malt. Recipes from the 1950s without it are rare.

The hopping is quite heavy for a mild, especially one this piss weak. The hops themselves were all English, from 1953 and 1954 crop.

1955 Lees Mild			
pale malt		3.00 lb	42.86%
mild malt		1.75 lb	25.00%
crystal malt 80 L		0.25 lb	3.57%
enzymic malt		0.25 lb	3.57%
flaked maize		0.25 lb	3.57%
No. 1 invert sugar		0.50 lb	7.14%
No. 2 invert sugar		1.00 lb	14.29%
Fuggles 95 mins		0.75 oz	
Fuggles 30 mins		0.75 oz	
OG		1031	
FG		1007	
ABV		3.18	
Apparent attenuation		77.42%	
IBU		23	
SRM		7	
Mash at		150° F	
Sparge at		170° F	
Boil time		95 minutes	
pitching temp		60° F	
Yeast	Wyeast 1318 London ale III (Boddingtons)		

1955 Lees Best Mild

A wonderfully contrary beer from Lees that, scorning the simplicity of most contemporary brews, throws the kitchen sink at their classy Mild.

My recipe has a crazy number of ingredients, but it doesn't show the true picture. The original contained five types of sugar, only one of which, glucose, appears exactly. No. 3 and No. 4 are my approximations of Invert, Carameline, P.S. Cr and M.S.P. And no, I've not the slightest idea what those last two are. Carameline I'm guessing is pretty dark. Hence the No. 4.

Then there all the coloured malts: brown, black, chocolate and crystal. Plus some oatmeal. It's pretty crazy. And really unlike most Dark Mild recipes of the time. It's unusual enough to have any malt darker than crystal, let alone three.

English hops again, though I know nothing else about them, other than that they were from the 1953 and 1954 harvest.

1955 Lees Best Mild		
pale malt	4.50 lb	66.08%
brown malt	0.125 lb	1.84%
black malt	0.06 lb	0.88%
chocolate Malt	0.25 lb	3.67%
crystal malt 80 L	0.25 lb	3.67%
oatmeal	0.125 lb	1.84%
glucose	0.25 lb	3.67%
No. 3 invert sugar	0.50 lb	7.34%
No. 4 invert sugar	0.75 lb	11.01%
Fuggles 90 mins	0.75 oz	
Fuggles 30 mins	0.75 oz	
OG	1035	
FG	1008	
ABV	3.57	
Apparent attenuation	77.14%	
IBU	20	
SRM	26	
Mash at	148° F	
Sparge at	170° F	
Boil time	105 minutes	
pitching temp	60° F	
Yeast	Wyeast 1318 London ale III (Boddingtons)	

1955 Lees Strong Ale

Immediately after WW II, Lees brewed "C" Ale, a strongish, dark bottled beer. They seem to have dropped that around 1954, originally replacing it with something called Golden Brew.

With an OG of 1078it was a good bit stronger than "C" Ale. But Golden Brew didn't last long. The very next year something simply called Strong Ale appeared with a slightly lower OG. This became a fixture in Lees range.

As with most Lees beers, there's a dizzying array of sugars. In this case: Invert, C.W.A., HX and C.D.M. I've replaced them with a combination of No. 2 and No. 3 invert.

The hops were English from 1953 and 1954 and a tiny amount of Styrians.

1955 Lees Strong Ale		
pale malt	9.00 lb	61.39%
mild malt	1.50 lb	10.23%
crystal malt 80 L	0.33 lb	2.25%
enzymic malt	0.33 lb	2.25%
flaked maize	1.50 lb	10.23%
No. 2 invert sugar	0.50 lb	3.41%
No. 3 invert sugar	1.50 lb	10.23%
Fuggles 180 mins	1.50 oz	
Fuggles 30 mins	1.50 oz	
OG	1068	
FG	1020	
ABV	6.35	
Apparent attenuation	70.59%	
IBU	34	
SRM	14	
Mash at	150° F	
Sparge at	170° F	
Boil time	180 minutes	
pitching temp	58° F	
Yeast	Wyeast 1318 London ale III (Boddingtons)	

1957 Lees Stout

Lees did a fair bit of tinkering with their Stout recipe in the 1950's and 1960's. A big one being adding lactose in 1956.

There have been other changes since 1952. Two malts – brown and chocolate – have been dropped. Plus flaked oats have replaced oatmeal. At least the percentage of oats is decent, unlike the tiny quantities employed by cheating London brewers.

The sugars have changed, too. Out go caremeline and Proteinex, in come HX and CDM. I've interpreted those latter two as No. 3 invert. There's also black invert, which is pretty obviously No. 4 invert.

No details on the hops again. I've gone for all Fuggles. But it could just have easily been a Fuggles/Goldings combination.

1957 Lees Stout		
pale malt	2.25 lb	33.33%
black malt	0.67 lb	9.93%
crystal malt 60 L	1.00 lb	14.81%
flaked oats	0.33 lb	4.89%
No. 3 invert sugar	1.00 lb	14.81%
No. 4 invert sugar	0.50 lb	7.41%
lactose	1.00 lb	14.81%
Fuggles 90 min	1.00 oz	
Fuggles 30 min	0.75 oz	
OG	1036	
FG	1014	
ABV	2.91	
Apparent attenuation	61.11%	
IBU	23	
SRM	32	
Mash at	152° F	
Sparge at	170° F	
Boil time	90 minutes	
pitching temp	60° F	
Yeast	Wyeast 1318 London ale III (Boddingtons)	

1957 Lees Bitter

Not a huge amount has changed with Lees Bitter since 1948.

OK, it's shed one point off its gravity. No big deal there. The tiny amount of black malt has gone and an adjunct has appeared in the form of flaked maize. A small amount of crystal malt has been added, too.

The original contained multiple types of sugar: 1 cwt. Invert, 1 cwt. C.M.E., 4 cwt. C.W.A., 1 cwt. HX. For all that lot, I've substituted No. 2 invert sugar. Though I've no idea how close that comes.

It's not very heavily hopped which is reflected in the fairly low IBU count.

1957 Lees Bitter		
pale malt	6.00 lb	75.00%
crystal malt 80 L	0.125 lb	1.56%
enzymic malt	0.125 lb	1.56%
flaked maize	0.50 lb	6.25%
No. 2 Invert	1.25 lb	15.63%
Fuggles 90 min	1.00 oz	
Fuggles 30 min	1.00 oz	
Goldings dry hops	0.50 oz	
OG	1040	
FG	1010	
ABV	3.97	
Apparent attenuation	75.00%	
IBU	25	
SRM	7.5	
Mash at	148° F	
Sparge at	170° F	
Boil time	90 minutes	
pitching temp	60° F	
Yeast	Wyeast 1318 London ale III (Boddingtons)	

1957 Lees Export

I'm not sure when Lees first introduced Export, but I doubt it's much earlier than when this beer was brewed. 29th May, if you're interested.

What was this beer? A strong draught Bitter? A special bottled Pale Ale? No idea. One thing I'm pretty certain of: it wasn't really exported. Lees was a small. Locally-oriented concern. They weren't shipping beer outside the UK. I doubt it got much further than Manchester.

The FG is a total guess as the brewers at Lees couldn't be arsed to note it down. All I know about the hops is that they were English and there's no mention of dry hops in the brewing log. Quite a bit of guesswork, then.

As with all Lees beers, it contained a cocktail of sugars. Only three in this case: 0.5 invert, 1 C.W.A., 0.5 HX. I've substituted No. 2 invert.

All I know about the hops is that they were English from the 1956 and 1957 crop.

1957 Lees Export		
pale malt	8.00 lb	73.80%
crystal malt 80 L	0.09 lb	0.83%
enzymic malt	0.25 lb	2.31%
flaked maize	0.75 lb	6.92%
No. 2 Invert	1.75 lb	16.14%
Fuggles 90 min	1.25 oz	
Fuggles 30 min	1.00 oz	
Goldings dry hops	0.50 oz	
OG	1053	
FG	1016	
ABV	4.89	
Apparent attenuation	69.81%	
IBU	26	
SRM	9	
Mash at	148° F	
Sparge at	170° F	
Boil time	90 minutes	
pitching temp	60° F	
Yeast	Wyeast 1318 London ale III (Boddingtons)	

1963 Lees Archer Stout

Lees were unusual in their use of many different coloured malts. And not just in Stout where you'd expect them.

By the 1960s most regional breweries' Stouts were pretty watery affairs. Archer Stout is by no means one of the worst culprits. Though a poor degree of attenuation leaves it just under 3% ABV. You can blame the lactose for that.

There's a lot of sugar in this beer – over 30% of the grist. The white sugar is my substitution for a sugar called HX. The No. 3 replaces CDM (Caramelised Dextro-Maltose) and the No. 4 black invert.

I suspect the finished product was pretty sweet. It's quite lightly hopped and the FG is pretty high.

1963 Lees Archer Stout			
pale malt		2.50 lb	36.60%
brown malt		1.00 lb	14.64%
black malt		0.67 lb	9.81%
flaked oats		0.33 lb	4.83%
white sugar		0.50 lb	7.32%
No. 3 invert sugar		0.33 lb	4.83%
No. 4 invert sugar		0.50 lb	7.32%
lactose		1.00 lb	14.64%
Fuggles 90 mins		0.25 oz	
Styrian Goldings 90 mins		0.25 oz	
Fuggles 60 mins		0.50 oz	
Goldings 30 mins		0.50 oz	
OG		1036	
FG		1014	
ABV		2.91	
Apparent attenuation		61.11%	
IBU		20	
SRM		31	
Mash at		154° F	
Sparge at		170° F	
Boil time		90 minutes	
pitching temp		60° F	
Yeast	Wyeast 1318 London ale III (Boddingtons)		

1963 Lees Mild

The 1950's version of Lees Best Mild has been a big hit with home brewers. Mostly, I think, because of its complex malt bill. This time, though, we're looking at its younger brother: simple Mild. What's most surprising to me, is that not only wasn't it parti-gyled with Best Mild, but it has a totally different grist.

There's one good reason for that: the two beers were different in colour. The usual convention was Ordinary Mild dark, Best Mild pale. For some reason, Lees did it the other way around. And with all the dark malt and dark sugar in Best Mild, there's no way they could parti-gyle Ordinary Mild with it.

I sometimes wonder why pubs sell several Bitters of only slightly differing gravities. This case is even crazier – Best Mild, at 1035°, was only 2 gravity points higher than this beer. It does make you wonder why they bothered. Though I suppose, at least, the different grists left beers with distinct characters.

Speaking of grists, Ordinary Mild contained crystal malt, which Best didn't. While Ordinary lacked the oak smoked and flaked oats that were in Best.

There's an even bigger difference when it comes to the sugars. Best: Invert, Black Invert, PS Crystals, D.C.S., HX and C.D.M. Ordinary: Invert, C.M.E., Stacons, Laverna, D.C.S, HX and a tiny amount of C.D.M. I won't even try to guess what all that lot were. I've substituted No. 1 and No. 2 invert.

Oddly, Ordinary Mild has a slightly higher hopping rate than Best. I've guessed Fuggles, but all I know for sure is that they were English. Around 10% of the hops were Styrian Goldings. But as that would only amount to 0.15 oz. at this scale, I didn't bother with it. Feel free to throw a few in if you feel like it.

Before I forget, the FG is also a guess. Lees didn't bother filling it in.

1963 Lees Mild		
pale malt	5.25 lb	76.98%
crystal malt 60 L	0.25 lb	3.67%
flaked maize	0.33 lb	4.84%
No. 1 invert sugar	0.33 lb	4.84%
No. 2 invert sugar	0.66 lb	9.68%
Fuggles 90 min	0.75 oz	
Fuggles 30 min	0.75 oz	
OG	1033	
FG	1007	
ABV	3.44	
Apparent attenuation	78.79%	
IBU	21	
SRM	6.5	
Mash at	148° F	
Sparge at	170° F	
Boil time	90 minutes	
pitching temp	60° F	
Yeast	Wyeast 1318 London ale III (Boddingtons)	

1963 Lees Best Mild

The recipes from Lees are quite a contrast with those of most other breweries. They're far more complicated, both in terms of grains and sugars.

The grist is a bit simpler than in 1955. The black and chocolate malt have been dropped. But, with two coloured malts, it's still much more complex than most Dark Mild recipes. Given just the list of ingredients, you could be forgiven for guessing this was a Stout. Especially with the presence of both flaked oats and lactose.

The sugars in the original were way more complicated, with six in total: Invert, Black Invert, PS Crystals, D.C.S., HX and C.D.M. That's quite a list. I've rationalised that to No. 3 and No. 4 invert.

The hops in the original were English from the 1961 and 1962 crops, plus a tiny quantity of Styrians from 1961.

1963 Lees Best Mild		
pale malt	4.00 lb	55.87%
brown malt	0.50 lb	6.98%
enzymic malt	0.125 lb	1.75%
crystal malt 80 L	0.33 lb	4.61%
flaked oats	0.125 lb	1.75%
lactose	0.25 lb	3.49%
No. 3 invert sugar	1.50 lb	20.95%
No. 4 invert sugar	0.33 lb	4.61%
Fuggles 90 mins	0.75 oz	
Goldings 30 mins	0.75 oz	
OG	1035	
FG	1008	
ABV	3.57	
Apparent attenuation	77.14%	
IBU	20	
SRM	19	
Mash at	148° F	
Sparge at	170° F	
Boil time	90 minutes	
pitching temp	60° F	
Yeast	Wyeast 1318 London ale III (Boddingtons)	

1963 Lees Bitter

There hasn't been a great deal happen to Lees Bitter since 1957. It still has the same OG and the recipe is quite similar.

The grist is the same. The only real change is a slightly lower level of hopping. Oh, and I've interpreted the sugars a bit differently.

As usual with Lees beers, there was a dizzying array of sugars: Invert, C.M.E., Stacons, C.W.A. and HX. I've interpreted that as a mixture of No. 1 and No. 2 invert.

1963 Lees Bitter		
pale malt	6.25 lb	75.03%
enzymic malt	0.125 lb	1.50%
crystal malt 80 L	0.125 lb	1.50%
flaked maize	0.50 lb	6.00%
No. 1 invert sugar	0.33 lb	3.96%
No. 2 invert sugar	1.00 lb	12.00%
Fuggles 90 mins	0.75 oz	
Fuggles 60 mins	0.50 oz	
Goldings 30 mins	0.50 oz	
Goldings dry hops	0.25 oz	
OG	1040	
FG	1010	
ABV	3.97	
Apparent attenuation	75.00%	
IBU	23	
SRM	7	
Mash at	148° F	
Sparge at	170° F	
Boil time	90 minutes	
pitching temp	60° F	
Yeast	Wyeast 1318 London ale III (Boddingtons)	

1963 Lees Export

Export was effectively a stronger version of Lees Bitter. Though was, as far as I can tell, exclusively a bottled product.

Despite being bottled, it was probably mostly sold in pubs. Just as the majority of beer was back then.

The very recipe is very similar to that from 1957. Just a little more enzymic malt and a bit more sugar. The hopping is about the same. With English hops from the 1961 crop and a tiny amount of Styrians, also from the 1961 harvest.

The FG, as for all Lees beers, is a guess. The brewing records don't include it and I have no analyses of Lees beers from other sources.

1963 Lees Export		
pale malt	7.75 lb	70.97%
enzymic malt	0.33 lb	3.02%
crystal malt 80 L	0.09 lb	0.82%
flaked maize	0.75 lb	6.87%
No. 1 invert sugar	1.00 lb	9.16%
No. 2 invert sugar	1.00 lb	9.16%
Fuggles 90 mins	0.75 oz	
Fuggles 60 mins	0.75 oz	
Goldings 30 mins	0.75 oz	
OG	1053	
FG	1015	
ABV	5.03	
Apparent attenuation	71.70%	
IBU	26	
SRM	8	
Mash at	148° F	
Sparge at	170° F	
Boil time	90 minutes	
pitching temp	59° F	
Yeast	Wyeast 1318 London ale III (Boddingtons)	

1963 Lees Strong Ale

There seems to have been quite a tradition of Strong Ales in the Manchester area. And ones that were properly strong, not just 5% ABV.

This beer from Lees is a good example. At over 7% ABV, it's strong by pretty much anyone's standards. So strong, that it almost certainly was exclusively a bottled. Though they did later produce Moonraker, a beer of a similar strength, on draught. So perhaps they did the same with this.

There's nothing too exciting or odd in the grist, which is all pale malt except for a tiny dash of crystal and enzymic malt. Plus flaked maize, of course. And a whole host of different types of sugar: 1 cwt Invert, 3 cwt Nut Brown, 1 cwt HX, 1 cwt Solprima and 20 lbs C.D.M. I've interpreted that as a mix of No. 2 and No. 3 invert.

The hops were mostly English from the 1961 crop, though there was also a small amount of 1961 Styrians. If you want to go for full accuracy, you could drop the 90-minute Fuggles addition to 0.75 oz and add 0.25 oz of Styrian Goldings.

1963 Lees Strong Ale		
pale malt	10.75 lb	71.29%
crystal malt 80 L	0.33 lb	2.19%
enzymic malt	0.25 lb	1.66%
flaked maize	1.00 lb	6.63%
No. 2 invert sugar	1.00 lb	6.63%
No. 3 invert sugar	1.75 lb	11.60%
Fuggles 90 mins	1.00 oz	
Fuggles 60 mins	1.00 oz	
Goldings 30 mins	1.00 oz	
OG	1076	
FG	1021	
ABV	7.28	
Apparent attenuation	72.37%	
IBU	31	
SRM	16	
Mash at	147° F	
Sparge at	170° F	
Boil time	90 minutes	
pitching temp	58° F	
Yeast	Wyeast 1318 London ale III (Boddingtons)	

1963 Lees Lager

Around 1960 a lot of smaller breweries suddenly got interested in Lager, which everyone in the industry reckoned would be the next Big Thing.

Rather than miss out on the fun, the set about brewing a Lager of their own. With wildly differing degrees of authenticity. Most breweries just didn't have the equipment to do the job properly. They could neither decoct nor lager properly. What they ended up doing was brewing a Golden Ale that was filtered and artificially carbonated.

Because some vital details are missing, it's impossible for me to tell how authentic Lees Lager was. For example, the pitching temperature isn't listed, nor is it clear exactly what yeast was being used. In the recipe below, I've given them the benefit of the doubt and gone for a cool fermentation with a genuine Lager yeast. There's a good chance it was really fermented warm with their standard yeast.

At least they did use proper lager malt, I know that for sure. Along with flaked rice and some enzymatic malt. The rice replaces the flaked maize used in Lees other beers. There are also two types of sugar: P.S. Crystals and Solprima. I've substituted No. 1 invert sugar.

The hops were something English and Styrian Goldings. I've guessed Fuggles for the former.

1963 Lees Lager		
pilsner malt	6.25 lb	78.13%
enzymic malt	0.25 lb	3.13%
flaked rice	0.75 lb	9.38%
No. 1 invert sugar	0.75 lb	9.38%
Fuggles 90 mins	0.75 oz	
Styrian Goldings 30 mins	0.75 oz	
OG	1037	
FG	1009	
ABV	3.70	
Apparent attenuation	75.68%	
IBU	20	
SRM	4	
Mash at	146° F	
Sparge at	170° F	
Boil time	90 minutes	
pitching temp	48° F	
Yeast	Wyeast 2042 Danish lager	

1952 Maclay PA 6d

Maclay's of Alloa was in many ways a typical Scottish brewery. Their beer range was pretty dull consisting of three Pale Ales of different strength plus a Strong Ale. All three were brewed from the same recipe and parti-gyled in various combinations.

PA 6d was their 60/-, or bottom-level Pale Ale. I drank a later version of it myself and though it was quite a nice Dark Mild. That's because the version I had was coloured dark brown. Which isn't necessarily the colour it always was. As with many Scottish brewers, Maclay coloured their beers up in a variety of ways, depending on which market it was intended for.

There's not a great deal to the recipe, which is also typically Scottish. Mostly pale malt with a bit of sugar and, oddly, some flaked rice. There's also a proprietary sugar called DCS. No idea what that is, so I've just increased the quantity of No. 1 invert.

1952 Maclay PA 6d		
pale malt	6.00 lb	87.68%
flaked rice	0.33 lb	4.82%
No. 1 invert sugar	0.50 lb	7.31%
caramel 5000 SRM	0.01 lb	0.19%
Fuggles 90 mins	0.50 oz	
Fuggles 60 mins	0.50 oz	
Goldings 30 mins	0.50 oz	
Goldings dry hops	0.50 oz	
OG	1030	
FG	1012	
ABV	2.38	
Apparent attenuation	60.00%	
IBU	22	
SRM	9	
Mash at	148° F	
Sparge at	165° F	
Boil time	90 minutes	
pitching temp	61° F	
Yeast	WLP028 Edinburgh Ale	

1952 Maclay Export

Parti-gyled with the PA 6d above was this Export. Or 80/-, as it was sometimes called.

There's not a huge amount to say, as, obviously, the recipe is identical. I should point out that I can only guess at how dark the caramel was. Scottish Pale Ales tended to be on the dark side, so my 5000 SRM guess might be correct. But it could also have been a less intense colour. Take your pick.

As with the PA 6d, it was doubtless coloured up to a variety of shades, anyway.

1952 Maclay Export		
pale malt	8.25 lb	87.30%
flaked rice	0.50 lb	5.29%
No. 1 invert sugar	0.50 lb	5.29%
caramel 5000 SRM	0.20 lb	2.12%
Fuggles 90 mins	0.75 oz	
Fuggles 60 mins	0.75 oz	
Goldings 30 mins	0.75 oz	
Goldings dry hops	0.50 oz	
OG	1041	
FG	1013	
ABV	3.70	
Apparent attenuation	68.29%	
IBU	31	
SRM	11	
Mash at	148° F	
Sparge at	165° F	
Boil time	90 minutes	
pitching temp	62° F	
Yeast	WLP028 Edinburgh Ale	

1952 Maclay SPA

I've often accuse Maclay of having the most boring brewing records ever. The same recipe, brewed over and over again for years on end. That's generally true. But they occasionally swapped things up. In quite confusing ways.

This beer is a case in point. SPA was there middle Pale Ale, or 70/-. The beer that filled the Ordinary Bitter slot. It was parti-gyled in every possible combination with their other beers. With the same recipe over and over again.

Then, in July 1952, some brews contain malted oats instead of flaked rice. It's a weird substitution. I can only think of one reason why they might have done it. They were making their Oat Malt Stout again. They needed the malted oats to be able to call it that.

There's no Oat Malt Stout in the brewing records, per se. But I've seen other Scottish brewers in this period create Stout from a Pale Ale parti-gyle. My guess is that's what's happening here. Why else would you randomly throw in malted oats. If you were being cheap, you'd go the flaked oats route.

How would that work? Throw in a shitload or caramel at the end of primary fermentation And maybe some proprietary sugar meant for Stout.

1952 Maclay SPA		
pale malt	7.00 lb	87.50%
malted oats	0.50 lb	6.25%
No. 1 invert sugar	0.50 lb	6.25%
Fuggles 90 mins	0.67 oz	
Fuggles 60 mins	0.67 oz	
Goldings 30 mins	0.67 oz	
Goldings dry hops	0.50 oz	
OG	1036	
FG	1013	
ABV	3.04	
Apparent attenuation	63.89%	
IBU	28	
SRM	4	
Mash at	149° F	
Sparge at	165° F	
Boil time	90 minutes	
pitching temp	61° F	
Yeast	WLP028 Edinburgh Ale	

1952 Maclay SA

Finishing off the set of Maclay beers is SA. Which stands for either Strong Ale or Scotch. Or quite possibly both. Scottish brewers tended to market beers of this type as Strong Ale in Scotland and Scotch Ale elsewhere.

If you like, you could scale this recipe down for the other Maclay beers. Or scale up one of the others to make this. Because they always parti-gyled their beers. This, for example, was brewed along with a PA 6d.

The big difference here is the greater quantity of caramel. Which produces a beer that's a good bit darker. Which I guess was the idea. There's also no flaked rice. Not sure why that might be. It could well be just random.

Even though between the wars there were some ridiculously strong draught beers in Scotland – I'm thinking Disher's – I'm pretty sure this was an exclusively bottled beer.

1952 Maclay SA		
pale malt	14.50 lb	91.60%
No. 1 invert sugar	1.25 lb	7.90%
caramel 5000 SRM	0.08 lb	0.51%
Fuggles 90 mins	1.25 oz	
Fuggles 60 mins	1.25 oz	
Goldings 30 mins	1.25 oz	
OG	1077	
FG	1028	
ABV	6.48	
Apparent attenuation	63.64%	
IBU	43	
SRM	27	
Mash at	148° F	
Sparge at	165° F	
Boil time	90 minutes	
pitching temp	61° F	
Yeast	WLP028 Edinburgh Ale	

1966 Maclay PA 6d

Despite 14 years having passed, not much has changed with Maclay 60/-. The OG and FG are identical. And there's not been much change in the recipe.

There's been a little tinkering with the recipe. There's flaked maize instead of flaked rice. And a touch of malt extract has been added. But it's really just a variation on a theme. There are also some Styrian Golding instead of 100% English hops.

As for colour, the one in the recipe is as brewed. The versions I drank were around 20-25 SRM. Feel free to colour it with caramel to any shade you fancy.

1966 Maclay PA 6d		
pale malt	5.00 lb	75.28%
flaked maize	0.75 lb	11.29%
malt extract	0.125 lb	1.88%
No. 1 invert sugar	0.75 lb	11.29%
caramel 5000 SRM	0.02 lb	0.26%
Styrian Goldings 90 mins	0.50 oz	
Fuggles 60 mins	0.50 oz	
Goldings 30 mins	0.50 oz	
Goldings dry hops	0.50 oz	
OG	1030	
FG	1012	
ABV	2.38	
Apparent attenuation	60.00%	
IBU	23	
SRM	11	
Mash at	148° F	
Sparge at	165° F	
Boil time	90 minutes	
pitching temp	61° F	
Yeast	WLP028 Edinburgh Ale	

1966 Maclay SPA

The 70/- recipe is exactly the same as that for 60/- with one exception: there's only half as much caramel.

Which doesn't leave me with a great deal to say. It's very similar in many ways to and English Ordinary Bitter. But with one difference: the degree of attenuation is much lower. I suspect this is why Scottish beers got the reputation for being sweet and malty. They had a much higher FG.

1966 Maclay SPA		
pale malt	5.75 lb	74.53%
flaked maize	1.00 lb	12.96%
malt extract	0.125 lb	1.62%
No. 1 invert sugar	0.75 lb	9.72%
caramel 5000 SRM	0.09 lb	1.17%
Styrian Goldings 90 mins	0.75 oz	
Fuggles 60 mins	0.75 oz	
Goldings 30 mins	0.50 oz	
Goldings dry hops	0.50 oz	
OG	1035	
FG	1013	
ABV	2.91	
Apparent attenuation	62.86%	
IBU	30	
SRM	8	
Mash at	148° F	
Sparge at	165° F	
Boil time	90 minutes	
pitching temp	62° F	
Yeast	WLP028 Edinburgh Ale	

1966 Maclay Export

No surprise to find that the recipe for Maclay 80/- was essentially the same as for 60/- and 70/-.

Again the only difference is in the caramel. In this beer there's none at all Otherwise it's exactly the same quantities of pale malt, flaked maize, No. invert sugar and something called DCS. No idea what that was so, as usual, I've bumped up the invert sugar a little.

1966 Maclay Export		
pale malt	7.00 lb	76.71%
flaked maize	1.00 lb	10.96%
malt extract	0.13 lb	1.37%
No. 1 invert sugar	1.00 lb	10.96%
Styrian Goldings 90 mins	1.00 oz	
Fuggles 60 mins	0.75 oz	
Goldings 30 mins	0.75 oz	
Goldings dry hops	0.50 oz	
OG	1040	
FG	1012	
ABV	3.70	
Apparent attenuation	70.00%	
IBU	39	
SRM	5	
Mash at	148° F	
Sparge at	165° F	
Boil time	90 minutes	
pitching temp	61° F	
Yeast	WLP028 Edinburgh Ale	

1966 Maclay Oat Malt Stout

Just when I thought Maclay's records were as exciting a wet February weekend in Skegness, they throw in something completely different. Not an Oatmeal Stout, but an Oat Malt Stout.

Maclay were the first to brew an Oat Stout, way back in the 1890s. They tried to patent Oat Malt Stout, but other brewers simply used flaked oats and called their beers Oatmeal Stout. It's weird that the two new types of Stout that appeared 1890 – 1910 both came from small, regional breweries. Oat Stout by Maclay, Milk Stout by Mackeson.

While London brewers threw in a token amount of flaked oats into their Oatmeal Stout, Maclay's version always contained a considerable proportion of oat malt. In this example, it makes up a full third of the grist.

1966 Maclay Oat Malt Stout		
pale malt	3.25 lb	42.15%
black malt	0.67 lb	8.69%
malted oats	2.50 lb	32.43%
No. 3 invert sugar	1.25 lb	16.21%
caramel 5000 SRM	0.04 lb	0.52%
Fuggles 90 mins	0.50 oz	
Fuggles 60 mins	0.50 oz	
Fuggles 30 mins	0.50 oz	
OG	1035	
FG	1012	
ABV	3.04	
Apparent attenuation	65.71%	
IBU	21	
SRM	34	
Mash at	145° F	
Sparge at	165° F	
Boil time	90 minutes	
pitching temp	62° F	
Yeast	WLP028 Edinburgh Ale	

1946 Shepherd Neame SXX

SXX, Shepherd Neame's Best Bitter, started WW II with a very respectable 1055° gravity. That had come down quite a way by 1946, but was still quite strong for the day.

The recipe is very unusual for a Shepherd Neame Pale Ale. Because they normally brewed them all malt. Well, apart from a touch of malt extract. The flaked barley in this beer is the result of wartime restrictions. As soon as they were lifted, Shepherd Neame went back to all malt. Not all breweries used adjuncts, but the use of sugar was near universal. Except at Guinness.

Other than that they were English and from the 1942, 1944 and 1945 crops, I know nothing about the hops. One thing that is surprising: how few hops Shepherd Neame used in their Pale Ales. You'd expect a brewery located in Kent to be a heavy hopper.

1946 Shepherd Neame SXX		
pale malt	8.25 lb	84.62%
flaked barley	1.25 lb	12.82%
malt extract	0.25 lb	2.56%
Fuggles 120 mins	0.75 oz	
Goldings 30 mins	0.75 oz	
Goldings dry hops	0.25 oz	
OG	1042	
FG	1009	
ABV	4.37	
Apparent attenuation	78.57%	
IBU	19	
SRM	4	
Mash at	152° F	
Sparge at	170° F	
Boil time	120 minutes	
pitching temp	62° F	
Yeast	WLP007 Dry English Ale	

1946 Shepherd Neame BA

Immediately after WW II Shepherd Neame had no fewer than five Pale Ales, which were parti-gyled together in various combinations. BA was the second strongest. And judging by the brewing records, one of the most popular.

See the SXX above for recipe comments.

1946 Shepherd Neame BA		
pale malt	7.00 lb	84.85%
flaked barley	1.00 lb	12.12%
malt extract	0.25 lb	3.03%
Fuggles 120 mins	0.75 oz	
Goldings 30 mins	0.50 oz	
Goldings dry hops	0.25 oz	
OG	1035	
FG	1008	
ABV	3.57	
Apparent attenuation	77.14%	
IBU	17	
SRM	4	
Mash at	152º F	
Sparge at	170º F	
Boil time	120 minutes	
pitching temp	63º F	
Yeast	WLP007 Dry English Ale	

1946 Shepherd Neame BB

Another popular beer was the Pale Ale one step down from BA, BB. Not sure what BB stands for. It could be Best Bitter. Or Bitter Beer. Or something else entirely. It doesn't really matter.

The dry hops, as with all Shepherd Neame's beers, are just a guess. Annoyingly few breweries bothered to note them down in their brewing records.

As this was parti-gyled with the two preceding beers, any comments on those recipes also apply here.

1946 Shepherd Neame BB			
pale malt		6.25 lb	86.21%
flaked barley		0.75 lb	10.34%
malt extract		0.25 lb	3.45%
Fuggles 120 mins		0.50 oz	
Goldings 30 mins		0.50 oz	
Goldings dry hops		0.125 oz	
OG		1031.5	
FG		1007	
ABV		3.24	
Apparent attenuation		77.78%	
IBU		14	
SRM		3	
Mash at		152° F	
Sparge at		170° F	
Boil time		120 minutes	
pitching temp		63° F	
Yeast	WLP007 Dry English Ale		

1946 Shepherd Neame AK

Weakest of all Shepherd Neame's Pale Ales was AK. Even before WW II it was pretty watery, with a gravity of just 1031°. By 1942 it was down to a mere 1027°. And from there, there was nowhere down left to go.

This must be one of the last brews, because by 1947 it had disappeared. Like most other AKs. Always a relatively light style, it had been one of the weakest Pale Ales at a brewery. When world wars caused gravities to fall, it was often an early victim. As beers higher up in the Pale Ale hierarchy fell to a similar strength, AK inevitably got the chop. Most didn't make it past WW I. Almost none past WW II.

Just for a change, there's a little black malt in this one. And the BA and BB it was parti-gyled with, obviously. Other than that, it's the same as their other Pale Ale recipes. All use exactly the same hops in the same proportions.

1946 Shepherd Neame AK		
pale malt	5.25 lb	84.00%
black malt	0.125 lb	2.00%
flaked barley	0.75 lb	12.00%
malt extract	0.125 lb	2.00%
Fuggles 120 mins	0.50 oz	
Goldings 30 mins	0.375 oz	
Goldings dry hops	0.125 oz	
OG	1027	
FG	1006	
ABV	2.78	
Apparent attenuation	77.78%	
IBU	12	
SRM	8	
Mash at	152° F	
Sparge at	170° F	
Boil time	120 minutes	
pitching temp	62° F	
Yeast	WLP007 Dry English Ale	

1946 Shepherd Neame LDA

LDA stands for Light Dinner Ale. I know that for certain because I've seen the labels. It was Shepherd Neame's Light Ale, so an exclusively bottled product.

It looks very similar to AK, but never seems to have been parti-gyled with it, for some reason. On the topic of parti-gyles, even though all the Pale Ales were brewed together in various combinations, the recipes weren't always exactly the same. You'll note that this recipe is different from the one above for BA, despite BA being the other beer in this parti-gyle. It's quite confusing.

What are the differences? This brew includes No. 3 invert and caramel. So, unsurprisingly, the BA from this brew came out darker.

LDA fared better than AK, surviving until at least the 1970s, though at some point its brewhouse name was shortened to just LA (Light Ale).

1946 Shepherd Neame LDA		
pale malt	4.25 lb	74.89%
flaked barley	0.50 lb	8.81%
No. 3 invert sugar	0.75 lb	13.22%
caramel 1000 SRM	0.13 lb	2.20%
malt extract	0.050 lb	0.88%
Fuggles 120 mins	0.50 oz	
Goldings 30 mins	0.375 oz	
Goldings dry hops	0.125 oz	
OG	1027	
FG	1007	
ABV	2.65	
Apparent attenuation	74.07%	
IBU	12	
SRM	14	
Mash at	154º F	
Sparge at	170º F	
Boil time	120 minutes	
pitching temp	63º F	
Yeast	WLP007 Dry English Ale	

1947 Shepherd Neame MB

Along with all those Pale Ales, Shepherd Neame also brewed a Mild. Assuming MB stands for Mild Beer.

I'm not at all sure about the colour on this one. I've two Whitbread Gravity Book analyses from 1950 and 1951, which list the colour as 16 and 6 SRM. So one fairly dark and one fairly pale. My guess is that they brewed one beer that was pale and coloured it up sometimes with caramel at racking. Timothy Taylor do something similar today with Golden Best/Dark Mild.

As with all their beers of this period, the bulk of the grist consists of pale malt and flaked barley. Which, oddly enough, were very similarly prices. The malt costing 107/- per quarter and the flaked barley 100/-. I'd have expected the barley to be significantly cheaper as it required a lot less processing.

One difference with their other beers is that there's considerably more malt extract. No idea why that might be.

Not totally surprisingly, as the brewery is located in Kent, Shepherd Neame had their own hop gardens. Which provided around half the hops for this beer. There's no indication of what variety they were, so I've made a fairly conservative guess.

1947 Shepherd Neame MB		
pale malt	3.75 lb	68.18%
flaked barley	0.75 lb	13.64%
no. 3 sugar	0.50 lb	9.09%
malt extract	0.50 lb	9.09%
Fuggles 120 mins	0.50 oz	
Goldings 30 mins	0.25 oz	
OG	1027.1	
FG	1005.5	
ABV	2.86	
Apparent attenuation	79.70%	
IBU	11	
SRM	7	
Mash at	156° F	
Sparge at	170° F	
Boil time	120 minutes	
pitching temp	63° F	
Yeast	WLP007 Dry English Ale	

1947 Shepherd Neame SS

I've come across some watery Stouts in my time, but this one takes the biscuit. With a gravity under 1030° it makes a total joke of the term. Stout did originally mean "strong", after all.

The grist is about as simple as it gets for a Stout: pale and black malt. Plus malted oats. The latter is rather unusual. Most breweries used flaked oats or oatmeal in their Stouts. Though the original, Maclays Oat Malt Stout, as the name implies, used the malted type.

Around half the hops were from Shepherd Neame's own hop garden. They were from the 1945 and 1946 harvests. The other half of the hops were pretty old: 1943. Which requires a reduction of the hopping rate in my recipe. On the other hand, there was also 3 lbs of humulone, a hop preparation. That's the equivalent of around 21 lbs of hops.

The sugars in the original were CD and JC. No idea what they were. But I can only get the colour to look anywhere near right if I substitute No. 4 invert for them.

With such a low gravity and a reasonable rate of attenuation, this Stout must have tasted pretty thin, even with the oats.

1947 Shepherd Neame SS			
pale malt		3.25 lb	59.09%
black malt		0.50 lb	9.09%
malted oats		0.50 lb	9.09%
No. 4 invert sugar		1.00 lb	18.18%
malt extract		0.25 lb	4.55%
Fuggles 120 mins		0.50 oz	
Goldings 30 mins		0.50 oz	
OG		1027.1	
FG		1006.1	
ABV		2.78	
Apparent attenuation		77.49%	
IBU		14	
SRM		30	
Mash at		159° F	
Sparge at		170° F	
Boil time		120 minutes	
pitching temp		62.75° F	
Yeast	WLP007 Dry English Ale		

1952 Shepherd Neame SM

Sometime in the late 1940s or early 1950s, Shepherd Neame changed the name of their Mild from MB (Mild Beer?) to SM (Special Mild?). Probably at the same time as they boosted the OG from 1027° to 1030°.

It looks like they also turned it into a truly dark mild at the same time. A healthy slug of both No. 3 invert and black malt take care of that. You'll note that, while their Pale Ales were all-malt their Mild and Stout weren't. Though none included any adjuncts. Even the oats for the Stout were in malted form.

The hops were the same mostly ancient ones that all their 1952 beers used. All from their own hop garden. They seem to have been self-sufficient in hops at this point.

1952 Shepherd Neame SM		
pale malt	5.50 lb	80.88%
black malt	0.75 lb	11.03%
No. 3 invert sugar	0.50 lb	7.35%
malt extract	0.05 lb	0.74%
Fuggles 120 mins	0.50 oz	
Goldings 30 mins	0.50 oz	
OG	1030	
FG	1006.5	
ABV	3.11	
Apparent attenuation	78.33%	
IBU	14	
SRM	25	
Mash at	149° F	
Sparge at	170° F	
Boil time	120 minutes	
pitching temp	62° F	
Yeast	WLP007 Dry English Ale	

1952 Shepherd Neame SXX

Quite a lot has changed in six years. Well, with regards to the recipe. Once the shackles were off, Shepherd Neame resorted to its pre-war habits.

Which were to brew all-malt Pale Ales. That doesn't leave much to discuss about the recipe. It's just a load of pale malt and a touch of malt extract. I assume that the latter was for extra enzymes in the mash tun. Though why you would need that in a beer without unmalted grains I'm not sure.

I find it strange that a brewery bang in the middle of England's main hop growing area should use so many old hops. In this case around 85% of the hops were from the 1949 crop. Though, as they were all from its own hop garden, that might explain why. Were they just using up hops that they'd been saving for a rainy day?

The gravity has dropped one point, but that's not really significant.

1952 Shepherd Neame SXX		
pale malt	9.50 lb	98.70%
malt extract	0.13 lb	1.30%
Fuggles 120 mins	1.00 oz	
Goldings 30 mins	1.00 oz	
Goldings dry hops	0.25 oz	
OG	1041	
FG	1008	
ABV	4.37	
Apparent attenuation	80.49%	
IBU	26	
SRM	4	
Mash at	149° F	
Sparge at	170° F	
Boil time	120 minutes	
pitching temp	62° F	
Yeast	WLP007 Dry English Ale	

1952 Shepherd Neame PA

As if they didn't have enough Pale Ales in their portfolio, Shepherd Neame introduced another in the early 1950s, simply called PA. It slotted into second place behind SXX.

This beer was parti-gyled with SXX and BB, but, for some reason, the recipe is different from their other Pale Ale brews. It's still all malt, but there's also some black malt. Looking at where it's placed in the brewing record, I suspect that it might have been added in the copper rather than the mash tun. It does leave this looking rather dark.

All their brews in late 1952 used the same combination of mostly pretty old hops from their own hop garden. As half were from the 1949 crop and hadn't even been in a cold store, I've reduced the hopping rate a fair bit.

1952 Shepherd Neame PA		
pale malt	7.75 lb	92.54%
black malt	0.50 lb	5.97%
malt extract	0.13 lb	1.49%
Fuggles 120 mins	0.75 oz	
Goldings 30 mins	0.75 oz	
Goldings dry hops	0.125 oz	
OG	1037.5	
FG	1008	
ABV	3.90	
Apparent attenuation	78.67%	
IBU	20	
SRM	19	
Mash at	152° F	
Sparge at	170° F	
Boil time	120 minutes	
pitching temp	62° F	
Yeast	WLP007 Dry English Ale	

1952 Shepherd Neame BB

This particular batch of BB is atypical, being a couple of gravity points stronger than usual. Not sure why, as it was parti-gyled with another BB that was the normal strength.

Like their other Pale Ales, BB was being brewed all-malt by this point. Which makes for a pretty boring recipe. And it really was just one type of pale malt. Which makes life easy for you home brewers.

1952 Shepherd Neame BB		
pale malt	7.50 lb	98.36%
malt extract	0.13 lb	1.64%
Fuggles 120 mins	0.75 oz	
Goldings 30 mins	0.75 oz	
Goldings dry hops	0.125 oz	
OG	1033	
FG	1007	
ABV	3.44	
Apparent attenuation	78.79%	
IBU	20	
SRM	3	
Mash at	150° F	
Sparge at	170° F	
Boil time	120 minutes	
pitching temp	62° F	
Yeast	WLP007 Dry English Ale	

1952 Shepherd Neame LDA

It turns out there was one Pale Ale that Shepherd Neame didn't brew all-malt: LDA. I wonder why that was?

There's one odd thing about LDA. In the brewing records LDA is always written in red. All the other beer names are in black ink. Red ink usually indicates something odd or something that has changed. So it seems strange that it's always in red.

As with the Mild, the OG has been increased by 3 points. Leaving LDA on the same gravity as BB. What's the difference between the two beers? No.3 invert sugar. The recipe still isn't exactly complicated. Other than the sugar there's just pale malt and a tiny amount of malt extract.

The hops are the same crappy ancient ones as in the other beers.

1952 Shepherd Neame LDA		
pale malt	6.00 lb	91.60%
No. 3 invert sugar	0.50 lb	7.63%
malt extract	0.05 lb	0.76%
Fuggles 120 mins	0.67 oz	
Goldings 30 mins	0.67 oz	
OG	1030	
FG	1007	
ABV	3.04	
Apparent attenuation	76.67%	
IBU	18	
SRM	6	
Mash at	152° F	
Sparge at	170° F	
Boil time	120 minutes	
pitching temp	63° F	
Yeast	WLP007 Dry English Ale	

1952 Shepherd Neame SS

This is a weird one. Something I've only seen Scottish brewers do before: parti-gyle a Stout with a Pale Ale.

How did they do that? By adding black malt and caramel to just one of the coppers. Hey presto! Pale Ale is now Stout. Though they did also end up with a Pale Ale that contained malted oats. I wonder if anyone ever noticed?

Compared to Shepherd Neame's other recipes, this one looks insanely complicated. A massive three types of malt, plus sugar and caramel. I've increased the quantity of black because, as it was added in the copper, it would have added more colour than if it were mashed.

1952 Shepherd Neame SS		
pale malt	5.75 lb	77.91%
black malt	0.75 lb	10.16%
malted oats	0.25 lb	3.39%
raw cane sugar	0.25 lb	3.39%
caramel 1000 SRM	0.33 lb	4.47%
malt extract	0.05 lb	0.68%
Fuggles 120 mins	0.75 oz	
Goldings 30 mins	0.75 oz	
OG	1030	
FG	1008	
ABV	2.91	
Apparent attenuation	73.33%	
IBU	21	
SRM	36	
Mash at	149° F	
Sparge at	170° F	
Boil time	120 minutes	
pitching temp	62° F	
Yeast	WLP007 Dry English Ale	

1954 Shepherd Neame Abbey Ale

Not content with the five Pale Ales they already brewed, Shepherd Neame introduced a new one, sometime around 1953. An exclusively bottled product, as far as I can tell.

Abbey Ale was parti-gyled with LDA and appears to just be a stronger version of that. Labels describe it as a Pale Ale.

In a radical departure from their normal practice, this didn't contain a single grain. This recipe also includes wheat. I'm not sure in which form, but, as they usually went all-malt, I've guessed at malted wheat. Why is it there? Usually a small quantity of wheat is added to help head retention, so that would be my guess.

Though there are also two types of sugar: No. 3 invert and something called Wortex. For the latter I've substituted No. 1 invert. Plus the obligatory tiny dash of malt extract.

Lots of old hops, as usual.

1954 Shepherd Neame Abbey Ale		
pale malt	10.00 lb	97.28%
wheat malt	0.25 lb	2.43%
malt extract	0.03 lb	0.29%
Fuggles 120 mins	0.75 oz	
Goldings 30 mins	0.75 oz	
OG	1044	
FG	1016	
ABV	3.70	
Apparent attenuation	63.64%	
IBU	19	
SRM	4	
Mash at	152° F	
Sparge at	170° F	
Boil time	105 minutes	
pitching temp	62° F	
Yeast	WLP007 Dry English Ale	

1956 Shepherd Neame DB

Here's a rarity – a genuine Brown Ale recipe. Two, actually, as there was also a single Brown Ale parti-gyled with it. Plus LDA and ESXA.

By this point Shepherd Neame's recipes were starting to get more complicated. In addition to the two grains, this beer has a whole cocktail of sugars. No. 3 invert, Wortex, Ale Priming, Dwax and caramel crystals. For the Wortex I've substituted No. 1 invert, the others more No. 3 invert.

DB probably stands for Double Brown. Though you may be asking yourself how a beer of under 1030° could be double anything. All I can say is: wait until you see the single Brown Ale.

Typically, over half the hops were from the 1953 crop.

1956 Shepherd Neame DB		
pale malt	4.25 lb	69.79%
wheat malt	0.25 lb	4.11%
No. 3 invert sugar	1.00 lb	16.42%
No. 1 invert sugar	0.50 lb	8.21%
caramel 1000 SRM	0.05 lb	0.82%
malt extract	0.04 lb	0.66%
Fuggles 105 mins	0.50 oz	
Goldings 60 mins	0.50 oz	
Goldings 30 mins	0.25 oz	
OG	1029.5	
FG	1010.5	
ABV	2.51	
Apparent attenuation	64.41%	
IBU	19	
SRM	12	
Mash at	153° F	
Sparge at	170° F	
Boil time	105 minutes	
pitching temp	61.25° F	
Yeast	a Southern English Ale yeast	

1956 Shepherd Neame Brown Ale

You've seen the "strong" Brown Ale, now time for the watery one. And believe me, it's watery.

Obviously, the recipe is identical as for Double Brown, just a little bit less of everything. Not really anything else to say, other than that it wasn't going to get you very pissed. I suppose if you drank it mixed with their Mild it might just about be intoxicating.

1956 Shepherd Neame Brown Ale		
pale malt	4.00 lb	73.94%
wheat malt	0.25 lb	4.62%
No. 3 invert sugar	0.75 lb	13.86%
No. 1 invert sugar	0.33 lb	6.10%
caramel 1000 SRM	0.04 lb	0.74%
malt extract	0.04 lb	0.74%
Fuggles 105 mins	0.50 oz	
Goldings 60 mins	0.25 oz	
Goldings 30 mins	0.25 oz	
OG	1026	
FG	1008	
ABV	2.38	
Apparent attenuation	69.23%	
IBU	15	
SRM	10	
Mash at	153º F	
Sparge at	170º F	
Boil time	120 minutes	
pitching temp	63º F	
Yeast	WLP007 Dry English Ale	

1956 Shepherd Neame EXSA

Top dog of the Brown Ale Parti-gyle was EXSA. Which I suppose makes it a strong Brown Ale. Or Old Ale.

I've been wondering what this beer was really called. I guessed Extra Strong Ale. Then I nosed around some label images and found one that actually said that: Bishop's Finger. Though, according to the brewery, that was only introduced in 1958. Breweries often get stuff like this wrong. I found a brewing record for Tally Ho! that was earlier than the creation date Adnams give.

This certainly looks about the right OG for Bishop's Finger. Possibly they only called it that in 1958, but had been brewing it under a different name for a couple of years.

It's considerably less well-attenuated than most of their beers, leaving it well under 5% ABV.

1956 Shepherd Neame EXSA		
pale malt	7.50 lb	71.70%
wheat malt	0.33 lb	3.15%
No. 3 invert sugar	1.75 lb	16.73%
No. 1 invert sugar	0.75 lb	7.17%
caramel 1000 SRM	0.07 lb	0.67%
malt extract	0.06 lb	0.57%
Fuggles 105 mins	1.00 oz	
Goldings 60 mins	0.50 oz	
Goldings 30 mins	0.50 oz	
OG	1053	
FG	1017.5	
ABV	4.70	
Apparent attenuation	66.98%	
IBU	32	
SRM	16	
Mash at	153° F	
Sparge at	170° F	
Boil time	105 minutes	
pitching temp	62° F	
Yeast	WLP007 Dry English Ale	

1956 Tennant's Best Bitter

The mid-1950's was a good time for British beer. Production was edging up a little and more stronger beers were available.

Tennant's Best Bitter is an example of a stronger type of Pale Ale that was introduced around this time by many breweries. Relative to the watery stuff that was around in the immediate post-war period, it's quite potent stuff. A high degree of attenuation leaves it with 4.3% ABV. Not bad for the time.

There are only two malts in the grist, one of which is a small quantity of enzymic malt, which is really just a special type of pale malt. The original contained four types of sugar, in addition to the No. 2 invert and lactose, there was SBS and CWA. I've substituted more No. invert for these.

The lactose is a bit of a surprise. I have seen it used in styles of beer other than Milk Stout - Scotch Ale, Mild and Brown Ale – but never in a Bitter before. I'm not sure what purpose it's serving as the quantity is pretty small. And the degree of attenuation is high.

The copper hops were Kent Fuggles (1954), Worcester Fuggles (1954) and Kent Goldings (1955) with Kent Goldings (1954) as dry hops. Tennant are one of the nice breweries that bothered to list the hop varieties. It takes out the guesswork.

It's odd to think that this is a beer that my dad might have drunk. The pub on our caravan site was tied to Tennant. And he was a Bitter drinker. They had those horizontal measure half pint electric pumps that were popular in the North. Which were probably dispensing bright beer rather than cask when he was drinking there in the mid-1960s.

1956 Tennant's Best Bitter		
pale malt	6.00 lb	70.88%
enzymic malt	0.25 lb	2.95%
flaked maize	1.00 lb	11.81%
No. 2 invert sugar	1.00 lb	11.81%
lactose	0.09 lb	1.06%
malt extract	0.125 lb	1.48%
Fuggles 95 mins	0.75 oz	
Goldings 40 mins	0.375 oz	
Goldings 20 mins	0.375 oz	
Goldings dry hops	0.25 oz	
OG	1040	
FG	1007.5	
ABV	4.30	
Apparent attenuation	81.25%	
IBU	20	
SRM	6	
Mash at	146° F	
Sparge at	165° F	
Boil time	95 minutes	
pitching temp	60° F	
Yeast	Wyeast 1099 Whitbread ale	

1956 Tennant's Queen's Ale

I'm going to stick my neck out here, but my guess is that Queen's Ale was first brewed in either 1952 or 1953.

It was a strong (by the standards of the day) Bitter which had a good reputation, at least in its early days. This is what one of Tennant's brewers thought of it:

> "Queen's Ale was a premium draught beer. It was a pale, hoppy beer with a good body. Its perfect balance of malty sweetness and the bitterness of the finest hops ensured that it was the best draught beer that I have ever tasted (and that is saying something)."
> "The Brewer's Tale" by Frank Priestley, 2010, page 11.

Praise indeed. By the time I started drinking Tennant brewed no cask beer. But in the early 1981 they did reintroduce cask and guess which beer it was? Queen's Ale. And at exactly the same gravity as this version.

Getting back to this beer, the grist is much the same as Best Bitter's. Except this contains No. 1 instead of No. 2 invert. Plus CWA, which I've interpreted as No. 2 invert. There's also no malt extract.

Note the lack of any malt other than pale and a touch of enzymic. As I keep saying, the use of crystal malt in Bitter is a pretty recent thing. Even after WW II, it was the exception rather than the rule.

The hops are all English: Kent Fuggles (1954), Worcester Fuggles (1954 CS) and Kent Goldings (1955 CS); plus Kent Goldings (1955) dry hops.

1956 Tennant's Queen's Ale		
pale malt	6.25 lb	67.57%
enzymic malt	0.25 lb	2.70%
flaked maize	1.25 lb	13.51%
No. 1 invert sugar	0.50 lb	5.41%
No. 2 invert sugar	0.75 lb	8.11%
lactose	0.25 lb	2.70%
Fuggles 90 mins	0.75 oz	
Goldings 90 mins	0.25 oz	
Goldings 40 mins	0.50 oz	
Goldings 20 mins	0.50 oz	
Goldings dry hops	0.125 oz	
OG	1044	
FG	1009	
ABV	4.63	
Apparent attenuation	79.55%	
IBU	26	
SRM	6	
Mash at	148º F	
Sparge at	165º F	
Boil time	95 minutes	
pitching temp	60º F	
Yeast	Wyeast 1099 Whitbread ale	

1956 Tennant's Rock Ale

Tennant's Mild had the rather odd name of Rock Ale. There was a simple explanation, according to Frank Priestley:

> "Tennant's produced four draught been and five bottled beers. The draught beers were: Bitter Beer (BB), Best Bitter Beer (BBB), Rock Ale, which was a dark, mild ale and Queen's Ale. Rock Ale probably originated at the Nottingham Brewery (see later). The Nottingham cellars had been excavated out of the solid rock on which the old town stood. Beers stored in the cellars were known as Rock Ales."
> "The Brewer's Tale" by Frank Priestley, 2010, page 11.

The beer itself is a pretty typical post-war Dark Mild. Not all that dark, with the colour all deriving from sugar. The high degree of attenuation must have left it tasting quite dry.

It's another simple grist, with just base pale malt and a dash of enzymic malt. Plus loads of sugar of various types. The No. 3 is my substitution for SBS and CWA. I've no idea how accurate that is.

The hops are all classic English varieties: Kent Fuggles (1954), Worcester Fuggles (1953 and 1954 CS), Worcester Goldings (1955 CS) copper hops, plus Kent Goldings (1955) dry hops.

The original mashing scheme started at 143° F, then raised to 148° F, presumably by an underlet, and held there for two hours.

1956 Tennant's Rock Ale		
pale malt	5.50 lb	76.44%
enzymic malt	0.25 lb	3.47%
malt extract	0.07 lb	0.97%
No. 2 invert sugar	0.125 lb	1.74%
No. 3 invert sugar	1.00 lb	13.90%
caramel 500 SRM	0.25 lb	3.47%
Fuggles 90 mins	0.50 oz	
Fuggles 40 mins	0.25 oz	
Goldings 20 mins	0.25 oz	
Goldings dry hops	0.125 oz	
OG	1033	
FG	1006	
ABV	3.57	
Apparent attenuation	81.82%	
IBU	13	
SRM	16	
Mash at	148° F	
Sparge at	165° F	
Boil time	90 minutes	
pitching temp	60° F	
Yeast	Wyeast 1099 Whitbread ale	

1956 Tennant's Lion Pale Ale

If it weren't for the fact that Tennant brewed a weaker Pale Ale called Light Dinner Ale, I would have guessed that this was their Light Ale. The gravity is certainly in the Light Ale range.

One thing I don't understand: why is it branded as Lion Pale Ale? It's not as if a Lion was their trademark, as it was for some other breweries, such as Matthew Brown or Camerons. It's got me stumped. Unless, like Rock Ale, it's a brand acquired from another brewer.

The grist is a little different from their draught Pale Ales. Principally in not containing any lactose. The other little idiosyncrasies like enzymic malt and malt extract are present, however. And there's some crystal malt. At least I think there is.

The records of many of the beers have a cryptic entry, below and apart from the rest of the grist. In the case of this beer, it says "90 gal. N of E crystal". It made no sense to me. Gallons implies something liquid to me. What the hell was liquid crystal?

I only twigged today when I looked further through my photos. In particular, a Glucose Stout record. Where something described as "N of E crystal" appears in the grist. It does mean crystal malt then. And that's volume gallons. They're measuring it in gallons often because it isn't a round number of bushels. At least that's my guess.

Nothing much else to say. Other than that there were 2 cwt. each of SBS and CWA, which I've added to the No. 2 invert.

1956 Tennant's Lion Pale Ale		
pale malt	4.25 lb	60.41%
crystal malt 60 L	0.33 lb	4.69%
enzymic malt	0.125 lb	1.78%
flaked maize	1.00 lb	14.21%
malt extract	0.33 lb	4.69%
No. 2 invert sugar	1.00 lb	14.21%
Fuggles 90 mins	0.25 oz	
Goldings 90 mins	1.50 oz	
Goldings 40 mins	0.25 oz	
Goldings 20 mins	0.25 oz	
OG	1034	
FG	1009	
ABV	3.31	
Apparent attenuation	73.53%	
IBU	34	
SRM	6	
Mash at	146° F	
Sparge at	165° F	
Boil time	145 minutes	
pitching temp	60° F	
Yeast	Wyeast 1099 Whitbread ale	

1956 Tennant's BB

As we've already learned, BB stands for Bitter Beer. Or Tennant's Ordinary Bitter.

It's a good bit weaker, understandably, than their Best Bitter. There used to be a lot of draught Bitters that were around the same strength as Mild. In the West Country, this type of beer was called Boy's Bitter. Sadly, it's all but died out.

I find Tennant's grists pretty odd. There are a lot of ingredients, many only in tiny amounts. I really can't see the point is some. For example, the lactose. It could hardly have had any impact on the flavour of the finished beer.

The recipe is very similar to the Best Bitter, unsurprisingly. Though Tennant don't seem to have ever gone in for parti-gyling. All the beers in this brewing book were produced single-gyle. To be honest, the level of hopping in this beer makes it more like a Light mild than a Bitter.

1956 Tennant's BB		
pale malt	5.00 lb	70.52%
enzymic malt	0.125 lb	1.76%
crystal malt 60 L	0.25 lb	3.53%
flaked maize	0.50 lb	7.05%
No. 2 invert sugar	1.00 lb	14.10%
lactose	0.09 lb	1.27%
malt extract	0.125 lb	1.76%
Fuggles 90 mins	0.50 oz	
Goldings 90 mins	0.125 oz	
Fuggles 40 mins	0.33 oz	
Goldings 20 mins	0.33 oz	
Goldings dry hops	0.125 oz	
OG	1033	
FG	1006.5	
ABV	3.51	
Apparent attenuation	80.30%	
IBU	17	
SRM	7	
Mash at	147° F	
Sparge at	165° F	
Boil time	90 minutes	
pitching temp	60° F	
Yeast	Wyeast 1099 Whitbread ale	

1956 Tennant's Lion Brown Ale

I imagine this beer must have been one of Tennant's biggest sellers in bottle. Brown Ale was all the rage in the 1950's.

Like Tennant's other recipes, it has a bit of everything in the grist. A couple of types of malt, flaked maize, sugar and caramel. The colour mostly deriving from the latter. The brewing record handily records the beer's colour. Handy, because it means I could work out what colour the caramel needed to be to get the correct colour.

Once again, there are two proprietary sugars, SBS and CWA, which I've interpreted as simply more No. 2 invert.

Bizarrely, this Brown Ale is more bitter than Tennant's draught Bitters. Though the poor degree of attenuation must have left plenty of residual sweetness. It's odd that while BB, Best Bitter and Queen's Ale all contain lactose, this beer doesn't. Despite Brown Ale being a style where lactose was sometimes present, unlike Bitter.

1956 Tennant's Lion Brown Ale		
pale malt	4.00 lb	57.60%
crystal malt 60 L	0.25 lb	3.60%
enzymic malt	0.25 lb	3.60%
flaked maize	1.75 lb	25.20%
malt extract	0.07 lb	1.01%
No. 2 invert sugar	0.50 lb	7.20%
caramel 2000 SRM	0.125 lb	1.80%
Fuggles 95 mins	1.00 oz	
Goldings 95 mins	0.25 oz	
Fuggles 40 mins	0.25 oz	
Goldings 20 mins	0.25 oz	
OG	1031	
FG	1010	
ABV	2.78	
Apparent attenuation	67.74%	
IBU	26	
SRM	20	
Mash at	148° F	
Sparge at	165° F	
Boil time	95 minutes	
pitching temp	60° F	
Yeast	Wyeast 1099 Whitbread ale	

1956 Tennant's Glucose Stout

Tennant is a very confusing brewery when it comes to ingredients. They seem to use some of them in the wrong beers.

Take Glucose Stout, for example. The name implies that it's a Sweet Stout. An obvious candidate for a dose of lactose, you'd think. Hang on. I think I'm missing something here. I've just taken a look at the Whitbread Gravity Book entries for Glucose Stout. And every example has an OG of around 1040° and an FG of around 1019°. I reckon Tennant used the Whitbread trick of adding the lactose after primary fermentation. I need to tinker with the recipe.

Right, that's it fixed. 1.5 lbs of lactose is what's needed. Without the Gravity Book to guide me, I would have got this terribly wrong.

Hang on again. The label goes on about the glucose content. I don't see any in the grist. And the Gravity Book doesn't mention the presence of lactose, which it often did. I reckon they've primed with glucose at the end of secondary conditioning and then pasteurised.

For some reason the enzymic malt and malt extract are missing in this case. As is the flaked maize. Perhaps that explains it. If the enzymic malt and malt extract are there to provide enzymes, they might not be needed here where there are no adjuncts.

It was mashed quite a bit warmer than their other beers. Presumably to produce a less fermentable wort.

Unlike all their other beers, there's a single hop addition at the start of the boil. As it's a bit more heavily hopped than most Tennant's beers, the (calculated) IBUs are quite high at 29.

1956 Tennant's Glucose Stout		
pale malt	5.50 lb	63.18%
crystal malt 60 L	0.33 lb	3.79%
black malt	0.125 lb	1.44%
amber malt	0.50 lb	5.74%
glucose	1.00 lb	11.49%
No. 2 invert sugar	0.25 lb	2.87%
caramel 1000 SRM	1.00 lb	11.49%
Fuggles 90 mins	1.75 oz	
OG	1040	
FG	1019	
ABV	2.78	
Apparent attenuation	52.50%	
IBU	29	
SRM	48	
Mash at	152° F	
Sparge at	165° F	
Boil time	90 minutes	
pitching temp	60° F	
Yeast	Wyeast 1099 Whitbread ale	

1956 Tennant's No. 1

It wasn't just the long list of ingredients in their grists that made Tennant unusual. They also brewed two Barley Wines over 1100º.

There were only a handful of beers of that strength in the UK at the time. Why did Tennant brew two? I've absolutely no idea. Though it looks as if Gold Label might have been a derivative of No. 1 Barley Wine. At one time both of them were called No. 1. My guess is that they decided to try a paler Barley Wine and it was a hit. This darker No. 1 was eventually dropped.

Unsurprisingly given the difference in colour, the grists of the two beers were quite different. The darker beer had No. 2 rather than No. 1 invert and contained two coloured malts, crystal and black.

The big difference in the hopping, is that the darker beer has three times the quantity of dry hops. Which is a sign to me that it, too, just like Gold Label, was matured for a long period before sale. It also says on the label "Specially brewed and long matured". Sort of a hint.

1956 Tennant's No. 1		
pale malt	16.75 lb	75.28%
crystal malt 60 L	0.50 lb	2.25%
black malt	0.50 lb	2.25%
enzymic malt	0.25 lb	1.12%
flaked maize	1.50 lb	6.74%
No. 2 invert sugar	2.75 lb	12.36%
Goldings 240 mins	3.00 oz	
Goldings 120 mins	1.75 oz	
Goldings 60 mins	1.75 oz	
Hallertau dry hops	0.75 oz	
OG	1101	
FG	1023.5	
ABV	10.25	
Apparent attenuation	76.73%	
IBU	78	
SRM	25	
Mash at	149º F	
Sparge at	165º F	
Boil time	240 minutes	
pitching temp	57º F	
Yeast	Wyeast 1099 Whitbread ale	

1956 Tennant's Gold Label

It's great to have recipes for some of the notable beers of the post-war period. Like Tennant's Gold Label.

Gold Label is interesting for several reasons. It was the first pale Barley Wine, for a start. But one that became so popular, that for quite a while I thought colour was the main difference between Old Ale and Barley Wine. Old Ale dark, Barley Wine pale.

It was also aged in wood for around a year at this point. Which tells me that there was almost certainly some Brettanomyces character to the end product. That also probably knocked the FG down by a few points.

Finally, it's much stronger than most beers brewed in the 1950s. There were only a handful of beers of a similar strength. Things like Barclay's Russian Stout and Benskins Colne Spring Ale.

It's not a particularly complicated recipe: pale malt, flaked maize and sugar. There's quite a lot of the latter two, presumably in order to keep the colour pale. And it helps the rate of attenuation, which is pretty high for a beer of this strength.

The hopping is pretty heavy and there's a long boil, which, in combination, leave the finished beer at over 70 calculated IBUs.

1956 Tennant's Gold Label			
pale malt		14.75 lb	67.82%
enzymic malt		0.25 lb	1.15%
flaked maize		4.00 lb	18.39%
No. 1 invert sugar		2.75 lb	12.64%
Fuggles 230 mins		2.50 oz	
Goldings 230 mins		0.75 oz	
Goldings 60 mins		3.25 oz	
Hallertau dry hops		0.67 oz	
OG		1103.5	
FG		1020	
ABV		11.05	
Apparent attenuation		80.68%	
IBU		72	
SRM		9	
Mash at		147° F	
Sparge at		165° F	
Boil time	230 minutes		
pitching temp		56° F	
Yeast	Wyeast 1099 Whitbread ale		

1953 Truman XX

Surprisingly, Truman's Burton brewery was still brewing three different Mild Ales after WW II. The weakest was XX.

The gravity isn't very impressive. But a high degree of attenuation boosts it to over 3% ABV.

Like most of Truman's beers, the bulk of the grist was pale malt, high dried malt and crystal malt. I'm never sure what the nearest modern equivalent to high dried is. Probably pale Munich malt.

I've guessed the hop varieties. All I Know for certain is that they were English and from the 1951 and 1952 harvests.

1953 Truman XX		
pale malt	3.00 lb	44.44%
high dried malt	3.00 lb	44.44%
crystal malt 60 L	0.50 lb	7.41%
raw cane sugar	0.25 lb	3.70%
Fuggles 90 mins	0.50 oz	
Fuggles 60 mins	0.25 oz	
Goldings 30 mins	0.25 oz	
OG	1029	
FG	1006	
ABV	3.04	
Apparent attenuation	79.31%	
IBU	14	
SRM	7	
Mash at	150° F	
Sparge at	170° F	
Boil time	90 minutes	
pitching temp	62.5° F	
Yeast	WLP013 London Ale (Worthington White Shield)	

1953 Truman No. 7

In the 19th century, Truman brewed a full range of numbered Ales, going all the way from 1 to 8. By the 1950s, only two remained, No. 1 Barley Wine and No. 7 Mild Ale.

I'm not sure that I understand Truman's naming system. Their weakest Mild was XX, their strongest XXX. And the middle one? No. 7. They were all parti-gyled together, meaning that all three have identical recipes in terms of percentages.

Again, a high degree of attenuation leaves the finished beer relatively strong for its gravity, at over 3.5% ABV.

1953 Truman No. 7		
pale malt	3.25 lb	43.33%
high dried malt	3.25 lb	43.33%
crystal malt 60 L	0.50 lb	6.67%
raw cane sugar	0.50 lb	6.67%
Fuggles 90 mins	0.50 oz	
Fuggles 60 mins	0.33 oz	
Goldings 30 mins	0.33 oz	
OG	1033	
FG	1006	
ABV	3.57	
Apparent attenuation	81.82%	
IBU	16	
SRM	7	
Mash at	150° F	
Sparge at	170° F	
Boil time	90 minutes	
pitching temp	61.5° F	
Yeast	WLP013 London Ale (Worthington White Shield)	

1953 Truman XXX

The strongest of Truman's Milds, XXX, was pretty strong for a 1950s Mild. I suppose it would count as a Best Mild.

I should mention something about the colour of these Milds. I've no idea what it was, to be honest. The colours in the recipes are the minimum they would have been. It's quite possible that they were sometimes, or always, coloured up at racking time. I've no Whitbread Gravity Book analyses for these beers so I've no way to check. Truman's London-brewed Mild was dark, around 20-25 SRM.

3.7% ABV was pretty pokey for a Mild Ale back in the early 1950s. There were plenty under 3% ABV.

1953 Truman XXX		
pale malt	3.50 lb	43.75%
high dried malt	3.50 lb	43.75%
crystal malt 60 L	0.50 lb	6.25%
raw cane sugar	0.50 lb	6.25%
Fuggles 90 mins	0.50 oz	
Fuggles 60 mins	0.50 oz	
Goldings 30 mins	0.25 oz	
OG	1036	
FG	1008	
ABV	3.70	
Apparent attenuation	77.78%	
IBU	17	
SRM	8	
Mash at	150° F	
Sparge at	170° F	
Boil time	90 minutes	
pitching temp	61.5° F	
Yeast	WLP013 London Ale (Worthington White Shield)	

1953 Truman P2

Truman brewed Bitter at both their London and Burton breweries. The London-brewed ones, LK and PA, were both fairly low gravity at 1031° and 1036°, respectively. The burton ones were stronger, even the weakest, P2, being 1037°.

I know from the Whitbread Gravity Book what this was called down the pub: Burton Ordinary Bitter. Which seems a fair enough description.

This particular P2 was parti-gyled with P1. Nothing shocking in that. It's the third guest at the party that's the surprise: XX Mild. I'm sometimes left scratching my head as to what the difference between Bitter and Mild is. This is one of those cases.

All English hops again, some from Truman's own hop gardens. The dry hopping is a guess, but probably about right, based on what I've seen at other breweries.

1953 Truman P2		
pale malt	7.00 lb	81.78%
high dried malt	1.25 lb	14.60%
crystal malt 60 L	0.06 lb	0.70%
No. 3 invert sugar	0.25 lb	2.92%
Fuggles 90 mins	0.50 oz	
Fuggles 60 mins	0.50 oz	
Goldings 30 mins	0.50 oz	
Goldings dry hops	0.25 oz	
OG	1037	
FG	1008.5	
ABV	3.77	
Apparent attenuation	77.03%	
IBU	20	
SRM	6	
Mash at	150° F	
Sparge at	170° F	
Boil time	90 minutes	
pitching temp	61° F	
Yeast	WLP013 London Ale (Worthington White Shield)	

1953 Truman P1

One step up from Ordinary Burton Bitter (P2) was Best Burton Bitter (P1).

Both P1 and P2 had a long history, appearing in the first preserved Truman Burton brewing book from 1877. Of course, they were both a fair bit stronger back then, at 1066.5° and 1062°. Just shows what a couple of world wars did to UK beer strengths.

In the early 1950's, 1044.5° was an impressive strength for a draught Bitter and there were few stronger. Draught Bass was about the same strength.

1953 Truman P1		
pale malt	8.25 lb	81.93%
high dried malt	1.50 lb	14.90%
crystal malt 60 L	0.07 lb	0.70%
No. 3 invert sugar	0.25 lb	2.48%
Fuggles 90 mins	0.75 oz	
Fuggles 60 mins	0.75 oz	
Goldings 30 mins	0.75 oz	
Goldings dry hops	0.75 oz	
OG	1044.5	
FG	1013	
ABV	4.17	
Apparent attenuation	70.79%	
IBU	28	
SRM	7	
Mash at	150° F	
Sparge at	170° F	
Boil time	90 minutes	
pitching temp	61° F	
Yeast	WLP013 London Ale (Worthington White Shield)	

1953 Truman P1 B

It's not the snappiest of names, P1 B. But that's not what the drinking public knew it as. For them, it was Ben Truman Pale Ale.

Though it later became a keg beer, in the 1950's Ben Truman was a classy bottled Pale Ale, intended to compete with Bass Red Triangle and Worthington White Shield, two other famous Burton Pale Ales. Though those two beers were a little stronger, around 1060°.

Strangely, Truman's poshest beer is the only one to contain an adjunct, in the form of flaked maize. I can only assume that this was intended to lighten the body. Otherwise, it's the standard pale malt, high dried malt, crystal malt and sugar combination.

1953 Truman P1 B		
pale malt	9.00 lb	77.65%
high dried malt	1.50 lb	12.94%
crystal malt 60 L	0.09 lb	0.78%
flaked maize	0.67 lb	5.78%
No. 1 invert sugar	0.33 lb	2.85%
Fuggles 90 mins	1.00 oz	
Fuggles 60 mins	1.00 oz	
Goldings 30 mins	1.00 oz	
Goldings dry hops	0.50 oz	
OG	1051	
FG	1014.5	
ABV	4.83	
Apparent attenuation	71.57%	
IBU	36	
SRM	6	
Mash at	150° F	
Sparge at	170° F	
Boil time	90 minutes	
pitching temp	60.5° F	
Yeast	WLP013 London Ale (Worthington White Shield)	

1964 Truman XX

Since 1953 there's been a small increase in the OG of XX, taking it over the magical 1030° level. The rate of attenuation has also gone up, giving this version a massive 3.3% ABV.

The grist is typical of this period Truman: pale and crystal malt, flaked maize and sugar. The latter includes a small amount of a sugar whose name is illegible in the records. I've just bumped up the No. 3 invert accordingly.

The biggest change is the dropping of high-dried malt. Which is good, because I'm never quite sure which modern malt is the best substitute.

Truman is always a bit vague with the hops, not even bothering to note the year of their harvest. My choice of Fuggles and Goldings is a pure guess.

1964 Truman XX		
pale malt	5.50 lb	77.68%
crystal malt 60 L	0.75 lb	10.59%
flaked maize	0.33 lb	4.66%
No. 3 invert sugar	0.50 lb	7.06%
Fuggles 95 mins	0.50 oz	
Fuggles 60 mins	0.50 oz	
Goldings 30 mins	0.25 oz	
OG	1030.5	
FG	1005.5	
ABV	3.31	
Apparent attenuation	81.97%	
IBU	17	
SRM	9	
Mash at	148° F	
Sparge at	160° F	
Boil time	95 minutes	
pitching temp	61.5° F	
Yeast	WLP013 London Ale (Worthington White Shield)	

1964 Truman No. 7

I can imagine a brewer at Truman saying: "What the hell are we doing parti-gyling two Milds at almost identical gravities?" It's a valid question.

You could also ask" "Why is this twat publishing two nearly identical recipes?" Also valid. As is my reply: because I can. My main motivation is showing you the full range of products of the brewery. No matter how nonsensical that might be.

This is, in effect, a marginally stronger version of XX. I wonder if any pub stocked both? Or two of any of them? It might sound weird having two draught Milds, but pubs did once do that. There was still even a few pubs in the 1970s that did.

1964 Truman No. 7		
pale malt	5.75 lb	78.44%
crystal malt 60 L	0.75 lb	10.23%
flaked maize	0.33 lb	4.50%
No. 3 invert sugar	0.50 lb	6.82%
Fuggles 95 mins	0.50 oz	
Fuggles 60 mins	0.50 oz	
Goldings 30 mins	0.25 oz	
OG	1032	
FG	1006	
ABV	3.44	
Apparent attenuation	81.25%	
IBU	17	
SRM	9	
Mash at	148º F	
Sparge at	160º F	
Boil time	95 minutes	
pitching temp	61.5º F	
Yeast	WLP013 London Ale (Worthington White Shield)	

1964 Truman XXX

You do have to wonder why Truman brewed three Milds with such a small spread of gravities. Probably just because they had for a few decades. Though surely at some point they must have culled the range.

This is about as strong as Mild got during the 1960s, around the same level as Ordinary Bitter.

1964 Truman XXX		
pale malt	6.25 lb	73.53%
crystal malt 60 L	1.00 lb	11.76%
flaked maize	0.50 lb	5.88%
No. 3 invert sugar	0.75 lb	8.82%
Fuggles 95 mins	0.50 oz	
Fuggles 60 mins	0.50 oz	
Goldings 30 mins	0.50 oz	
OG	1036	
FG	1009	
ABV	3.57	
Apparent attenuation	75.00%	
IBU	20	
SRM	10	
Mash at	148° F	
Sparge at	160° F	
Boil time	90 minutes	
pitching temp	60° F	
Yeast	WLP013 London Ale (Worthington White Shield)	

1964 Truman P1

In the eleven years since 1953, a few things have changed with P1, Truman's Burton Best Bitter.

A couple of points have been shaved off the OG. In the grist, high dried malt has been dropped and flaked maize added. While the invert sugar has changed from No. 3 to No. 1. The percentage of crystal malt has also been increased quite a bit. There's also a small amount of a proprietary sugar whose name I can't read. I've just bumped up the No.1.

The hopping rate has also been reduced a little, knocking off a couple of (calculated) IBUs. The hops were all English.

1964 Truman P1		
pale malt	8.00 lb	84.21%
crystal malt 60 L	0.25 lb	2.63%
flaked maize	0.50 lb	5.26%
No. 1 invert sugar	0.75 lb	7.89%
Fuggles 100 mins	0.75 oz	
Fuggles 60 mins	0.75 oz	
Goldings 30 mins	0.50 oz	
Goldings dry hops	0.50 oz	
OG	1043	
FG	1009.5	
ABV	4.43	
Apparent attenuation	77.91%	
IBU	26	
SRM	6	
Mash at	150° F	
Sparge at	170° F	
Boil time	100 minutes	
pitching temp	62° F	
Yeast	WLP013 London Ale (Worthington White Shield)	

1964 Truman P2

Truman produced a lot of their Bitter not in their Brick Lane brewery, but in Burton.

By 1964, Truman had owned their Burton brewery for around a century, though it had never operated at full capacity.

At this point, three Bitters were produced in Burton: P1, P1 B and P2. The latter being their Ordinary Bitter. I'm not quite sure what it was called down the pub. Possibly Titan or Special. At least they're the names of Truman Bitters of around the right period that I have analyses for.

The grist is a reasonable enough mix of pale malt, crystal malt, flaked maize and No. 1 invert sugar. Only one substitution this time: more No. 1 for some sort of proprietary sugar whose name I can't read. That's typical. The brewers at Truman's Burton brewery mostly had terrible handwriting.

The hops were English, some grown by Truman itself. Other than that, I know nothing. I've gone for the safe bet of Fuggles and Goldings.

1964 Truman P2		
pale malt	7.00 lb	85.31%
crystal malt 60 L	0.125 lb	1.52%
flaked maize	0.33 lb	4.02%
No. 1 invert sugar	0.75 lb	9.14%
Fuggles 100 mins	0.50 oz	
Fuggles 60 mins	0.50 oz	
Goldings 30 mins	0.50 oz	
Goldings dry hops	0.25 oz	
OG	1037	
FG	1008	
ABV	3.84	
Apparent attenuation	78.38%	
IBU	20	
SRM	5	
Mash at	150° F	
Sparge at	170° F	
Boil time	100 minutes	
pitching temp	62.5° F	
Yeast	WLP013 London Ale (Worthington White Shield)	

1964 Truman P1 B

In the intervening decade or so since the previous Ben Truman recipe there have been changes here, too.

It's possible that by this point it was no longer exclusively a bottled beer. A keg version was definitely around in the 1970s.

As with P1 and P2 the high dried malt has been dropped. As has the crystal malt. It's made the recipe a good deal simpler. In fact it's very much like a late 19th-century Pale Ale in terms of ingredients.

As Truman never bothered with much in the way of descriptions for the hops it used, I've had to guess again. Going with the two classic English hops, Fuggles and Goldings.

1964 Truman P1 B		
pale malt	9.75 lb	88.64%
flaked maize	0.75 lb	6.82%
No. 1 invert sugar	0.50 lb	4.55%
Fuggles 95 mins	0.75 oz	
Fuggles 60 mins	0.75 oz	
Goldings 30 mins	0.75 oz	
Goldings dry hops	0.50 oz	
OG	1049.5	
FG	1012	
ABV	4.96	
Apparent attenuation	75.76%	
IBU	27	
SRM	5	
Mash at	150° F	
Sparge at	170° F	
Boil time	95 minutes	
pitching temp	61° F	
Yeast	WLP013 London Ale (Worthington White Shield)	

1964 Truman S1

No. 1 was a popular designation for Barley Wine, especially in Burton. And the S prefix here tells you that this was the Stock version.

Truman brewed a Stock No. 1 in Burton and aged it for a year or so. It was then shipped down to London, where a weaker Running version was made and the two blended together. One of the main purposes of blending being to get the level of acidity right. The Runner you'll need is the next recipe.

The recipe is quite simple: pale malt, crystal malt a No. 3 invert sugar. And a shitload of hops. Really loads of hops. But that's exactly what you would expect in a Stock Ale. S1 was aged for at least a year. It needed all those hops to protect it during that long ageing.

1964 Truman S1		
pale malt	22.00 lb	92.63%
crystal malt 60 L	0.50 lb	2.11%
No. 3 invert sugar	1.25 lb	5.26%
Fuggles 150 mins	3.25 oz	
Fuggles 60 mins	3.25 oz	
Goldings 30 mins	3.25 oz	
Goldings dry hops	0.50 oz	
OG	1105.5	
FG	1035	
ABV	9.33	
Apparent attenuation	66.82%	
IBU	87	
SRM	14	
Mash at	148° F	
Sparge at	160° F	
Boil time	150 minutes	
pitching temp	57.5° F	
Yeast	WLP013 London Ale (Worthington White Shield)	

1964 Truman R1

If you're wanting to faithfully recreate Truman No. 1 Barley Wine, you'll need to brew this beer, too. This is the unaged Runner with which the Stock version in the previous recipe was blended.

I'm surprised at how different the two recipes are. This has No. 1 instead of No. 3 invert and some flaked maize. Leaving this quite a good bit paler than S1. R1 is also 12 gravity points weaker. Quite a difference.

The hopping is lower in R1, too. But that's what you would expect. When they still made Running and Keeping Porter in London, the OGs and recipes were identical, except for the hopping rate. Which was 50% higher in the Keeper.

Derek Prentice told me that the Runner was brewed in London. But that wasn't the case here. This was a Burton-brewed beer. Maybe things changed in the late 1960s and they shifted production to London.

1964 Truman R1		
pale malt	19.00 lb	87.68%
crystal malt 60 L	1.00 lb	4.61%
flaked maize	1.00 lb	4.61%
No. 1 invert sugar	0.67 lb	3.09%
Fuggles 150 mins	1.75 oz	
Fuggles 60 mins	1.75 oz	
Goldings 30 mins	1.75 oz	
OG	1093.5	
FG	1027	
ABV	8.80	
Apparent attenuation	71.12%	
IBU	50	
SRM	11	
Mash at	150° F	
Sparge at	160° F	
Boil time	150 minutes	
pitching temp	61° F	
Yeast	WLP013 London Ale (Worthington White Shield)	

1961 Thomas Usher P 1/4

If you're wondering about the cryptic name for this beer, it's quite simple, really. P stands for Pale Ale and 1/4 is the retail price per pint. It's very Scottish to name beers by their price. I wonder why?

The system isn't great in times of inflation. By 1965 the name was P 1/8, the price having gone up by 4d per pint. And it didn't stop there.

Usher's records for this period are wonderfully detailed. Before WW II they were in the typical Scottish format, with multiple brews spread across two pages. But these are two pages per brew, one with the brewing details, the other logging the progress of the fermentation.

As the malt extract was added to the mash tun, I assume that its purpose is enzymatic.

Typically, the grist is just pale malt, flaked maize and sugar. The last, in this case, being invert and DAS. Which I've interpreted as No. 1 and No. 3 invert, respectively.

The hops were English, more I don't know.

1961 Thomas Usher P 1/4		
pale malt	5.25 lb	70.42%
flaked maize	0.50 lb	6.71%
malt extract	0.125 lb	1.68%
No. 1 invert sugar	1.25 lb	16.77%
No. 3 invert sugar	0.33 lb	4.43%
Fuggles 120 mins	0.50 oz	
Fuggles 60 mins	0.50 oz	
Goldings 30 mins	0.50 oz	
Goldings dry hops	0.125 oz	
OG	1036	
FG	1006.5	
ABV	3.90	
Apparent attenuation	81.94%	
IBU	22	
SRM	7	
Mash at	150° F	
Sparge at	157° F	
Boil time	120 minutes	
pitching temp	60° F	
Yeast	WLP013 London Ale (Worthington White Shield)	

1961 Thomas Usher GSA

Usher's records from this period are some of the dullest I've come across. I can only find two beers: their 70/- and this Strong Ale. Or was it a Scotch Ale? One of the two. It was certainly strong and brewed in Scotland.

Which is a bit odd, as I've seen labels for Export, Amber Ale, Sweet Stout, Brown Ale and Pale Ale labels from this period. Were all of those beers really just P 1/4? I suppose if they blended GSA with it they could make a stronger Export-style beer. But how would you make the Stout?

There's only one sugar in this, DAS. Could that be Dark Amber Syrup? Maybe. I've gone for No. 3 invert, in any case. The colour is close to the one in the brewing record so it can't be that far off. The final colour was almost certainly quite a bit darker, around 20-25 SRM. Probably achieved through a caramel addition at racking time.

I know from the weekly totals on materials that Usher used considerable amounts of caramel. But it doesn't appear in the brewing records of the individual beers. It must have been added at a later stage in the brewing process.

1961 Thomas Usher GSA		
pale malt	15.25 lb	86.35%
flaked maize	1.75 lb	9.91%
malt extract	0.33 lb	1.87%
No. 3 invert sugar	0.33 lb	1.87%
Fuggles 120 mins	2.25 oz	
Fuggles 60 mins	0.75 oz	
Goldings 30 mins	0.75 oz	
OG	1077	
FG	1025	
ABV	6.88	
Apparent attenuation	67.53%	
IBU	43	
SRM	8	
Mash at	150° F	
Sparge at	157° F	
Boil time	120 minutes	
pitching temp	57.5° F	
Yeast	WLP013 London Ale (Worthington White Shield)	

1959 Ushers (Trowbridge) IPA

Did I mention that I'd created my own new style? English Watery IPA I've called it. I needed a new definition because the standard BJCP definition of English IPA doesn't really fit any IPA brewed in the UK before 1996. Unfortunately, Usher's IPA doesn't fit either mine of the BJCP's definition of an English IPA.

What it looks most like to me is a classic post-war Best Bitter. But who really cares? IPA has been used to describe beers of very different characters in the past. So much so that the term is essentially meaningless, unless limited to beers like Worthington White Shield and Bass Red Triangle. Beers which retained some similarity to the IPAs from before WW I.

Returning to Usher's IPA, the grist is simplicity itself, consisting of just one type of malt, sugar and malt extract. Not sure exactly what type of invert sugar was used, as the log isn't specific. No. 2 is just my guess, but it could just have easily been No. 1 invert. Use whichever suits you best.

The caramel is there for colour adjustment. Without any crystal to darken it, the finished beer would have been pretty pale otherwise. Not sure what the point of the malt extract is. Probably for the enzymes. Though that does seem odd in a beer with no unmalted adjuncts in the mash.

Not sure what purpose the ginger serves. It's a tiny amount, about a fifth of a gram for the 6 US gallons, 5 UK gallons that's the batch size of the recipe below.

The hop varieties are again guesses. All I know is that the copper hops were from Kent and the dry hops from East Kent. Bramling Cross or Northern Brewer would be just as appropriate. But do please stick with English hops.

1959 Usher (Trowbridge) IPA		
pale malt	8.75 lb	90.83%
No. 2 invert	0.75 lb	7.79%
malt extract	0.125 lb	1.30%
caramel	0.01 lb	0.08%
ginger	pinch	
Fuggles 75 min	2.00 oz	
Goldings 30 min	2.00 oz	
Goldings dry hops	0.25 oz	
OG	1044	
FG	1013	
ABV	4.10	
Apparent attenuation	70.45%	
IBU	23	
SRM	10	
Mash at	154° F	
Sparge at	160° F	
Boil time	75 minutes	
pitching temp	61° F	
Yeast	White Labs WLP099 Super High Gravity	

1959 Ushers (Trowbridge) X Mild

After their takeover by Watney Ushers brewed both their own beers and some of Watneys. My guess is that as time progressed Watney discontinued the Ushers beers in favour of their own. starting with the bottled range.

For a while they brewed their own X Ale and Watney XX Mild. You'd expect a XX to be stronger than an X, but that wasn't the case. Ushers Mild was 3 gravity points stronger.

It's another Dark Mild with a relatively complicated grist. There's black and crystal in addition to the base malt. Topped up with invert sugar and caramel. The record says simply "invert". No. 3 is my guess.

The hops were from Kent from the 1958 crop. Fuggles is a pretty safe guess.

1959 Ushers (Trowbridge) X Mild		
pale malt	5.75 lb	80.20%
black malt	0.125 lb	1.74%
crystal malt	0.67 lb	9.34%
No. 3 invert sugar	0.33 lb	4.60%
malt extract	0.125 lb	1.74%
caramel 1000 SRM	0.17 lb	2.37%
ginger	pinch	
Fuggles 90 min	0.75 oz	
Fuggles 60 min	0.75 oz	
OG	1031	
FG	1008	
ABV	3.04	
Apparent attenuation	74.19%	
IBU	19	
SRM	20	
Mash at	156° F	
Sparge at	165° F	
Boil time	75 minutes	
pitching temp	60° F	
Yeast	WLP023 Burton Ale	

1959 Ushers (Trowbridge) KK

If IPA was Ushers Best Bitter, KK certainly looks like it fits into the Ordinary Bitter slot.

Ushers were enthusiastic part-gylers and this is part of a three-way brew, along with BPA and LB. Though the recipe is identical to IPA, except that the hopping rate is a little bit lower. My guess would be that this was their biggest selling Bitter.

The invert is a guess again, as are the hop varieties. Using my usual method: Kent and Mid Kent I interpret as Fuggles, East Kent as Goldings. They may not have been those exact varieties, but were probably something similar.

1959 Ushers (Trowbridge) KK		
pale malt	7.50 lb	92.19%
No. 2 invert	0.50 lb	6.15%
malt extract	0.125 lb	1.54%
Caramel 1000 SRM	0.01 lb	0.12%
Fuggles 75 mins	1.00 oz	
Goldings 30 mins	0.50 oz	
Goldings dry hops	0.125 oz	
OG	1037	
FG	1011	
ABV	3.44	
Apparent attenuation	70.27%	
IBU	19	
SRM	6	
Mash at	149° F	
Sparge at	160° F	
Boil time	75 minutes	
pitching temp	61° F	
Yeast	WLP023 Burton Ale	

1959 Ushers (Trowbridge) BPA

The next beer in the three-way parti-gyle is BPA. Which probably stands for Bottling Pale Ale. Making this Ushers Light Ale. Especially if you look at the OG.

Light Ale is another beer you rarely come across, at least under that name, in brewing records. It's usually called some sort of Pale Ale. A bottled Pale Ale of this strength would inevitably been ordered as Light Ale in the pub, no matter what was on the label.

Obviously, it's simply a weaker version of KK.

1959 Ushers (Trowbridge) BPA		
pale malt	6.25 lb	90.78%
No. 2 invert sugar	0.50 lb	7.26%
malt extract	0.125 lb	1.82%
caramel 1000 SRM	0.01 lb	0.15%
Fuggles 75 mins	0.75 oz	
Goldings 30 mins	0.50 oz	
Goldings dry hops	0.25 oz	
OG	1032	
FG	1008.5	
ABV	3.11	
Apparent attenuation	73.44%	
IBU	17	
SRM	6	
Mash at	149° F	
Sparge at	160° F	
Boil time	75 minutes	
pitching temp	61° F	
Yeast	WLP023 Burton Ale	

1959 Ushers (Trowbridge) LB

Last in the parti-gyle trio is LB, which is surely Light Bitter. I'll plump for this being a draught beer. In the class Boy's Bitter.

The brewery was certainly in the right part of the country, the Southwest. That's where the style of very Light Bitter, with gravities of 1027° - 1032°, was popular. Beers of the same strength as Ordinary Mild and presumably a cheap drink. Certainly lower in price than Ordinary Bitter.

Looking in an old Good Beer Guide, I see that in 1977 Ushers had two Bitters: PA at 1031° and Best Bitter at 1038°. That's spookily similar to LB and KK. I'm sure they were their direct ancestors.

1959 Ushers (Trowbridge) LB		
pale malt	6.00 lb	90.43%
No. 2 invert sugar	0.50 lb	7.54%
malt extract	0.125 lb	1.88%
caramel 1000 SRM	0.01 lb	0.15%
Fuggles 75 mins	0.75 oz	
Goldings 30 mins	0.50 oz	
Goldings dry hops	0.25 oz	
OG	1031	
FG	1009.5	
ABV	2.84	
Apparent attenuation	69.35%	
IBU	17	
SRM	6	
Mash at	149° F	
Sparge at	160° F	
Boil time	75 minutes	
pitching temp	61° F	
Yeast	WLP023 Burton Ale	

1959 Watneys XX Mild

Watney – now there's a name to conjure with. The bogeyman of brewing in the 1970's. This wasn't brewed in their own Mortlake brewery but at Ushers of Trowbridge in the West Country. Watney owned the brewery and clearly made them brew some of their own lovely brands.

If I remember correctly, Ushers was one of the few Watney plants that never completely got rid of cask. Their beers were OK, if nothing particularly special. When Watney started to unravel, Ushers regained its independence with its own estate of tied houses. This arrangement only lasted around a decade, when the brewery was closed and it continued as a pure pub company. The brewing equipment ended up in North Korea.

Returning to the beer, XX belongs to the wateriest class of Milds, whose origins can be traced back to the Government Ale of WW I. After war's end, a new, very low-gravity type of Mild called 4d Ale continued to be brewed. At a time when standard Mild was 1035 – 1043°, 4d Ale was usually under 1030°. When WW II forced down gravities of standard Mild to a similar level, 4d Ale mostly disappeared.

Some brewers, particularly in the West Country, continued to brew their Mild at very low gravities, even after most had bounced back to the low 1030's. It's no coincidence that the gravity is 1028°. There was no point dropping below 1027° as no matter how low the gravity, the minimum duty chargeable was as if a beer were 1027°.

There's nothing too horrible about the grist: mostly mild ale malt with a bit of crystal and flaked maize, plus a bit of sugar. As with Watney's Brown Ale, it's the other shit thrown in that's the problem. This was added to the gyles (332 barrels) to make 383 barrels:

BB 18 barrels
Bottoms 18 barrels
RB 11 barrels
finings 4 barrels

A bit better than the Brown Ale – at least this is only 15% crap.

I wouldn't recommend trying to recreate that gyling. I can't imagine the leftover beer added anything positive to the finished product.

1959 Watneys XX Mild		
MA malt	4.75 lb	79.76%
crystal malt 40 L	0.25 lb	4.20%
flaked maize	0.33 lb	5.54%
roast barley	0.25 lb	4.20%
No. 2 invert	0.25 lb	4.20%
caramel	0.125 lb	2.10%
ginger	pinch	
Fuggles 45 min	1.00 oz	
OG	1028	
FG	1007	
ABV	2.78	
Apparent attenuation	75.00%	
IBU	14.5	
SRM	30	
Mash at	152º F	
Sparge at	170º F	
Boil time	45 minutes	
pitching temp	60º F	
Yeast	WLP023 Burton Ale	

1959 Watneys Dairy Maid Sweet Stout

What typifies the 1950s more than a piss-weak, ridiculously sweet Stout? This beer certainly fits that bill.

I'm lucky to have this brewing. For a start, I didn't collect it myself. And it doesn't come from Watneys themselves. Well, not directly. Because it's in a brewing book of Ushers of Trowbridge. A brewery Watneys had purchased and which made some of their beers.

Once again, I'm thankful for having some Whitbread Gravity Book analyses. Because they tell me that the OG and FG were quite different from those in the brewing record. The OG is 3 points higher and the FG 6.5 points. Which doesn't make a lot of sense.

Candy primings were added at the end of primary fermentation. But, assuming the OG of the primings is 1150°, they add 7 gravity points, according to my calculations. What's going on? Well, my guess is that all the other shit they mixed in at racking time is bringing down the OG. 667 barrels were brewed and a further 106 barrels of various types of ullage blended in. That's around 14% of the total.

I'm guessing that the candy sugar raised the effective OG by six or seven points and the ullage brought it down by four. Watneys beers are so much fun. Not quite sure how you would replicate that on a homebrew scale.

Based on the name, you'd assume there was lactose in this beer. But there doesn't seem to be. I can't see any in the recipe and not of the Gravity Book analyses mention its presence. As owners of the biggest Milk Stout brand, Whitbread took a particular interest in lactose in Stout.

The recipe contains just one coloured malt, black malt. Though that's in quite a large amount. Then lots of sugar. The No. 3 invert is my substitution for CDM (Caramelised Dextro-Maltose). There's just one type of hops, described simply as "Kent". They were from the 1958 crop.

1959 Watneys Dairy Maid Sweet Stout		
mild malt	4.75 lb	65.11%
black malt	0.67 lb	9.18%
flaked maize	0.25 lb	3.43%
malt extract	0.125 lb	1.71%
No. 4 invert sugar	0.67 lb	9.18%
cane sugar	0.33 lb	4.52%
candy sugar	0.50 lb	6.85%
ginger	pinch	
Fuggles 45 mins	0.75 oz	
Fuggles 30 mins	0.50 oz	
OG	1034	
FG	1012	
ABV	2.91	
Apparent attenuation	64.71%	
IBU	14	
SRM	39	
Mash at	154° F	
Sparge at	170° F	
Boil time	45 minutes	
pitching temp	60° F	
Yeast	WLP023 Burton Ale	

1963 Watneys Special Mild

It's weird sometimes writing a recipe for a beer that you just know was awful. And this almost certainly was, after they'd finished filtering and pasteurising the life out of it.

At the end of primary fermentation, it was primed and blended with all sorts of "reprocessed beer". That is, returns and other crap. To a maximum of 10%. The cheeky bastards. I've upped the No. 3 invert to account for the priming sugar, which increased the effective OG by 3 points.

The grist doesn't look that bad. It is about 75% malt and the percentage of adjuncts is quite low. Though I'm not so sure about the wheat flour.

The hops were definitely all Fuggles and all added at the start of the boil.

Not so sure what's so special about this beer. Unless it's special in the sense of school.

1963 Watneys Special Mild		
mild malt	4.75 lb	68.30%
crystal malt 60 L	0.33 lb	4.74%
black malt	0.25 lb	3.59%
flaked maize	0.25 lb	3.59%
wheat flour	0.25 lb	3.59%
No. 3 invert sugar	0.75 lb	10.78%
malt extract	0.25 lb	3.59%
caramel 2000 SRM	0.125 lb	1.80%
Fuggles 60 mins	1.50 oz	
OG	1032	
FG	1010	
ABV	2.91	
Apparent attenuation	68.75%	
IBU	21	
SRM	25	
Mash at	158° F	
Sparge at	175° F	
Boil time	60 minutes	
pitching temp	60.5° F	
Yeast	WLP023 Burton Ale	

1963 Watneys Brown Ale

The recipe of this beer is pretty much identical to Special Mild and the Watney Quality Manual, from which these details are taken, recommends parti-gyling the two beers.

The biggest difference are that the gravity is a little higher here and the hopping a little lighter.

It doesn't mention it in the Watney Quality Manual, but my guess is that mixed in all sorts of crap at the end of primary fermentation. Certainly the version brewed at Usher in 1959 was 19% ullage of various types. Lovely. It's no wonder they had such a bad reputation.

I wouldn't try to recreate that at home. The beer as brewed, Looks OK. There are a couple of coloured malts and the percentage of adjuncts in quite low. Very dark and sweet is how I guess it tasted. Probably with a lactic note in the background from all the ullage.

1963 Watneys Brown Ale		
mild malt	5.00 lb	68.63%
crystal malt 60 L	0.50 lb	6.86%
black malt	0.33 lb	4.53%
flaked maize	0.33 lb	4.53%
wheat flour	0.25 lb	3.43%
No. 3 invert sugar	0.50 lb	6.86%
malt extract	0.25 lb	3.43%
caramel 2000 SRM	0.125 lb	1.72%
Fuggles 60 mins	1.00 oz	
Goldings 60 mins	0.125 oz	
OG	1033	
FG	1012	
ABV	2.78	
Apparent attenuation	63.64%	
IBU	16	
SRM	28	
Mash at	158° F	
Sparge at	175° F	
Boil time	60 minutes	
pitching temp	60.5° F	
Yeast	WLP023 Burton Ale	

1963 Watneys Pale Ale

I suspect that this beer, despite its Pale Ale name, was probably ordered as Light Ale down the pub. As far as I can tell, this was exclusively a bottled beer.

The grist doesn't look particularly odd, other than the wheat flour. A quite typical weaker Pale Ale/Light Ale recipe. With the crystal malt presumably adding a little body.

As this recipe is taken from the Watneys Quality Manual rather than brewing records I know some extra details. Like the hop additions. Or addition, I should say. There was just the one, right at the start of the boil.

1963 Watneys Pale Ale		
pale malt	6.50 lb	86.67%
crystal malt 60 L	0.25 lb	3.33%
wheat flour	0.25 lb	3.33%
No. 3 invert sugar	0.25 lb	3.33%
malt extract	0.25 lb	3.33%
Fuggles 90 mins	1.25 oz	
Goldings 90 mins	0.75 oz	
Goldings dry hops	0.125 oz	
OG	1033	
FG	1009	
ABV	3.18	
Apparent attenuation	72.73%	
IBU	31	
SRM	6	
Mash at	156° F	
Sparge at	175° F	
Boil time	90 minutes	
pitching temp	60° F	
Yeast	WLP023 Burton Ale	

1965 Watneys Keg Red Barrel

I'd forgotten that I had this Red Barrel recipe. Probably because it's one that comes indirectly via Usher's.

They really did seem to try with Red Barrel. For a start, it doesn't have all the ullage and other crap mixed in at racking time. And it has a grist of just malt and sugar. But – and this is a big but – the processing it received after primary fermentation would have had a big impact on the flavour. That's when it was filtered, fizzed up and heavily pasteurised. Not good.

I regret now never having given any of Watneys keg beers a try back in the 1970s. Then I'd know for sure if they were as awful as I imagine. Someone must have liked it, as it sold in massive quantities at one point. Before it became a laughing stock.

The hops are all English: Kent, East Kent and Mid Kent, all from the 1963 crop.

1965 Watneys Keg Red Barrel		
pale malt	8.50 lb	94.81%
crystal malt 60 L	0.33 lb	3.68%
No. 3 invert sugar	0.13 lb	1.39%
caramel	0.01 lb	0.11%
Fuggles 105 min	1.75 oz	
Goldings 15 min	0.50 oz	
Goldings dry hops	0.125 oz	
OG	1038.5	
FG	1008	
ABV	4.03	
Apparent attenuation	79.22%	
IBU	29	
SRM	6	
Mash at	150° F	
Sparge at	175° F	
Boil time	105 minutes	
pitching temp	60° F	
Yeast	WLP023 Burton Ale	

1948 Whitbread Stout

Whitbread were unusual in brewing three Stouts, Whitbread Stout being the weakest. And not very Stout at all.

You find quite a few Stouts of this strength – or even weaker – in the aftermath of WW II. Average OG was in the low 1030s, after all.

I assume this was coloured darker with caramel. As brewed, it's way too pale.

1948 Whitbread Stout		
pale malt	4.25 lb	55.56%
mild malt	1.50 lb	19.61%
brown malt	0.50 lb	6.54%
chocolate malt	0.50 lb	6.54%
malted oats	0.07 lb	0.92%
No. 3 invert sugar	0.50 lb	6.54%
No. 2 invert sugar	0.33 lb	4.31%
Spalt 60 mins	0.50 oz	
Goldings 60 mins	0.75 oz	
Goldings 30 mins	1.00 oz	
OG	1035	
FG	1010	
ABV	3.31	
Apparent attenuation	71.43%	
IBU	27	
SRM	21	
Mash at	150° F	
Sparge at	170° F	
Boil time	90 minutes	
pitching temp	64° F	
Yeast	Wyeast 1099 Whitbread ale	

1949 Whitbread Extra Stout

Extra Stout, a staple product of Whitbread's, was discontinued in 1940. I think I know the reason why: it was brewed for the Belgian market. They weren't going to sell much beer there after the Germans occupied it. Extra Stout reappeared again in 1948.

It's a pretty standard Whitbread Stout recipe, with a combination of mild, brown and chocolate malt. Plus a couple of types of sugar, No. 3 invert and Duttsons. I've substituted No. 2 invert for the latter.

The hops were all Mid Kent, from the 1947, 1948 and 1949 harvests.

1949 Whitbread Extra Stout			
mild malt		9.25 lb	75.51%
brown malt		1.00 lb	8.16%
chocolate Malt		1.00 lb	8.16%
No. 3 invert sugar		0.50 lb	4.08%
No. 2 invert sugar		0.50 lb	4.08%
Fuggles 60 min		1.00 oz	
Fuggles 40 min		1.00 oz	
Fuggles 20 min		1.00 oz	
OG		1056	
FG		1017	
ABV		5.16	
Apparent attenuation		69.64%	
IBU		28	
SRM		32	
Mash at		150° F	
Sparge at		170° F	
Boil time		60 minutes	
pitching temp		64° F	
Yeast	Wyeast 1099 Whitbread ale		

1948 Whitbread Mackeson Stout

Stout remained an important part of Whitbread's business. Especially Mackeson, which was hugely popular just after WW II.

So popular, in fact, that score of other breweries made their own Milk Stouts. The history of Milk Stout in the UK is rather odd. Hugely fashionable in the 1940s and 1950s, almost totally disappeared by 1990 and now making a comeback. Maybe it will be Brown Ale's turn next.

The recipe is identical to Extra Stout, with which it was parti-gyled. How can that be? Because they didn't add the lactose until the ned of primary fermentation. Which means lactose doesn't appear at all in the brewing record. Luckily, I have Whitbread Gravity Book analyses of the finished beer. By looking at the difference between the OG there and the one in the brewing record, I can work out how much lactose they added.

The No. 2 invert is a substitution for Duttsons, presumably a yype of proprietary sugar.

1948 Whitbread Mackeson Stout		
pale malt	4.50 lb	48.65%
mild malt	2.25 lb	24.32%
brown malt	0.50 lb	5.41%
chocolate malt	0.67 lb	7.24%
No. 3 invert sugar	0.50 lb	5.41%
No. 2 invert sugar	0.33 lb	3.57%
lactose	0.50 lb	5.41%
Fuggles 60 min	1.00 oz	
Saaz 30 min	1.00 oz	
OG	1044	
FG	1017.5	
ABV	3.51	
Apparent attenuation	60.23%	
IBU		
SRM		
Mash at	148° F	
Sparge at	170° F	
Boil time	60 minutes	
pitching temp	64° F	
Yeast	Wyeast 1099 Whitbread ale	

1954 Whitbread Extra Stout

Belgium was an important export market for British brewers. 59,127 barrels of the total exports of 248,024 barrels were destined for Belgium.[9] That's not far of a quarter. Unsurprisingly, many brewers had products specifically destined for the Belgian market. Whitbread Extra Stout was such a beer.

It's very unlike most of the Stouts sold in the UK at the time. I'll tell you what it looks like: pre- WW II Guinness Extra Stout. Both the OG and FG are very similar. It was introduced in 1921 at 1055° and my guess is that it was intended to be a rival for Guinness. That it changed so little between 1921 and 1955 is a sure sign it was an export beer.

The grist is the classic Whitbread combination of mild, brown and chocolate malt. Plus sugar: No. 3 invert and something called Duttson, which I've replaced with No. 2 invert.

The hops were Mid Kent from 1952 and 1953 and East Kent from 1952. It doesn't take a genius to guess that they were Fuggles and Goldings, respectively.

1954 Whitbread Extra Stout			
mild malt		8.75 lb	73.96%
brown malt		0.75 lb	6.34%
chocolate malt		1.00 lb	8.45%
No. 3 invert sugar		1.00 lb	8.45%
No. 2 invert sugar		0.33 lb	2.79%
Fuggles 60 min		1.25 oz	
Fuggles 40 min		1.00 oz	
Goldings 20 min		1.00 oz	
OG		1056.5	
FG		1013.5	
ABV		5.69	
Apparent attenuation		76.11%	
IBU		35	
SRM		32	
Mash at		150° F	
Sparge at		170° F	
Boil time		60 minutes	
pitching temp		64° F	
Yeast	Wyeast 1099 Whitbread ale		

[9] "1962 Brewers' Almanack", pages 56-57.

1954 Whitbread Stout

Whitbread's Stout for the domestic market was a good deal more watery than Extra Stout. Though, to be fair, it's stronger than most English Stout of the time.

Most of the time Whitbread parti-gyled their three Stouts in various combinations. But this particular example was brewed single-gyle

1954 Whitbread Stout		
mild malt	6.00 lb	72.73%
brown malt	0.50 lb	6.06%
chocolate malt	0.75 lb	9.09%
No. 3 invert sugar	0.67 lb	8.12%
No. 2 invert sugar	0.33 lb	4.00%
Fuggles 60 min	1.00 oz	
Fuggles 40 min	1.00 oz	
Goldings 20 min	1.00 oz	
OG	1039	
FG	1011	
ABV	3.70	
Apparent attenuation	71.79%	
IBU	36	
SRM	26	
Mash at	150° F	
Sparge at	170° F	
Boil time	60 minutes	
pitching temp	64° F	
Yeast	Wyeast 1099 Whitbread ale	

1954 Whitbread XXX Mild

This is a good one. I'd wondered about this beer, which is a bit of an oddity. I meant to post this during May, but got distracted. Another of my recipes, by the way. Sorry about that.

It's a strong Mild introduced by Whitbread in 1954. I'd wondered what exactly it was and why they suddenly released it. Having found some adverts for it, I'm now a little wiser.

There were stronger Milds, but it many cases Best Mild was only 1032° or 1033°, while Ordinary Mild was 1028-1030°. Milds as strong as XXX were a real rarity and seem to have mostly been limited to the West Midlands, a Mild stronghold.

> "Try this today at your local Whitbread house
> Take a pal to your local Whitbread house and have a "Treble X" apiece. This new brew is a draught mild ale of exceptional quality it really has something you'll be sure to enjoy. The strongest and richest mild ale in your district."
> Luton News and Bedfordshire Chronicle - Thursday 15 April 1954, page 7.

The last sentence was probably true. Very few Milds were over 1035°.

Sadly, XXX didn't last long. The first brew was 21st January 1954 (today's recipe) and the last I have photographed is 24th October 1955. So two years at most. But it's nice to see a big brewer like Whitbread push Mild, especially a strong one.

XXX was parti-gyled with Whitbread's standard Mild, Best Ale. That was just 1031°, but because its attenuation was under 70%, it was a mere 2.75% ABV. The one parti-gyled with this beer had a higher finishing gravity: 1010°.

The recipe is simplicity itself: mild malt as base, a touch of crystal and dark sugar. The original isn't all No. 3 invert. There's also something called Hay Six. Some sort of proprietary sugar. No idea what the composition of that was. But as it isn't in any of the pale beers, my guess is that it was dark. To get the specified colour, you'll need to add caramel colouring.

Whitbread consistently used mild ale malt as the base for their Milds and Forest Brown, while their Pale Ales used PA malt. Mild ale malt was around 10% cheaper than PA malt. There were four different types of pale malt back then: PA malt, SA malt, MA malt and plain old pale malt. MA malt was generally made from slightly lower quality barley and was kilned a bit darker than PA malt. As for SA malt – who knows? I've never been able to find any details about its manufacture or composition.

1954 Whitbread XXX Mild		
MA malt	6.25 lb	80.65%
crystal malt 40 L	0.50 lb	6.45%
No. 3 sugar	1.00 lb	12.90%
Fuggles 90 min	1.00 oz	
Fuggles 60 min	1.00 oz	
OG	1037.4	
FG	1007.5	
ABV	3.96	
Apparent attenuation	79.95%	
IBU	30	
SRM	40	
Mash at	147° F	
Sparge at	165° F	
Boil time	90 minutes	
pitching temp	65° F	
Yeast	WLP007 Dry English Ale	

1953 Whitbread Best Ale

Whitbread's X Ale underwent a couple of names changes in the 1940s. In 1940 it became XX Ale and in 1949 Best Ale. Not that there was anything particularly good about it. Though the gravity did increase in 1950 from 1027.7° to 1030.6°.

Whitbread didn't go in for complicated recipes. And didn't fart around with malt extract and enzymic malt as many brewers did. Malt and sugar, that was it. Though not all the sugar was No. 3 invert. Around a third was Hay's M, a proprietary sugar.

The caramel is my addition. No way they could have hit that colour without it. Must have been some sort of primings.

The hopping is heavier than for most provincial Mild Ales. In fact, it's around the level of most provincial Ordinary Bitters. The hops all from Mid Kent from the 1951 and 1952 harvests.

1953 Whitbread Best Ale		
mild malt	5.75 lb	81.21%
crystal malt 60 L	0.50 lb	7.06%
No. 3 invert sugar	0.50 lb	7.06%
caramel 1000 SRM	0.33 lb	4.66%
Fuggles 60 min	0.50 oz	
Fuggles 40 min	0.50 oz	
Goldings 20 min	0.50 oz	
OG	1031	
FG	1008.5	
ABV	2.98	
Apparent attenuation	72.58%	
IBU	19	
SRM	25	
Mash at	150° F	
Sparge at	168° F	
Boil time	60 minutes	
pitching temp	65° F	
Yeast	Wyeast 1099 Whitbread ale	

1953 Whitbread Double Brown

Whitbread's first Brown Ale, as the name implies, was a beer with a decent strength. It's a shame that, about year after this beer was brewed, it was discontinued. As they concentrated on the watery Forest Brown. Which, I suppose, fitted better with 1950s drinkers' expectations of a Brown Ale.

Whitbread's two Brown ales had very different recipes. As you'll see with the Forest Brown recipe that follows this.

1953 Whitbread Double Brown		
pale malt	10.50 lb	90.32%
chocolate Malt	0.125 lb	1.08%
No. 3 invert sugar	1.00 lb	8.60%
Fuggles 60 mins	1.00 oz	
Fuggles 40 mins	1.00 oz	
Fuggles 20 mins	1.00 oz	
OG	1053	
FG	1017.5	
ABV	4.70	
Apparent attenuation	66.98%	
IBU	30	
SRM	12	
Mash at	154° F	
Sparge at	168° F	
Boil time	90 minutes	
pitching temp	62° F	
Yeast	Wyeast 1099 Whitbread ale	

1955 Whitbread Forest Brown

Double Brown was the first Brown Ale that Whitbread brewed, back in the 1920's. Forest Brown only appeared later, after the Forest Hill brewery had been purchased.

One of the reasons Whitbread wanted to get their hands on Forest Hill was that they had the technology to produce brewery-conditioned bottled beer. Whitbread had stubbornly stuck with bottle conditioning much longer than their rivals.

Whitbread were already brewing Forest Brown before WW II. Sadly, it doesn't turn up in the brewing records. Presumably because it was a tweaked version of X Ale. That's what this beer was. Though thankfully it was properly recorded in the logs.

The grist is identical to their Mild, Best Ale. Mild malt, crystal malt and sugar in the same proportions. All very straightforward. The only slight complication is that not all the sugar in the original was No. 3 invert. Just under 20% was Hay's M, a type of proprietary sugar.

The hops were a combination of Kent from 1954 and Mid Kent from 1953. I've guessed Fuggles.

The caramel is my addition to get the colour to match the one on the brewing record.

1955 Whitbread Forest Brown		
mild malt	5.25 lb	75.00%
crystal malt 60 L	0.50 lb	7.14%
No. 3 invert sugar	1.00 lb	14.29%
caramel 1000 SRM	0.25 lb	3.57%
Fuggles 60 min	0.50 oz	
Fuggles 40 min	0.50 oz	
Fuggles 20 min	0.50 oz	
OG	1032.5	
FG	1010	
ABV	2.98	
Apparent attenuation	69.23%	
IBU	17	
SRM	23	
Mash at	150° F	
Sparge at	168° F	
Boil time	60 minutes	
pitching temp	65° F	
Yeast	Wyeast 1099 Whitbread ale	

1954 Whitbread IPA

Whitbread had brewed an IPA since 1900. It had never been a particularly strong beer. But that was typical for a certain type of English IPA.

By the 1920's, Whitbread's IPA had become an exclusively bottled beer. Which I'm pretty sure it still was in the mid-1950s. Serving as their Light Ale, an essential for any pub, especially in London where Light and Bitter was a popular mix. Later it would become a draught beer under a name the older amongst you might recall: Trophy.

There's not much to say about the grist. It really is what the recipes says: pale malt (actually PA malt, the poshest kind of pale malt), crystal malt and No. 1 invert sugar.

The hops were Mid Kent from 1952 and something simply described as H, also from 1952. I've gone out on a limb and guessed that H stands for Hallertau. I could be wrong. But it does make the recipe more fun.

One common feature of Whitbread's Ales in the 1950s is a short boil. Best Ale and Forest Brown just got 60 minutes. The Pale Ales got a little bit longer, but not much.

1954 Whitbread IPA		
pale malt	6.50 lb	83.87%
crystal malt 60 L	0.50 lb	6.45%
No. 1 invert sugar	0.75 lb	9.68%
Fuggles 75 mins	1.00 oz	
Hallertau 30 mins	1.25 oz	
Goldings dry hops	0.25 oz	
OG	1034	
FG	1004	
ABV	3.97	
Apparent attenuation	88.24%	
IBU	29	
SRM	7	
Mash at	150° F	
Sparge at	165° F	
Boil time	75 minutes	
pitching temp	64° F	
Yeast	Wyeast 1099 Whitbread ale	

1954 Whitbread PA

The PA from Whitbread had an even longer history than their IPA. It was the very first Pale Ale they brewed, way back on 1st November 1865.

What I love about the Whitbread recipes from the 1950s is that many of them can be converted for home brewing without any substitutions. There are no weird ingredients like proprietary sugars which are unavailable to the home brewer. The only slight inconvenience is having to make your own invert sugar.

The grist is just pale malt, crystal malt and No. 2 invert sugar. 1950s recipes don't come simpler than that. Outside wartime when they had no choice, Whitbread never used adjuncts. That's very unusual, especially for a large brewery. That is, until 1963, when flaked barley appeared in some of their Pale Ales. In the 1970a, most of their beers include torrefied barley or flaked maize.

The hops in the original were Mid Kent for the 1953 harvest and Kent hops from 1952. I've guessed Fuggles for both.

1954 Whitbread PA		
pale malt	6.50 lb	76.47%
crystal malt 60 L	0.50 lb	5.88%
No. 1 invert sugar	1.50 lb	17.65%
Fuggles 75 mins	0.75 oz	
Fuggles 30 mins	0.75 oz	
Goldings dry hops	0.25 oz	
OG	1039.5	
FG	1012	
ABV	3.64	
Apparent attenuation	69.62%	
IBU	19	
SRM	8	
Mash at	150° F	
Sparge at	165° F	
Boil time	75 minutes	
pitching temp	64° F	
Yeast	Wyeast 1099 Whitbread ale	

1958 Whitbread KKKK

You may remember that back in the 18th century, London had ranges of X and K Ales. The K's, or Keeping Ales, usually went: KK, KKK and KKKK. The last being a mighty beer of over 1100°. After WW I, the stronger varieties mostly disappeared, but KK kept going strong and, called Burton, it was one of the standard draught beers in a London pub.

Barclay Perkins did brew a KKKK between the wars, but only as a winter seasonal. It was still a strong beer, with a gravity of around 1080°. From adverts, it appears this was a draught beer, dispensed from a pin on the bar. That sort of thing still went on in the 1970's and 1980's. A pin of Marston's Owd Rodger would appear when the weather got cold.

Whitbread did a fair bit of messing around with their Burton. Before WW I, they brewed three K Ales: KK at 1071°, 2KKK at 1077° and KKK at 1082°. By the middle of 1917, all three had been dropped. KK reappeared in 1921 at the reduced gravity of 1055°. In 1931, no doubt prompted by the big tax increase that year, it was replaced by a beer called XXX at just 1045°. When the tax dropped again in 1933, they introduced another new beer called 33 at an impressive 1060°. That lasted until 1940, when it was in turn replaced by XXXX at 1053°, falling to 1043° by 1945. Between 1947 and 1958, surprisingly, Whitbread didn't brew a Burton. Then they introduced KKKK.

There's an elegant simplicity about Whitbread's beers of this period. Mostly pale malt, sugar and English hops. Daringly, this recipe includes a little chocolate malt, something they only normally used in their Stouts. There was a proprietary sugar called Hays M, but only a relatively small amount. I've just upped the No. 3 quantity.

It doesn't actually give the hop varieties, just their origin. I've assumed the Mid Kents were Fuggles and the East Kents Goldings. It seems a fair enough guess, given that those two varieties made up the vast majority of hops grown in England.

Almost forgot. To get the right colour you'll need to add caramel.

1958 Whitbread KKKK		
pale malt	8.50 lb	81.93%
chocolate malt	0.13 lb	1.20%
no. 3 sugar	1.75 lb	16.87%
Fuggles 75 min	2.00 oz	
Goldings 20 min	1.75 oz	
OG	1050.5	
FG	1011.5	
ABV	5.16	
Apparent attenuation	77.23%	
IBU	44	
SRM	30	
Mash at	150º F	
Sparge at	168º F	
Boil time	90 minutes	
pitching temp	62º F	
Yeast	Wyeast 1099 Whitbread ale	

1960 Whitbread PA (Tankard)

I'm not sure exactly when Whitbread PA became Tankard. Sometime in the late 1950s. The first Whitbread Gravity Book entry that mentions it by name is from 1959.

Interestingly, there still seems to have been something simply called Whitbread Bitter, which is the same strength. Though there is one difference between the two beers: the price. The Tankard is 1s 10d per pint and the Bitter just 1s 5d. A sure sign that the former was keg and the latter cask.

The recipe remains the same combination of pale malt, crystal malt and No. 1 invert sugar. Nothing much to see there.

The hopping rate on PA is very low for a Bitter at 5.5 lbs per quarter of malt. That's the same as their Mild, Best Ale. And considerably less than WPA (formerly IPA), their other Pale Ale at this point, which had 8.5 lbs per quarter.

The hops were all English, a combination of Kent, Mid Kent and East Kent from the 1958 and 1959 crops. I've interpreted the East Kent as Goldings and the others as Fuggles.

1960 Whitbread PA (Tankard)		
pale malt	6.75 lb	77.14%
crystal malt 60 L	0.50 lb	5.71%
No. 1 invert sugar	1.50 lb	17.14%
Fuggles 60 min	0.50 oz	
Fuggles 40 min	0.50 oz	
Goldings 20 min	0.50 oz	
Goldings dry hops	0.25 oz	
OG	1039	
FG	1013	
ABV	3.44	
Apparent attenuation	66.67%	
IBU	17	
SRM	8	
Mash at	150° F	
Sparge at	165° F	
Boil time	65 minutes	
pitching temp	63° F	
Yeast	Wyeast 1099 Whitbread ale	

1960 Whitbread Best Ale

The hundreds of hours I spent photographing and analysing Whitbread's brewing records have been well worth it. Because I have their beers for every year from 1805 to 1973, when Chiswell Street closed.

Remember that photo I posted recently showing Best Ale being racked into casks? I was able to work from the gyle number that was stencilled onto the casks (348) that the beer was brewed around 19th May. I don't have a photo of that particular brewing record, but I do have one from 9th June, gyle number 391. That's close enough for me.

Other than that, there isn't anything particularly special about this beer. And it's certainly nowhere near what I'd describe as "best"[10]. It's a totally run of the mill post- WW II Mild. With a gravity around 1030°, and a simple grist of mild malt, crystal malt and No. 3 invert. Though in the original some of the sugar was Hay M. Pretty sure that's a dark proprietary sugar, so I've just upped the No. 3.

It's also a very typical London Mild, in that it's quite dark and poorly attenuated. London Milds after WW II developed their own identity. At least until they started to die off in the 1960's. By the late 1970's, I believe Fullers Hock was the last cask Mile regularly brewed in London.

That's it. I only really wanted to let you know what the beer they were filling in that picture was like.

1960 Whitbread Best Ale			
mild malt		4.75 lb	76.00%
crystal malt 120 L		0.50 lb	8.00%
no. 3 invert sugar		1.00 lb	16.00%
Fuggles 60 min		0.50 oz	
Fuggles 40 min		0.50 oz	
Fuggles 20 min		0.50 oz	
OG		1030.3	
FG		1008.5	
ABV		2.88	
Apparent attenuation		71.95%	
IBU		17	
SRM		25	
Mash at		150° F	
Sparge at		168° F	
Boil time		60 minutes	
pitching temp		64° F	
Yeast	Wyeast 1099 Whitbread ale		

[10] Come to think of it, as Whitbread only brewed one Mild they couldn't even call it Better Ale, let alone Best Ale.

1964 Whitbread Ex PA

Now here's an interesting beer. I'm pretty sure that this is the Pale Ale Whitbread brewed for the Belgian market. I think it might even still be available over there. Though, obviously, brewed by someone else.

It's a very different beer from Whitbread's domestic PA. The OG is a lot higher, for a start. And it's much more heavily hopped, at almost 9 lbs per quarter of malt instead of 5.5 lbs. That's reflected in the calculated IBUs, which are considerably higher.

The basic recipe, however, is much the same: pale malt, crystal malt and No. 1 invert sugar.

1964 Whitbread Ex PA		
pale malt	10.50 lb	85.16%
crystal malt 60L	1.50 lb	12.17%
No. 1 invert sugar	0.33 lb	2.68%
Fuggles 90 min	1.25 oz	
Styrian Goldings 90 min	0.25 oz	
Fuggles 60 min	1.25 oz	
Fuggles 30 min	1.25 oz	
Goldings dry hop	0.50 oz	
OG	1056.5	
FG	1009.5	
ABV	6.22	
Apparent attenuation	83.19%	
IBU	45	
SRM	8	
Mash at	153° F	
Sparge at	165° F	
Boil time	90 minutes	
pitching temp	62° F	
Yeast	Wyeast 1099 Whitbread ale	

1964 Whitbread Oatmeal Stout

This Oatmeal Stout has a recipe very similar to Whitbread's 1954 Stout, with one obvious difference in the presence of oats.

Whitbread often threw some oats into their Stout parti-gyles. Even ones including Mackeson. I wonder if anyone realised they were drinking an Oatmeal Milk Stout? Probably not, as the amounts were usually tiny. The quantity here is quite large by Whitbread's standards. Often it was little more than 1%.

Indeed, Mackeson and Extra Stout (which I think was for the Belgian market) were the other two beers in this parti-gyle.

1964 Whitbread Oatmeal Stout			
mild malt		8.00 lb	76.19%
brown malt		0.75 lb	7.14%
chocolate malt		0.75 lb	7.14%
malted oats		0.50 lb	4.76%
No. 3 invert sugar		0.25 lb	2.38%
No. 2 invert sugar		0.25 lb	2.38%
Fuggles 60 mins		1.50 oz	
Goldings 30 mins		1.50 oz	
OG		1038	
FG		1011	
ABV		3.57	
Apparent attenuation		71.05%	
IBU		40	
SRM		25	
Mash at		150° F	
Sparge at		170° F	
Boil time		60 minutes	
pitching temp		64° F	
Yeast	Wyeast 1099 Whitbread ale		

1965 Whitbread Best Ale

Best Ale hasn't changed a great deal since 1960. The OG is a tiny bit higher and the percentages of the ingredients are slightly different. But essentially, it's the same beer.

Quite a watery one, as it doesn't quite make 3% ABV. I drank a later version on keg and I can attest that it was bland and watery. Perhaps on cask it was a little more exciting. Or maybe not.

1965 Whitbread Best Ale		
mild malt	5.50 lb	83.59%
crystal malt 60 L	0.33 lb	5.02%
No. 3 invert sugar	0.75 lb	11.40%
Fuggles 60 min	0.50 oz	
Fuggles 40 min	0.50 oz	
Fuggles 20 min	0.50 oz	
OG	1031	
FG	1009	
ABV	2.91	
Apparent attenuation	70.97%	
IBU	17	
SRM	25	
Mash at	150° F	
Sparge at	168° F	
Boil time	60 minutes	
pitching temp	64° F	
Yeast	Wyeast 1099 Whitbread ale	

1965 Whitbread Forest Brown

Over the years, Forest Brown came to be one of the cornerstones of Whitbread's range. When they took over a brewery, its Brown Ale was doomed, destined to be replaced by Forest Brown.

It's not exactly what you'd call an extreme beer. Not quite 3% ABV and with a very modest degree of hopping.

The grist is slightly odd, with a high percentage of flaked barley. What's even odder, is that this example was parti-gyled with Best Ale, which, when brewed alone had quite a different grist. As you can see above.

The No.3 invert is a substitute. In the original all the sugar is Hay's M, a proprietary sugar. I've no idea of its composition but, as it's only appears in dark beers, I assume it's dark. In any case, to hit the colour of the real beer, you'll need to add caramel. As brewed, it was only 9-10 SRM, depending on how dark the crystal malt was.

1965 Whitbread Forest Brown		
mild malt	5.25 lb	70.00%
crystal malt 60 L	0.50 lb	6.67%
flaked barley	1.50 lb	20.00%
No. 3 invert sugar	0.25 lb	3.33%
Fuggles 60 min	0.50 oz	
Fuggles 40 min	0.50 oz	
Fuggles 20 min	0.25 oz	
OG	1032	
FG	1009.5	
ABV	2.98	
Apparent attenuation	70.31%	
IBU	15	
SRM	30	
Mash at	150° F	
Sparge at	168° F	
Boil time	60 minutes	
pitching temp	64° F	
Yeast	Wyeast 1099 Whitbread ale	

1965 Whitbread W (Trophy)

Whitbread's trick in getting a national Ordinary Bitter brand, was to simply rename the appropriate beer in the range of every brewery they took over Trophy.

At one time there were 20-odd beers called Trophy, with quite different characters. Yet if you just looked at the TV adverts, you'd have assumed it was one uniform product across the country. "Whitbread big head Trophy Bitter, the pint that thinks it's a quart." That's how the jingle went.

Whitbread took some strange turns in their later years, when they become a national group. After 1880, they were relatively unusual in not using adjuncts as most other UK breweries did. They brewed from malt and sugar, except for during WW II when they were forced, as all brewers were, to use adjuncts. In the later war years, this was flaked barley.

But as early as 1946, they dropped it again. Presumably as soon as they were allowed to. They reverted to brewing from malt and sugar alone. Flaked barley returned in 1963. But only in their Pale Ales. Though by 1965 it also featured in Best Ale and Forest Brown.

1965 Whitbread W		
pale malt	7.00 lb	82.35%
crystal malt 60 L	0.50 lb	5.88%
flaked barley	1.00 lb	11.76%
Fuggles 75 min	0.75 oz	
Goldings 40 min	0.75 oz	
Goldings 20 min	0.75 oz	
Goldings dry hops	0.25 oz	
OG	1036.5	
FG	1007	
ABV	3.90	
Apparent attenuation	80.82%	
IBU	29	
SRM	6	
Mash at	148° F	
Sparge at	165° F	
Boil time	75 minutes	
pitching temp	64° F	
Yeast	Wyeast 1099 Whitbread ale	

1965 Whitbread PA (Tankard)

I'm not sure if Whitbread PA, or Tankard, still existed in cask form at this point. I suspect it did, because it's not until 1970 that it's called Tankard in the brewing records. My guess is that the name Tankard was reserved for the keg version.

The whole naming thing with draught only really comes in with keg beer. Before that, names were generic: Bloggs Best Bitter, Tetley Mild or even Draught Bass. But in the snazzy new world of keg – where marketing was paramount – beers needed to be properly branded. Double Diamond, Tavern, E, Tartan, Starlight and, of course, Tankard and Trophy.

There's nothing wrong with this beer, per se. Pale malt, crystal malt, invert sugar and English hops. It's a fairly classic post-war Best Bitter recipe. Though not particularly well hopped, which perhaps betrays its main function as a Keg Bitter. It's interesting that the weaker Trophy is more bitter.

Tankard was heavily promoted through TV advertising. "It's Tankard that helps me excel, after one I do *anything* well!" was the slogan. Pretty sure that wouldn't be allowed today.

In line with earlier versions, the hopping is relatively light. You'll note that the (calculated) IBUs are quite a bit lower than in Trophy.

1965 Whitbread PA			
pale malt		7.00 lb	82.35%
crystal malt 60 L		0.50 lb	5.88%
No. 1 invert sugar		1.00 lb	11.76%
Fuggles 65 min		0.75 oz	
Goldings 40 min		0.50 oz	
Goldings 20 min		0.50 oz	
Goldings dry hops		0.25 oz	
OG		1039.5	
FG		1008	
ABV		4.17	
Apparent attenuation		79.75%	
IBU		21	
SRM		7	
Mash at		149° F	
Sparge at		165° F	
Boil time		65 minutes	
pitching temp		62° F	
Yeast	Wyeast 1099 Whitbread ale		

1960 Robert Younger 54/-

In 1960 Robert Younger brewed a total of five Pale Ales. All parti-gyled in various combinations. Though you have to wonder why they bothered to brew so many.

By this point most Scottish breweries had settled on three Pale Ales: 60/- (1030°), 70/- (1036°) and 80/- (1042°). Robert Younger managed to squeeze in an extra beer at each end of the gravity range. 54/- is the weakest of the bunch.

54/- had been reasonably common before WW II, when it had an OG in the low 1030's. The war forced its gravity down to below 1030°. Most brewers dropped 54/- in the early 1950s when times started improving.

The recipe is pretty typical of Scottish Pale Ale: pale malt, flaked maize and sugar. Plus the obligatory dash of malt extract. The sugar in this case was half "Hydrol" and half "invert". I've interpreted that as No. 2 invert.

The brewing record is pretty vague about the hops, not even listing the year they were harvested. Two types, both English. I've guessed Fuggles and Goldings. Dry hops aren't records, but I've assumed that there were some.

1960 Robert Younger 54/-		
pale malt	4.25 lb	69.27%
flaked maize	1.25 lb	20.37%
malt extract	0.13 lb	2.04%
No. 2 invert sugar	0.50 lb	8.15%
caramel 1000 SRM	0.01 lb	0.16%
Fuggles 120 mins	0.50 oz	
Goldings 60 mins	0.50 oz	
Goldings dry hops	0.125 oz	
OG	1028	
FG	1012	
ABV	2.12	
Apparent attenuation	57.14%	
IBU	16	
SRM	5	
Mash at	150° F	
Sparge at	170° F	
Boil time	120 minutes	
pitching temp	60° F	
Yeast	Wyeast 1728 Scottish ale (McEwans)	

1960 Robert Younger 60/-

Next Pale Ale up is 60/-. This was universally produced by Scottish brewers, though it wasn't always called 60/-. William Younger's, for example, had the brew house name of XXP.

At only two gravity points more, there's little difference between this and 54/-. The rate of hopping, typically for Scotland, is very low. 4.5 lbs per quarter of malt compared to 5.5 lbs per quarter for Whitbread's Mild, Best Ale. You could say that this more resembles a Light Mild than an Ordinary Bitter.

Though, it being a Scottish beer, you need to be careful when it comes to colour. There's a good chance this was often coloured quite dark, to 20 or 25 SRM, as was Maclays 60 Bob. Which would have left it doing a pretty good impersonation of Dark Mild.

1960 Robert Younger 60/-		
pale malt	4.75 lb	71.59%
flaked maize	1.25 lb	18.84%
malt extract	0.13 lb	1.88%
No. 2 invert sugar	0.50 lb	7.54%
caramel 1000 SRM	0.01 lb	0.15%
Fuggles 120 mins	0.50 oz	
Goldings 60 mins	0.50 oz	
Goldings dry hops	0.125 oz	
OG	1030	
FG	1012	
ABV	2.38	
Apparent attenuation	60.00%	
IBU	16	
SRM	5	
Mash at	150º F	
Sparge at	170º F	
Boil time	120 minutes	
pitching temp	60º F	
Yeast	Wyeast 1728 Scottish ale (McEwans)	

1960 Robert Younger 70/-

At least there's a reasonable jump in gravity between 60/- and 70/-. A whole five points.

Not surprising, as both those beers were part of a normal set of Scottish Pale Ales. 70/- was the equivalent of an English Ordinary Bitter. Though with a lower hopping rate and a higher FG.

By the 1970s 70/-, or Heavy as it was usually called in the pub, was the most popular style in Scotland (though it was quickly overtaken by Lager). But at this point it was still massively outsold by the weaker 60/-.

1960 Robert Younger 70/-		
pale malt	5.50 lb	72.56%
flaked maize	1.50 lb	19.79%
malt extract	0.07 lb	0.92%
No. 2 invert sugar	0.50 lb	6.60%
caramel 1000 SRM	0.01 lb	0.13%
Fuggles 120 mins	0.75 oz	
Goldings 60 mins	0.50 oz	
Goldings dry hops	0.125 oz	
OG	1035	
FG	1011	
ABV	3.18	
Apparent attenuation	68.57%	
IBU	19	
SRM	5.5	
Mash at	150° F	
Sparge at	170° F	
Boil time	120 minutes	
pitching temp	60° F	
Yeast	Wyeast 1728 Scottish ale (McEwans)	

1960 Robert Younger 80/-

Top spot in the standard Scottish trilogy of Pale Ales was 80 Bob. Or Export. Or was it always called Export? (See next recipe.)

80/- - according to a fairly random sample of a couple of weeks in March 1960 – was their second-best selling beer. After 60/-, of course. It's not totally representative because I didn't take every beer from every page. The three beers at the bottom will be overrepresented. For the first five Pale Ales, it should be about right.

Robert Younger beer brewed March & July 1960	
beer	**barrels**
54/-	140.25
60/-	437
70/-	111
80/-	187.75
Ex	187
OEA	37.5
SA	80.5
SS	67.5
Source: Robert Younger brewing record held at the Scottish Brewing Archive, document number RY/6/1/3.	

80/- is more highly attenuated than the weaker Pale Ales, leaving it a pretty reasonable 4.2% ABV.

1960 Robert Younger 80/-		
pale malt	6.75 lb	72.27%
flaked maize	1.75 lb	18.74%
malt extract	0.09 lb	0.96%
No. 2 invert sugar	0.75 lb	8.03%
Fuggles 120 mins	0.75 oz	
Goldings 60 mins	0.75 oz	
Goldings dry hops	0.25 oz	
OG	1043	
FG	1011	
ABV	4.23	
Apparent attenuation	74.42%	
IBU	22	
SRM	6	
Mash at	150° F	
Sparge at	170° F	
Boil time	120 minutes	
pitching temp	60° F	
Yeast	Wyeast 1728 Scottish ale (McEwans)	

1960 Robert Younger Export

Robert Younger wasn't unique in having a beer called Export that was just stronger than their 80/-. Drybrough did, too. And at exactly the same gravities.

It's odd, because I was brought up to believe that 80/- and Export were names for the same thing. Evidently that wasn't always the case. I can of one explanation: the ones actually called Export in the brewery were bottled beers and 80/- draught beers. That I can find labels for Robert Younger Export Pale Ale tends to confirm that.

Just the 80/- with slightly more of anything.

1960 Robert Younger Export		
pale malt	7.00 lb	70.99%
flaked maize	2.00 lb	20.28%
malt extract	0.10 lb	1.01%
No. 2 invert sugar	0.75 lb	7.61%
caramel 1000 SRM	0.01 lb	0.10%
Fuggles 120 mins	1.00 oz	
Goldings 60 mins	0.75 oz	
Goldings dry hops	0.25 oz	
OG	1045	
FG	1011.5	
ABV	4.43	
Apparent attenuation	74.44%	
IBU	25	
SRM	7	
Mash at	150° F	
Sparge at	170° F	
Boil time	120 minutes	
pitching temp	57° F	
Yeast	Wyeast 1728 Scottish ale (McEwans)	

1960 Robert Younger Sweet Stout

Here's another of those oddities: a Stout parti-gyled with a Pale Ale. Which makes formulating a recipe tricky.

They used the normal trick of throwing all the coloured stuff into just one of the worts at boil time. With a bit of fiddling about, I've managed to come up with this recipe. It should be about right. I've assumed this beer got its proportion of all the standard ingredients, plus all the stuff thrown into the one wort.

Unsurprisingly, given how it was brewed, the recipe is very similar to their other beers, just with black malt and loads of caramel thrown in. And some liquorice.

Like many Scottish Stouts of the time, the combination of low OG and high FG leaves it barely alcoholic.

1960 Robert Younger Sweet Stout		
pale malt	4.50 lb	63.38%
black malt	0.25 lb	3.52%
flaked maize	1.25 lb	17.61%
malt extract	0.10 lb	1.41%
No. 2 invert sugar	0.50 lb	7.04%
caramel 1000 SRM	0.50 lb	7.04%
liquorice	1.00 oz	
Fuggles 120 mins	0.50 oz	
Goldings 60 mins	0.50 oz	
OG	1031	
FG	1015	
ABV	2.12	
Apparent attenuation	51.61%	
IBU	16	
SRM	34	
Mash at	150° F	
Sparge at	170° F	
Boil time	120 minutes	
pitching temp	60° F	
Yeast	Wyeast 1728 Scottish ale (McEwans)	

1960 Robert Younger Old Edinburgh Ale

This beer was a bit of a surprise. Loads of Pale Ales, dodgily produced Stout and a Strong Ale. That was the usual run of play.

I've no idea how this beer was marketed. My guess is that it's a bottled beer in the William Younger No. 3 category. But I could be totally wrong. That's the problem when you've no information on the finished beer.

Though the large amount of caramel does make it pretty dark. The colour below is as brewed. Achieved by throwing all the caramel in the wort intended for this beer. I think. That looks like what it says in the brewing record. There's always some magic in the parti-gyling together very different styles.

Note the presence of liquorice. Never seen that in anything but Porter or Stout before.

1960 Robert Younger Old Edinburgh Ale		
pale malt	7.00 lb	72.09%
flaked maize	1.50 lb	15.45%
malt extract	0.10 lb	1.03%
No. 2 invert sugar	0.75 lb	7.72%
caramel 1000 SRM	0.33 lb	3.40%
liquorice	0.03 lb	0.31%
Fuggles 120 mins	0.75 oz	
Goldings 60 mins	0.75 oz	
OG	1044	
FG	1016	
ABV	3.70	
Apparent attenuation	63.64%	
IBU	22	
SRM	23	
Mash at	150° F	
Sparge at	170° F	
Boil time	120 minutes	
pitching temp	60° F	
Yeast	Wyeast 1728 Scottish ale (McEwans)	

1960 Robert Younger Strong Ale

Yes, Robert Younger managed to make eight beers from that one recipe of theirs. The oddest thing is, that wasn't even unusual in Scotland.

A Strong Ale spun out of a Pale Ale parti-gyle was common in Scotland. And why not? It was an efficient way of brewing a small-volume, high-gravity beer.

Colour is always a tricky topic with Scottish beer. Luckily, I've a Whitbread Gravity Book analysis for this beer from 1953. It's about 25 SRM. The colour in the recipe below is as brewed. The difference would have been made up with caramel after primary fermentation.

1960 Robert Younger Strong Ale		
pale malt	11.00 lb	72.68%
flaked maize	2.75 lb	18.17%
malt extract	0.125 lb	0.83%
No. 2 invert sugar	1.25 lb	8.26%
caramel 1000 SRM	0.01 lb	0.07%
Fuggles 145 mins	1.25 oz	
Goldings 60 mins	1.25 oz	
OG	1070	
FG	1024	
ABV	6.09	
Apparent attenuation	65.71%	
IBU	31	
SRM	9	
Mash at	150° F	
Sparge at	170° F	
Boil time	145 minutes	
pitching temp	60° F	
Yeast	Wyeast 1728 Scottish ale (McEwans)	

1958 William Younger XXPQ

You know what we need? A nice watery 1950's Bitter. Not done one of those for a while. And this William Younger job from 1958 is suitably feeble.

It was brewed at their Holyrood Brewery, the younger of their two plants at the bottom end of the Royal Mile. Originally, it was built to brew Pale Ale and was fitted out with Burton unions.

What the hell does XXPQ stand for? Well, XXP is the beer name. It started as the stronger of their two IPAs, but a century or so of gravity erosion had knocked it down from 1060° to 1033°. And the name changed from IPA to 60/-.

What about the Q? That's the colour indicator. According to an internal brewery document, it's 47° Lovibond or about 12 SRM. I suspect you'll need to use dark candy sugar to hit that.

It's not a very complicated grist: pale malt, flaked maize and sugar. Though high compared to most English beers, the percentage of maize looks very reasonable compared to the 40% grits Younger's pre-WW II recipes contained. The hopping is extremely light. Lighter than in many Mild Ales.

The poor degree of attenuation probably left it with a little body, despite the very modest gravity. The Scots had a habit of having quite similar FGs for all their Pale Ales, whatever the OG.

1958 William Younger XXPQ		
pale malt	4.50 lb	62.07%
flaked maize	1.75 lb	24.14%
cane sugar	0.75 lb	10.34%
candy sugar	0.25 lb	3.45%
Fuggles 90 mins	0.50 oz	
Fuggles 60 mins	0.25 oz	
Goldings 30 mins	0.25 oz	
Goldings dry hops	0.125 oz	
OG	1033	
FG	1012	
ABV	2.78	
Apparent attenuation	63.64%	
IBU	15	
SRM	3	
Mash at	149° F	
Sparge at	160° F	
Boil time	90 minutes	
pitching temp	61° F	
Yeast	WLP028 Edinburgh Ale	

1958 William Younger XXPSL

Up one from XXPQ is XXPSL. 70/-, as it was sometimes called. This was one of Younger's best-selling beers. Though they continued to brew a bafflingly large range.

The recipe differs slightly from XXPQ in that there's a third sugar, simply listed as invert. No. 2 is my guess.

Talking of guesses, the 90 minute boil time is another one. Younger couldn't be arsed to record the boil times at this point. The records get even worse in the 1960s, without even the ingredients properly listed.

You'll note that none of these Pale Ales is very bitter. That's through a combination of a low hopping rate – around 4 lbs per quarter of malt – and some not very fresh hops. To put that hopping rate into perspective, Whitbread Pale Ale from the same year, a beer with an OG of 1035°, had almost 8 lbs of hops per quarter.

As with all Younger's Pale Ales, it came in a variety of shades, depending on which town you bought it in.

1958 William Younger XXPSL		
pale malt	5.00 lb	60.02%
flaked maize	2.25 lb	27.01%
No. 2 invert sugar	0.25 lb	3.00%
candy sugar	0.33 lb	3.96%
cane sugar	0.50 lb	6.00%
Fuggles 90 mins	0.33 oz	
Fuggles 60 mins	0.33 oz	
Goldings 30 mins	0.33 oz	
OG	1038	
FG	1012.5	
ABV	3.37	
Apparent attenuation	67.11%	
IBU	13	
SRM	4	
Mash at	149° F	
Sparge at	160° F	
Boil time	90 minutes	
pitching temp	62° F	
Yeast	WLP028 Edinburgh Ale	

1958 William Younger Export

Unlike most Scottish breweries, William Younger didn't parti-gyle. All their beers were single-gyle. Which means, in theory, they could have quite different recipes. In practice, they were all much the same.

About the only difference was in the sugars. So while their Ordinary Bitter, XXPQ, contained candy and cane sugar, Export had invert and cane. I've guessed for No. 2 invert. But could have been No. 1.

As always, there's a very high percentage of flaked maize. I'm surprised that they didn't have problems with converting it all, there's that much.

The colour is as brewed. Doubtless it was coloured up a variety of shades with caramel at racking time.

1958 William Younger Export		
pale malt	6.00 lb	60.00%
flaked maize	3.00 lb	30.00%
No. 2 invert sugar	0.33 lb	3.30%
cane sugar	0.67 lb	6.70%
Fuggles 90 mins	0.50 oz	
Fuggles 60 mins	0.50 oz	
Goldings 30 mins	0.50 oz	
OG	1046	
FG	1009.5	
ABV	4.83	
Apparent attenuation	79.35%	
IBU	18	
SRM	4.5	
Mash at	149° F	
Sparge at	160° F	
Boil time	90 minutes	
pitching temp	60° F	
Yeast	WLP028 Edinburgh Ale	

1958 William Younger XXX

What's the difference between XXX and XXPQ? Not very much, despite one being a Mild and the other a Bitter. William Younger were always a funny bunch.

The OG, FG and hopping rate of the two beers are identical. The only difference is the lack of candy sugar and a little more flaked maize in XXX. The only really big difference between the two beers isn't visible in the brewing records: the colour. I know from Whitbread Gravity book analyses that the colour of XXX was around 19 SRM. Presumably this was achieved by the addition of caramel at racking time.

William Younger is unusual for a Scottish brewery in making a Mild at all. Most had dropped Mild before WW II. With coloured up 60/- Pale Ale operating as a substitute. I assume the reason Younger still brewed one was that they had quite a large amount of trade in England, where Mild was still king in the 1950's.

1958 William Younger XXX		
pale malt	4.00 lb	57.14%
flaked maize	2.25 lb	32.14%
cane sugar	0.75 lb	10.71%
Fuggles 90 mins	0.50 oz	
Fuggles 60 mins	0.25 oz	
Goldings 30 mins	0.25 oz	
Goldings dry hops	0.125 oz	
OG	1033	
FG	1012	
ABV	2.78	
Apparent attenuation	63.64%	
IBU	15	
SRM	3	
Mash at	149° F	
Sparge at	160° F	
Boil time	90 minutes	
pitching temp	63.5° F	
Yeast	WLP028 Edinburgh Ale	

1958 William Younger No. 3 L

They weren't the most exciting brewery when it came to recipes, William Younger. Their No.3 Scotch Ale looks very similar to the Bitter XXPQ and the Mild XXX.

But why change a recipe when you have a good one? And why change what you've done for a century or more? William Younger's recipes always looked creepily familiar, whatever the supposed style.

The colour of the finished beer would have been much darker than the calculated colour in the recipe below. Probably not just one shade either, if I know Scottish brewing. Anywhere between 15 and 50 SRM would be my guess. Depending on which market the beer was intended for. Colour it up with caramel as dark as you like.

1958 William Younger No. 3 L		
pale malt	6.25 lb	64.10%
flaked maize	3.00 lb	30.77%
cane sugar	0.50 lb	5.13%
Fuggles 90 mins	0.50 oz	
Fuggles 60 mins	0.50 oz	
Goldings 30 mins	0.50 oz	
Goldings dry hops	0.125 oz	
OG	1044	
FG	1014	
ABV	3.97	
Apparent attenuation	68.18%	
IBU	20	
SRM	3	
Mash at	149° F	
Sparge at	160° F	
Boil time	90 minutes	
pitching temp	61° F	
Yeast	WLP028 Edinburgh Ale	

1958 William Younger Brown Ale

It's no surprise that William Younger brewed a Brown Ale in its own right. That's how they made everything.

Though the recipe is eerily similar to their other beers: pale malt, flaked maize and sugar. Though something is obviously missing: something to colour the beer. BeerSmith tells me that this is 2.5 SRM, based on the recipe. But I know from a Whitbread Gravity Book analysis from 1956 that it was 17.5 SRM.

Caramel is the answer. Presumably added at the end of primary fermentation. A quarter pound of 1000 SRM caramel will get you to the correct colour. 1950s brewing is such fun. Not at all what I'd expected. That's what's so satisfying about primary research: discovering the unexpected.

1958 William Younger Brown Ale		
pale malt	3.75 lb	57.69%
flaked maize	2.00 lb	30.77%
cane sugar	0.75 lb	11.54%
Fuggles 90 mins	0.75 oz	
Fuggles 30 mins	0.25 oz	
OG	1031	
FG	1005	
ABV	3.44	
Apparent attenuation	83.87%	
IBU	16	
SRM	17.5	
Mash at	149° F	
Sparge at	160° F	
Boil time	90 minutes	
pitching temp	62° F	
Yeast	WLP028 Edinburgh Ale	

1958 William Younger Edinburgh Brown Ale

William Younger didn't just brew one Brown Ale, they had two. Edinburgh Brown Ale being the stronger of the two.

I think I know the reason why: they did a lot of trade in the Northeast of England, where there was a market for stronger Brown Ales. Newcastle Breweries, Vaux and Federation – all located in the region – all had one in their range.

And what an exciting recipe. It has another type of malt in it. No flaked maize, either. That's a really radical departure from their usual practice. That's really rather a lot of crystal malt. So much that the colour is just about right without any caramel adjustment. Though the two analyses I have list quite different colours. The 1956 one is 19S RM, the 1957 one 14 SRM.

I can guess what happened to this beer. Phased out in favour of Newcastle Brown after Scottish Brewers merged with Newcastle Breweries to form Scottish & Newcastle.

1958 William Younger Edinburgh Brown Ale		
pale malt	7.00 lb	68.29%
crystal malt 60 L	2.25 lb	21.95%
cane sugar	1.00 lb	9.76%
Fuggles 90 mins	0.50 oz	
Fuggles 60 mins	0.50 oz	
Fuggles 30 mins	0.50 oz	
OG	1047	
FG	1012	
ABV	4.63	
Apparent attenuation	74.47%	
IBU	21	
SRM	13	
Mash at	149° F	
Sparge at	160° F	
Boil time	90 minutes	
pitching temp	59.5° F	
Yeast	WLP028 Edinburgh Ale	

1958 William Younger Double Century Ale

Double Century Ale was introduced in 1949 to commemorate 200 years of William Younger. Except, as Martyn Cornell has pointed out, the date is a few decades too early.

I'm not sure what style it's meant to be. Strong Brown Ale? Old Ale? Scotch Ale? Who really cares?

One odd feature of Double Century is that, despite containing lactose, it has a higher degree of attenuation than most William Younger beers. A bit weird, that. The grist isn't complicated, just pale malt, flaked maize and sugar. Once again, the percentage of adjunct is very high

1958 William Younger Double Century Ale		
pale malt	8.00 lb	61.54%
flaked maize	4.00 lb	30.77%
lactose	0.50 lb	3.85%
cane sugar	0.25 lb	1.92%
caramel 1000 SRM	0.25 lb	1.92%
Fuggles 90 mins	1.00 oz	
Fuggles 60 mins	0.50 oz	
Goldings 30 mins	0.25 oz	
OG	1057	
FG	1014	
ABV	5.69	
Apparent attenuation	75.44%	
IBU	21	
SRM	19	
Mash at	149° F	
Sparge at	160° F	
Boil time	90 minutes	
pitching temp	59° F	
Yeast	WLP028 Edinburgh Ale	

1959 William Younger No. 1 BW

Younger's No. 1 was one of the company's longest-lived products, having debuted in the 1860s. Originally it was one of a series of numbered Ales, from 1 to 4. Though by the 1950s, 2 and 4 were long gone.

The recipe is typical Younger: pale malt, loads of maize and a little dash of sugar. Not the slightest trace of coloured malt, despite this being a dark beer. There must have been some extra colouring going on at racking time, as an analysis in the Whitbread Gravity Book gives the colour as 20 SRM.

All I know about the hops is that they were from Kent, harvested in 1956 and 1957, making them a bit on the old side. That and a relatively low hopping rate leave a finished beer that isn't particularly bitter for its strength.

1959 William Younger No. 1 BW		
pale malt	11.50 lb	59.74%
flaked maize	6.25 lb	32.47%
No. 3 invert sugar	1.50 lb	7.79%
Fuggles 90 mins	1.00 oz	
Goldings 60 mins	1.00 oz	
Goldings 30 mins	1.00 oz	
Goldings dry hops	0.33 oz	
OG	1089	
FG	1027.5	
ABV	8.14	
Apparent attenuation	69.10%	
IBU	29	
SRM	14	
Mash at	151° F	
Sparge at	160° F	
Boil time	90 minutes	
pitching temp	57.5° F	
Yeast	WLP028 Edinburgh Ale	

1958 William Younger 200/- Barley Wine

WW I basically did for the strong Shilling Ales of Scotland. With one exception: William Younger 200/-. A beer that continued to be brewed occasionally right through the 1950s.

Meaning Younger had two Barley Wines. No. 1 and the even stronger 200/-. I know that No. 1 was sold in the UK, but I'm not so sure about 200/-. It's possible that it was an export beer.

The recipe is a little different from its other recipes in that the proportion of flaked maize is lower, under 20% of the total. There's not much else to the recipe, just pale malt and something simply described as "invert". I've guessed No. 3 invert.

The hops were all Kent from the 1957 crop. Fuggles seems a fair enough bet.

1958 William Younger 200/- Barley Wine		
pale malt	17.25 lb	76.67%
flaked maize	4.00 lb	17.78%
No. 3 invert sugar	1.25 lb	5.56%
Fuggles 90 mins	1.00 oz	
Fuggles 60 mins	1.00 oz	
Goldings 30 mins	0.75 oz	
Goldings dry hops	0.33 oz	
OG	1100	
FG	1025	
ABV	9.92	
Apparent attenuation	75.00%	
IBU	25	
SRM	12	
Mash at	149° F	
Sparge at	160° F	
Boil time	90 minutes	
pitching temp	57.5° F	
Yeast	WLP028 Edinburgh Ale	

1958 William Younger Sweet Stout

I'd have put money on William Younger's Sweet Stout having more than one type of malt. But it doesn't.

In fact, the only colouring is from sugar in the form of CDM (Caramelised Dextro-Maltose). I've replaced it No. 3 invert. Though maybe it should be No. 4 invert.

The recipe in the brewing log produces a beer that's way too pale. I know from a Whitbread Gravity Book analysis from 1959 that the colour was 300 EBC, a standard colour for Stout. There's only one way they could have got it the right colour: a stack of caramel. So I've added enough to get it to the right colour

That it contains lactose is no surprise. This is a Sweet Stout, after all. And Younger used it in several of their beers, not just Stout. It's made even sweeter in this case by a minimal level of hopping – under 2.5 lbs of hops per quarter of malt. That's extremely low.

1958 William Younger Sweet Stout		
pale malt	3.75 lb	48.89%
flaked maize	1.50 lb	19.56%
lactose	0.67 lb	8.74%
No. 3 invert sugar	0.67 lb	8.74%
cane sugar	0.33 lb	4.30%
caramel 1000 SRM	0.75 lb	9.78%
Fuggles 90 mins	0.33 oz	
Fuggles 30 mins	0.33 oz	
OG	1034	
FG	1011	
ABV	3.04	
Apparent attenuation	67.65%	
IBU	8	
SRM	39	
Mash at	149° F	
Sparge at	160° F	
Boil time	90 minutes	
pitching temp	63° F	
Yeast	WLP028 Edinburgh Ale	

Appendix I – weights and measures

Not everyone went to school in pre-metric days as I did. So an overview of Imperial measures is in order.

Weight

16 oz (ounces) = 1 lb (pound)
112 lbs = 1 cwt (hundredweight)

1 lb = 0.4535 kilograms

Volume

8 gallons = 1 bushel
8 bushels = 1 quarter
1 quarter pale malt = approx. 324 lbs
1 quarter black malt = approx. 224 lbs
1 quarter brown malt = approx. 224 lbs

1 bushel = 36.369 litres

Liquid

20 fl. oz (fluid ounce) = 1 pint
8 pints = 1 gallon
36 gallons = 1 barrel
54 gallons = 1 hogshead

1 pint = .568 litre
1 barrel = 163.584 litres

Money

12d (pence) = 1s (shilling)
20s = 1 pound

Temperature

Fahrenheit to Celsius			
° F	° C	° F	° C
50	10	150	65.6
51	10.6	151	66.1
52	11.1	152	66.7
53	11.7	153	67.2
54	12.2	154	67.8
55	12.8	155	68.3
56	13.3	156	68.9
57	13.9	157	69.4
58	14.4	158	70.0
59	15.0	159	70.6
60	15.6	160	71.1
61	16.1	161	71.7
62	16.7	162	72.2
63	17.2	163	72.8
64	17.8	164	73.3
65	18.3	165	73.9
66	18.9	166	74.4
67	19.4	167	75.0
68	20.0	168	75.6
69	20.6	169	76.1
70	21.1	170	76.7
71	21.7	171	77.2
72	22.2	172	77.8
73	22.8	173	78.3
74	23.3	174	78.9
75	23.9	175	79.4
76	24.4	176	80.0

Index

www.ingramcontent.com/pod-product-compliance
Lightning Source LLC
Chambersburg PA
CBHW072008270326
41928CB00009B/1583
* 9 7 8 9 4 9 0 2 7 0 3 3 9 *